# WHAT HORSES
# REALLY WANT

# WHAT HORSES REALLY WANT

### Unlocking the Secrets to Trust, Cooperation and Reliability

## Lynn Acton

Photographs by Jerry Acton

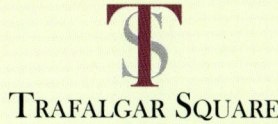

TRAFALGAR SQUARE

First published in 2020 by
Trafalgar Square Books
an imprint of The Stable Book Group
32 Court Street Suite 2109
Brooklyn, New York 11201
www.trafalgarbooks.com

Copyright © 2020 Lynn Acton

All rights reserved. No part of this book may be reproduced, by any means, without written permission of the publisher, except by a reviewer quoting brief excerpts for a review in a magazine, newspaper, or website.

**Disclaimer of Liability**
The author and publisher shall have neither liability nor responsibility to any person or entity with respect to any loss or damage caused or alleged to be caused directly or indirectly by the information contained in this book. While the book is as accurate as the author can make it, there may be errors, omissions, and inaccuracies.

Trafalgar Square Books encourages the use of approved safety helmets in all equestrian sports and activities.

ISBN: 978 1 57076 945 0
Library of Congress Control Number: 2020930156

Photographs by Jerry Acton except 20.1 (by Charles Schock)
Book design by Lauryl Eddlemon
Cover design by RM Didier
Index by Andrea Jones (JonesLiteraryServices.com)
Typefaces: Charter, Proxima Nova

Printed in Hong Kong
10 9 8 7 6 5 4 3

*Dedicated to my wonderful family, all four
generations, for their enthusiastic support*

*and*

*to everyone who wants to make
life better for horses.*

# Contents

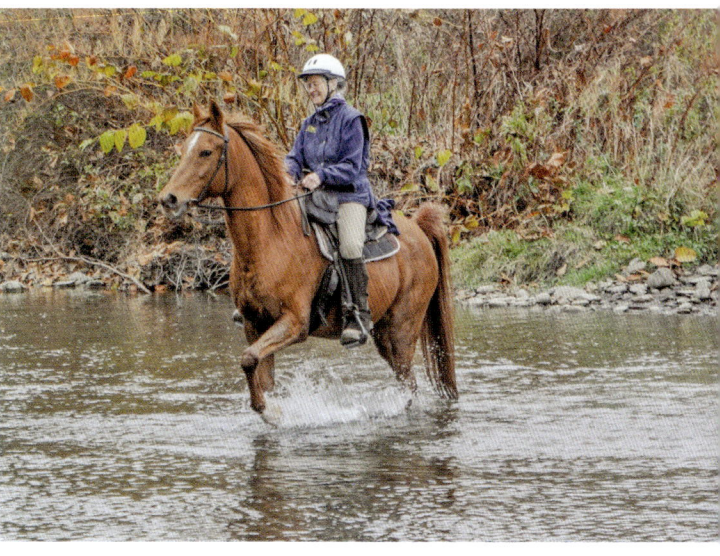

**Acknowledgments**     xi

## Part One: Horses Want a Leader They Trust     1

### Chapter 1: A Tale of Two Ponies     7
Snickers, Pony Einstein?     7
What I Discovered About Leadership     10
Brandy the Uncatchable     11
Protector Leadership     12
Safety     14
Things to Try     15

### Chapter 2: Earning Trust     16
Catching the Uncatchable Horse     18
Earning Brandy's Trust     19
Becoming a Protector Leader to My Own Horses     28

## Part Two: Horses Want Security and Social Bonds     31

### Chapter 3: Free-Roaming Herds: Complex Social Networks     34
Lifestyle of Free-Roaming Herds     34
Protector Leadership Validated     42

### Chapter 4: Domestic Horses: Social Networks Disrupted     43
Lifestyle of Domestic Herds     43
Stress-Related Behaviors     46

### Chapter 5: Brandy's New Herd     51
Our Semi-Dysfunctional Herd     51
Brandy Changes Herd Dynamics     53
Changes in Relationships with Us     60
Sapphire's Point of View     61

## Part Three: Interpreting Behavior Accurately     63

### Chapter 6: Positive Behaviors Misinterpreted     66
Initiating an Action in an Attempt to Communicate with You     66
Pausing or Experimenting to Figure Out What You Want     69

    Anticipating What You Are
        Going to Ask         70

    Volunteering an Action That
        Has Been Rewarded in the Past    71

    Disobeying for What the Horse
        Believes to Be a Good Reason    72

    Showing Signs of Trust
        and Attachment    74

## Chapter 7: Interpreting the Causes of Unwanted Behavior    77

    Pain    79
    Insecure Balance    81
    Confusion and Misunderstandings    83
    Inconsistent Expectations    83
    Punishment    84
    Fatigue and Boredom    84
    Living Conditions and Diet    85
    Pressure the Horse Cannot Relieve    86
    Stressful Situations    87
    Anxiety    87

## Chapter 8: Brandy and Friends: "Bad" Behavior Reinterpreted    90

    Bronzz: Spooking and Bucking    90
    Shiloh: Lazy with a Bad Attitude    92
    Brandy: Dangerously Unpredictable    94
    In Retrospect    98

## Part Four: Communicate Like a Horse    99

## Chapter 9: The Power and Pitfalls of Pressure    102

    How Horses Use Pressure
        with Each Other    102

    How People Inadvertently
        Turn Pressure into Stress    104

    The Pitfalls of Pressure    107

    The Power of Pressure
        as Positive Communication    109

## Chapter 10: Friendly Body Language    113

    Synchronizing: Body Language That
        Promotes Trust and Leadership    114

    How Synchronizing Is Different
        from Learning Through Pressure    114

    Brandy Demonstrates
        Synchronizing with Me    115

    Standing Still: Influencing
        Energy and Emotions    120

    Recall    121
    An Exciting New Perspective    123

    The Benefits of Friendly
        Body Language    124

    Training Myself    125

    Expanding Your Fluency in
        Friendly Body Language    126

## Chapter 11: Rewards are Positive Feedback    128

    Is Your Approval a Reward?    129
    Basic Facts About Rewards    129

Typical Rewards — 131
Making the Most of Rewards — 135
Limitations of Rewards — 137

## Part Five: Investigative Behavior Expands Horses' Comfort Zone — 139

## Chapter 12: How Horses Explore the World — 141
Why Confidence Matters — 141
The Investigative Behavior Sequence — 143
Obedience vs. Learning — 146
Horses See Things That Humans Do Not — 146
Horses See Things in a Different Context Than We Do — 147
Investigative Behavior Study: Retraining Jumpers — 149
Long-Term Benefits of Investigative Behavior — 151

## Chapter 13: Encouraging Investigative Behavior — 154
Your Role as Protector Leader — 154
Investigative Behavior: General Guidelines — 155
Investigative Behavior on the Lead — 155
Investigative Behavior Under Saddle — 158
Investigative Behavior Compared to Desensitizing, Bomb-Proofing, Spook-Busting, and Flooding — 161
Why Investigative Behavior Is Underused — 164

## Chapter 14: Adventures with Investigative Behavior — 166
Enlisting Assistance: Alien on Wheels — 166
More Assistance: The Fly Fisherman — 167
Special Incentives: The Lean Mean Green Machine — 167
Jackpot: The Sky is Falling — 167
Three-Day Wonder: The Big Wide Scary Creek — 168
Positive Associations: Introducing Bugs on Wheels — 169
Observing from Afar: The Not-Quite-a Horse — 170
Protecting the Leader: The Big Bad Recycle Mess — 170
Protector Leader vs. The Monster in the Woods — 171
New Species: Pint-Sized Humans — 172
Taming the Trailer Terror — 173
Is There a Downside to Investigative Behavior? — 173

## Part Six: Positive Experiences Build Confidence and Reliability — 175

## Chapter 15: Systematic Confidence Building — 178
A Systematic Confidence Building Program — 179
Flexibility: Six Ways to Introduce Crossing a Tarp — 186
Long-Term Benefits of Confidence Building — 187

| | | | |
|---|---|---|---|
| Obstacle Clinics and Competitions | 188 | **Part Seven: Reducing Stress** | **221** |
| Making Progress | 188 | | |
| The Ultimate Measure of Success | 190 | **Chapter 18: Problem-Solving Strategies** | **224** |

### Chapter 16: Brandy's Confidence Blossoms — 192

Role Playing for Health Care — 192
Confidence Building and Horse Agility — 196
Practical Application: Brandy Plays Super Pony — 202
My Pony, My Teacher — 208

### Chapter 17: Freedom and Liberty — 209

Four Ways to Give Freedom Safely — 210
Liberty and Protector Leadership — 215

### Chapter 18: Problem-Solving Strategies — 224

Identifying the Underlying Problem — 225
New Horses Need Extra Reassurance that You Will Be a Protector Leader — 230
Good Horse and Bad Match — 232

### Chapter 19: Being a Considerate Rider — 236

13 Ways to Become the Rider Horses Want to Carry — 237

### Chapter 20: Our Horses' Low-Stress Lifestyle — 247

Mealtime Routines — 247
Turnout — 250
Jobs, Responsibilities, and Social Time — 253

Conclusion — 256
Endnotes — 259
Reading and References — 269
Index — 271

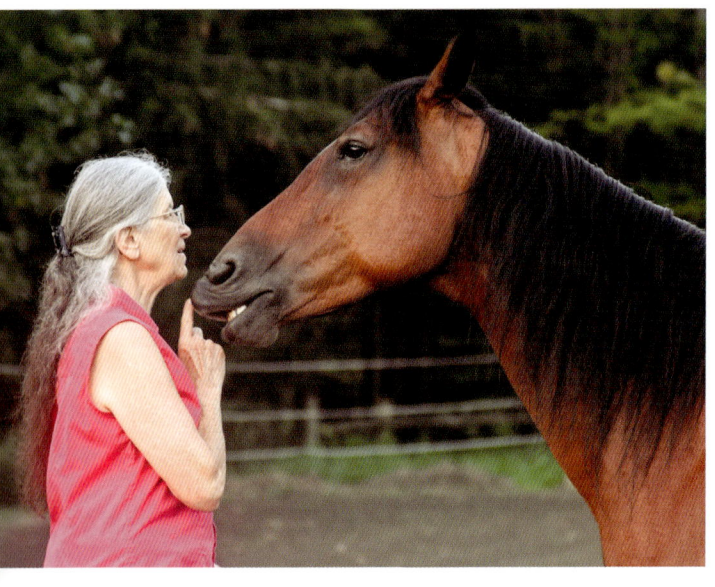

# Acknowledgments

I am especially grateful to:

The many people who provided ideas, encouragement, and feedback.

My friends and sister who allowed me to share photographs of their horses.

The late Frederick "Fritz" Paul of Dry Brook Arabians who bred and raised my dear Bronzz, and modeled Protector Leadership.

Meadowgate Equine Rescue (Newfield, New York) who rescued Brandy and Snickers, cared for them, and entrusted us with those two very special ponies.

The wonderful people at Trafalgar Square Books for their guidance and their faith in me.

# PART ONE:
# Horses Want a Leader They Trust

> "*Every single time we interact with a horse, we are teaching him.* We are either teaching him that he can trust us or that he cannot...That we will listen to his side of the story or that the relationship will be only one-sided."
>
> —Kim Walnes, "Being a Leader/Protector for Your Horse"

We all wish for a horse who meets us at the pasture gate, works because his heart is in it, approaches new situations with confidence, and seeks our guidance when he is scared. All too often horse-human relationships fall short of this cooperative ideal. Horses are hard to catch, resist or do only what is required, appear to take advantage, regress in their training, are anxious and unreliable in new situations, and seem to forget we exist when they are scared.

One reason for these problems is too much focus on what we expect from our horses and too little on what they need from us. "Partnership" and "mutual respect" are often mentioned, but what makes the horse feel respected? What makes him feel like a partner? Most important to the horse, what tells him he can trust us to keep him safe?

When the focus is on what we want from the horse, his compliance becomes the measure of success, and what he thinks and feels may be overlooked. Is he calm, confident, and trusting? Or anxiously wishing he could escape? His behavior, performance, and reliability depend on the answers to those questions.

This book is about a way of relating to horses and providing leadership that has been successful since ancient times because it makes intuitive sense to horses.

Horses want security and social bonds. They want leaders they trust to protect them, not only from danger, but from stress. When we provide this security, they accept our rules. This not only puts us in charge, it makes our leadership *more* effective because we do not force it on them; they *seek* it. The result is less anxiety, fewer behavior problems, better relationships with people, more efficient learning, and better reliability. Research consistently validates this.

I refer to this relationship as *Protector Leadership* because being the protector is the foundation of our leadership. Time-honored riding, handling, and training principles are integral parts of it. Great trainers show how well it works. Scientific research explains *why*. Unfortunately, this wonderful information often appears in bits and pieces, making it hard to see how the pieces relate to each other. Explanations of how we can apply it with our own horses are rare.

I have gathered information from many sources to show how and why Protector Leadership works, and how to make it work for you. To the best of my knowledge this is the first book to fit these separate pieces together, illustrating the connections with practical examples of real horses in everyday life.

My examples are situations I have personally experienced or witnessed, and recorded in my journal. They include my own adventures as I have learned, experimented, and listened to my horses. You will meet my horses Sapphire

# Meet My Horses

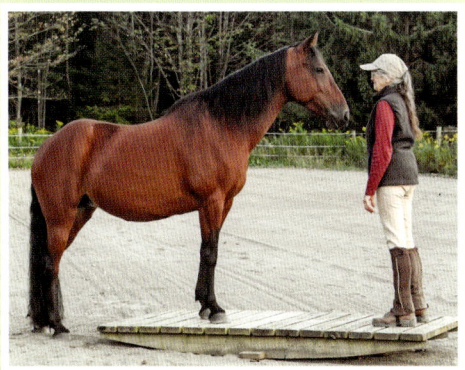

**Brandy,** breed unknown: "Wild" pony turned international agility competitor, kid-partner, and cover girl.

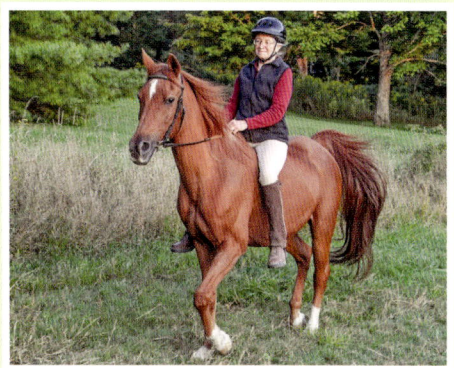

**Bronzz,** Arabian: My partner for many years and adventures. Bold, brave, easily bored, but never boring. The International Horse Agility Club's 2018 Equagility World Champion.

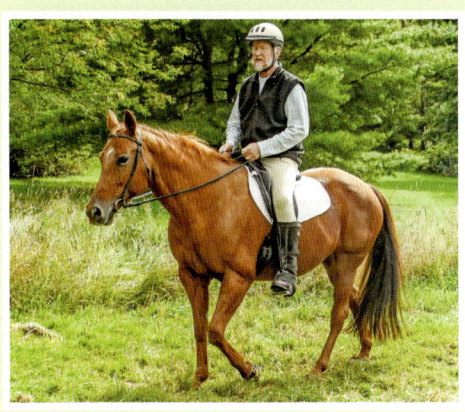

**Shiloh,** Quarter Horse-cross: My husband's current partner. Her mellow personality suits his favorite sort of ride (a bird-watching stroll through the woods).

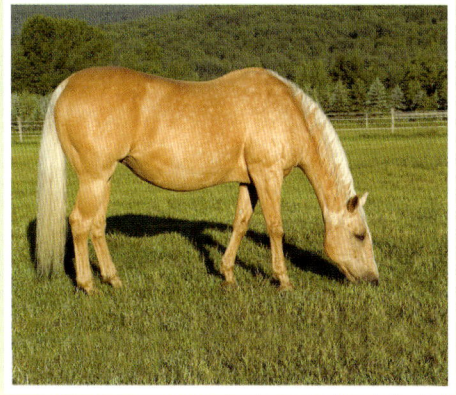

**Sapphire,** breed unknown: My husband's first horse. A sensitive mare with a strong personality, she just wanted to be someone's special partner. She and Jerry took good care of each other for 12 years of trekking rugged trails together.

(1981–2015), Bronzz, and Shiloh, as well as a few horses belonging to family and friends. You will meet the foster pony who first made me rethink my ideas about leadership. Most of all, you'll follow the adventures of Brandy, a little bay mare whose profound transformation illustrates the power of Protector Leadership.

Protector Leadership is not a training system. It is a relationship. Every interaction you have with a horse tells him what kind of leader you are, whether he wants to trust and follow you, or whether he would rather be somewhere else. This is true whether you ride, drive, do groundwork, or keep horses as companions; whether you compete or not; whether your connection with a horse lasts five minutes or his whole life.

Wonderful possibilities are open to you when you provide the leadership horses want. My experience shows that anyone can learn to be a Protector Leader without being a world-class trainer. I use a variety of riding, training, and handling examples to demonstrate how they work in the context of Protector Leadership. I do not suggest that the way I do things is the best or the only way, but more ideas give you more options to choose from. I share mistakes as well as successes, because we learn from mistakes. The resources I found most helpful are listed in the bibliography and mentioned as I go along.

Each of the seven parts in this book is devoted to a different element of Protector Leadership, showing how and why it works, what research supports it, and how you can apply it. The horse's need for security and social bonds is at the core of everything you do, and that is what makes Protector Leadership so powerful.

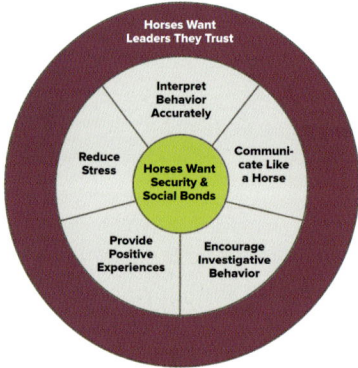

- **Part One** (p. 1) describes Protector Leadership, why horses seek a leader they trust to protect them, and how you can begin earning that trust.

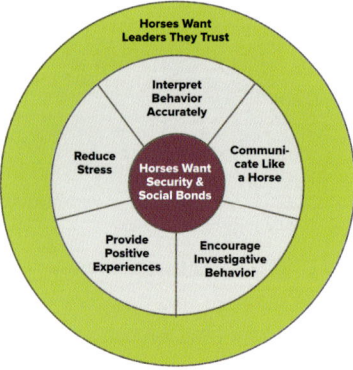

- **Part Two** (p. 31) contrasts the behavior of wild and domestic horses, showing how important security and social bonds are, why this may not be obvious in domestic horses, and how typical domestic living conditions can cause problems.

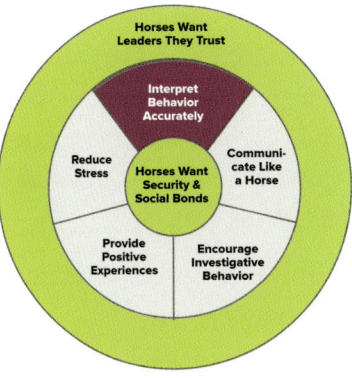

- **Part Three** (p. 63) is a guide to equine behaviors that are frequently misinterpreted, so you can better understand what your horse is trying to tell you.

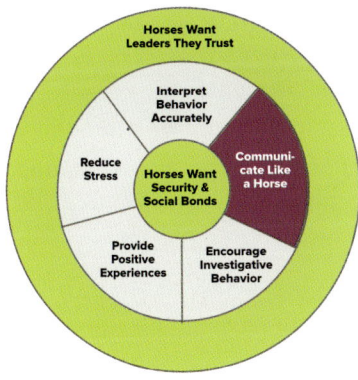

- **Part Four** (p. 99) describes the pressure-based communication that is commonly used with horses, how it can cause problems, and how to use it constructively. Then I show you ways to communicate with your horse using less pressure, or none at all.

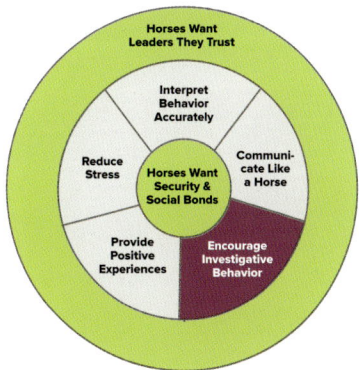

- **Part Five** (p. 139) demonstrates horses' innate curiosity and how you can use it to help your horse overcome fear and anxiety quickly.

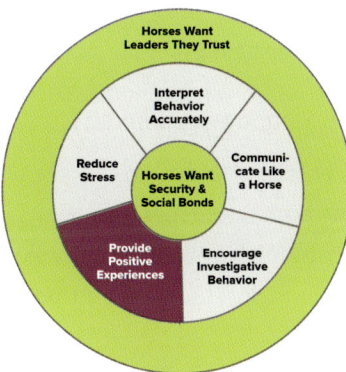

- **Part Six** (p. 175) shows how to build your horse's confidence and reliability with positive experiences that assure him he can trust you. It also describes how to safely allow your horse to express his personality and feelings, and finally how to work with him at liberty.

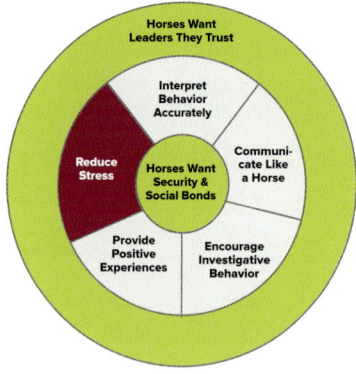

- **Part Seven** (p. 221) focuses on ways you can reduce stress in your horse's lifestyle, thus improving his welfare, behavior, and performance.

Protector Leadership is not a guaranteed solution to all problems; there are no guarantees. But focusing on being a horse's protector helps you to see things from the horse's perspective, which prevents many unnecessary problems and points you to solutions when they do occur.

Many people use Protector Leadership or elements of it. I hope you will get ideas for changes that will improve your relationship with your horse, and make him happier and more productive.

If this sounds too good to be true maybe that is because we have settled for too little for too long. The relationship we hope for with our horses is the same one many of us take for granted with our dogs. Dog training has undergone a revolution in the last few decades. Authoritarian handling techniques that used to be the norm have been replaced with positive ones that speed training, improve relationships and reliability, and make everyone happier and more productive.

The horse world is due for such a transformation. You and your horse can be on the leading edge of it.

**Part One Key Points:**
- Horses want to feel safe; this is more important to them than who is in charge.
- They look for leaders they trust to protect them: Protector Leaders.
- Trusted leaders inspire more cooperation, faster learning, and better reliability.
- Trust must be *earned* through your actions; it cannot be demanded or "taught."

**You will learn how to:**
- Earn a horse's trust starting from the moment you meet him.
- Discourage unwanted behavior without punishment.
- Catch an "uncatchable" horse by showing him he will be safe with you.

## chapter 1
# A Tale of Two Ponies

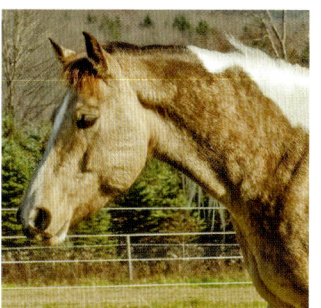

> "...the first question in their mind is not who is boss, it's 'Who is the protector, and who is being protected?'...In the horse's mind, it is an automatic agreement that the protector becomes the leader."
>
> —Kim Walnes ("Being a Leader/Protector for Your Horse")

Snickers, our first foster pony, was a charming tri-colored pinto, rescued by court order as a starved yearling. After four years at a rescue farm he was healthy, sound, and handsome, but his adoption prospects were low because he was not trained for riding.

We were looking for a companion to keep my husband's retired mare company when we rode our other two horses. Fostering a horse from a rescue meant no long-term obligation, or so we imagined. I love to train, and my first focus is the kind of safe, reliable behavior that helps horses find and keep long-term homes. Snickers appeared to be a fun project whose future prospects would be improved with such training.

### Snickers, Pony Einstein?

It soon became apparent that beneath Snickers' cheerfully friendly exterior lurked a significant amount of anxiety. Since an anxious horse is neither safe nor reliable, this posed a dilemma: how to reduce his anxiety and build his confidence?

Our communication with horses relies heavily on pressure, whether it is a pull on a lead line, the squeeze of a leg, or our body language. Theoretically, that pressure is a cue that tells the horse what you want, and it is released when he complies. To a horse who has not been taught what it means, however, it is just pressure, and that can create anxiety even in horses who are not anxious to start with. Picture the frantic reaction of a horse who puts his head down, steps on his own lead line, and doesn't know what to do about it.

"Corrections" are usually a big part of horse training: when a horse does something wrong, he is often notified with sharp words, or more pressure, such as a tug on his lead line. Since even a stern tone of voice sent Snickers' head up in alarm, this was another source of anxiety I wanted to avoid.

I made a plan I hoped might build Snickers' self-confidence so he would become anxious less readily in the future. I couldn't avoid pressure; I didn't know how else to train a horse. But I tried to use it as gently as possible, and back off any time he looked anxious. I capitalized on all the positive training techniques I knew, expanding on anything that elicited cooperation and enthusiasm. I risked avoiding corrections, even though that seemed radical to me at the time. Instead I ignored misbehaviors except when they were immediately dangerous, such as barging into my space. Even then I tried to anticipate problems and quietly redirect him *before* he got in trouble.

For example, Snickers had a habit of using his stall door as a starting gate, shooting out the instant it opened. In the past I would have brought him up short and scolded him sternly. Instead, I headed him off. I slipped in and shut the door behind me, haltered him, and backed him up a few steps to get his mind on me instead of going full speed ahead. If he started forward when I opened the door, I backed him up again, and asked him to wait for my cue to walk forward. This meant that every time he left his stall he was getting a friendly two-minute lesson in, "Back up, head down for halter, stand still, walk forward on cue." Daily repetition in this logical context reinforced the skills. He soon understood that the opening of his stall door meant "Back up."

I used the same principles for all of Snickers' training. I showed him what I wanted, praised him for trying, ignored mistakes, and reassured him when he looked anxious. When introducing something new, I gave him time to think things through and experiment until he found the right answer. My consistently clear expectations emphasized that I was the leader; my quiet manner reassured him that he could trust me. My relationship with him was more like a friendly teacher than a dominant leader. Many trainers would have predicted that Snickers would test, disobey, and run roughshod over me. He did nothing of the sort.

Snickers whizzed through his lessons so quickly he confused me. There was little resistance and no regression. Rude behaviors disappeared. He stood like a statue at the mounting block. He responded to light cues for speed up, slow down, turn, stop, and then for lateral moves. When I taught him to stop on his own if I leaned off balance, a safety feature for young and novice riders, he understood immediately. His spooks went from a wild bucking charge across the arena to spook-in-place. His confidence blossomed, anxiety creeping in only in stressful situations. He met me at the pasture gate every day as if he looked forward to his training sessions (fig. 1.1).

There had to be a catch. This was not *normal*. Certain I was missing something, I went through a spell of being downright nervous about riding him, but the explosion I feared never came. His skills were solid, and his attitude positive—for *me*. Would he fall apart when he was ridden by someone else? I had one of my advanced students ride him. He never missed a beat.

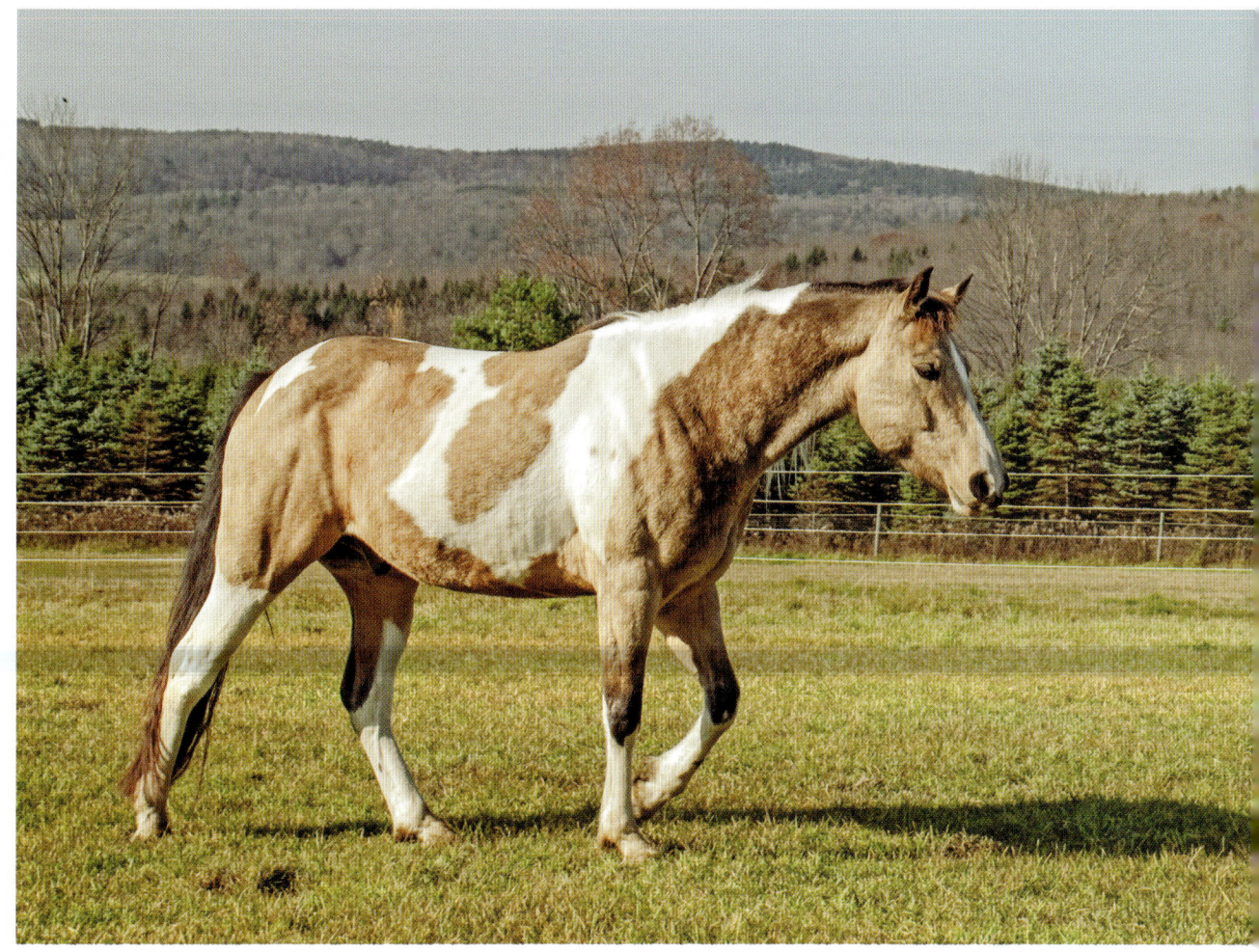

1.1 Snickers routinely came to meet me at the pasture gate, ready for his lessons.

The first prospective adopter was a skilled riding instructor who brought along two very different riders, one gentle and timid, the other bold and determined. It was a real test for Snickers, and he passed with flying colors, adjusting gracefully to each new rider. They adopted him.

Snickers left me wondering, what just happened here? How did this previously anxious pony learn so quickly, then figure out for himself how to adapt to three new and completely different riders, and do it all with calm, cheerful confidence? Was he a Pony Einstein? Or was I onto principles that not only help horses learn more efficiently, but promote the confident, willing attitude that makes them most reliable?

I researched what different trainers said, and what scientific studies have to tell us. I began to suspect that Snickers' success had more to do with my change in *leadership* than changing training techniques. Instead of emphasizing my authority, I had focused on making him feel safe. Several other surprising discoveries emerged from my research.

## What I Discovered About Leadership

• **This Leadership approach has been around a long time** and is still used by world-class trainers. The following quotes reflect the recognition that horses want leaders they trust to protect them:

Kim Walnes, partner of The Gray Goose (Eventing Hall of Fame, 2012), says the most important thing in horses' minds is survival. When they encounter someone new "…the first question in their mind is not who is boss, it's 'Who is the protector, and who is being protected?'…*In the horse's mind, it is an automatic agreement that the protector becomes the leader.*"[1]

Magali Delgado and Frédéric Pignon, founding stars of the spectacular Cavalia show, explain it this way in *Gallop to Freedom*. Although human leaders are the decision-makers, we must also be the horse's protector because "…a horse seeks freedom from fear and stress above all else…"[2]

Vanessa Bee, founder of the sport of Horse Agility, says, "[Horses] don't want to be 'on duty' all the time, so when you turn up and take responsibility for their safety for a while, they're delighted!" Her horses prove it by negotiating complex obstacles at liberty and in large grassy fields where they are free to leave.[3]

Protector Leaders inspire bonds of trust that go both ways.

Over 2,000 years ago, Xenophon advised his fellow cavalry officers, "Make your horse your friend because in battle your life depends on him."[4]

Harry deLeyer, owner of Snowman, the legendary show jumper of the 1950s and 60s, summed it up in the saying, "If you take care of your horse, your horse will take care of you."[5]

- **Research shows that Protector Leadership is based on horse behavior**: the way horses think, learn, and relate to each other and to humans.

Studies of behavior in free-roaming herds (those with little or no human intervention—see p. 34) consistently show that horses care more about security than rank, and security means having "friends" (close associations with other horses).[6] Other research indicates that horses who feel a close attachment to their person have a stronger sense of security, making them calmer and more focused, thus more reliable.[7] This is significant because anxiety is more prevalent than most people realize and, along with pain, accounts for many behavior problems, including many perceived as aggression.[8]

Research shows significant differences in domestic versus free-roaming herds. Free-roaming herds actually have fascinatingly complex social dynamics. They are not led by a single dominant individual, nor do they have a clearly linear ranking. Domestic groups, which often appear to have a dominant leader, do not represent normal social dynamics.[9] (These herd characteristics are the subjects of chapters 3 and 4—pp. 34 and 43.)

In the past, horse people tended to be skeptical of "scientific evidence," and rightly so. Horses were described as unintelligent creatures who operated solely on instinct and learned only by rote memory. Equine researchers now recognize that the intelligence and behavior of horses, like other species, are best understood in the context of what matters to them, not what matters to people. Many new studies, focused on practical application, provide truly useful insights.

## Brandy the Uncatchable

Considering Snickers' success, I was eager to see if the same approach produced similar results with a horse of a different personality. Donna, the director of the rescue farm, was happy to introduce us to another pony in need of training.

Brandy was a dark bay mare built more like a small horse than a large pony. Found wandering loose in upstate New York where we are not supposed to have free-roaming horses, she was so feral it had taken months to lure her into a pasture so she could be herded into a trailer for transport to a rescue farm. I cringe to imagine how traumatic that must have been for her. It was many more months before she could be touched.

Scars showed she'd had serious wounds. Her eyes, though now healthy, showed signs of an untreated infection. Her udder indicated she'd had a foal. All this happened before she was captured at the age, according to her teeth, of three. Like Snickers, she had been handled kindly at the rescue farm but, unlike

*Studies consistently show that horses care more about security than rank.*

Snickers, she had spent 30 days with a professional trainer and returned more fearful than ever. At age six, her adoption prospects hovered around zero.

When my husband and I first saw Brandy in a paddock with a small group of mares, she seemed fairly calm. Donna turned Brandy loose in a large arena so we could observe her by herself. Brandy instantly darted away, kept her distance from us, and then dodged all of Donna's attempts to catch her. We saw no aggression, only fear. Since Brandy had not objected to Donna catching her in the paddock, I supposed that it was the presence of strangers that had triggered her flight reflex. Now every step Donna took toward her heightened her anxiety.

I have always been good at catching horses. I have been doing it the same way for so long I don't remember when or how I learned, but it works. Donna, satisfied to let me have a try, joined my husband at the gate, and I moseyed into the ring.

What happened next surprised even me, and that was just the first of many surprises Brandy had in store for us. Her story will continue in the next chapter as I describe how I learned to be her protector, leader, friend, and source of security (see p. 16).

## Protector Leadership

As I studied the kind of leadership I aspired to, I could not find a consistently used term for it. Mark Rashid describes elements of it as "passive" leadership—"passive leaders" being followed willingly because they lead by example, not force.[10]

Human leaders who offer friendship and protection *do* lead by example, but also take initiative. Frederic Pignon describes us as "the decider." We are passive only in the sense of being quiet and patient. As a result, horses tend to be calm and quiet, creating little drama and thus rather tame training demonstrations.

After many discussions, my husband and I agreed on "Protector Leadership" as the most descriptive term we could think of. The very next day, I happened upon an article in which Kim Walnes gave a wonderfully clear description of the relationship. The title of the article was "Being a Leader/Protector for Your Horse."[11] That clinched it.

## Training vs. Relationship

Leadership is not a technique. It is a *relationship*, and we are the ones responsible for making it whatever it is. Good training teaches horses *how* to meet our expectations, but good leadership is what makes them *want* to. It is independent of riding style, skill level, or training style. As Mark Rashid says, "I have found that tools and techniques don't matter all that much unless they are applied with the right attitude."[12]

Horses' actions are influenced by their feelings, just as ours are, no matter how much training they have. Thus, controlling a horse's body is only part of the equation. We must also have a positive influence on his thoughts and emotions. When horses associate people with unpleasantness, their focus naturally turns to how they can most effectively avoid whatever unpleasantness they anticipate. When they have a positive attitude about us and the things we want them to do, they learn new skills readily and apply them reliably. In order to develop that willing attitude we must have communication going *both* ways, so that we are listening to our horses just as we want them to listen to us. After all, how long do we want to listen to people who do not listen to us?

## Empathy vs. Anthropomorphism

Consideration for horses' feelings is sometimes dismissed as anthropomorphic (ascribing human characteristics to animals), but there is an important distinction between anthropomorphism and empathy.

*Anthropomorphism* means projecting *human* motivation, feelings, or behavior onto an animal.

*Empathy* is the ability to recognize and respect the emotions experienced by another being of any species. It is an indispensable quality of a good leader. Recognizing a horse's emotions is essential to humane treatment; we cannot relieve pain, fear, or other distress if we don't recognize them. Failing to relieve distress jeopardizes our own safety because horses' feelings are important predictors of their actions.

Empathy also impacts performance. When a horse is seen only as an obedient servant or a piece of sports equipment, there is no partnership. A real partnership requires understanding a horse as an individual with personality and feelings. Margie Goldstein Engle (American Grand Prix Association Rider of the Year 10 times) described this nicely in an article titled "Empathy, the Secret Ingredient for Success."[13]

## Being in Charge

Protector Leadership is a responsibility position. You accept responsibility for your horses' safety and welfare, and for showing them what you expect of them. In order to fulfill these responsibilities, you must be clearly and reliably in charge.

You are attentive to your horse's needs, and take them into account as you make decisions, but *you make the decisions*. Then you carry them out in ways that are consistent and friendly, so that you are the leader, not enforcer. This is like a teacher whose students work because they recognize her caring for them and respect her rules, not because they are intimidated by her authority or fear unpleasant consequences.

Respecting your horse's needs and wishes never means indulging him. Permissiveness is not kindness. I hold my horses to a high standard of reliably good behavior. They have latitude to express their personalities and opinions, but not to be rude or unsafe. When my farrier was recovering from a broken leg and still on crutches, my horses were the first he chose to work on. That was because, he said, they were the ones he trusted most. They did not disappoint us.

## Mentors and Role Models

It is a fact of life that we are influenced by the actions and attitudes of those around us. If our main horse time is spent with people whose view of horsemanship is authoritarian, it is easy to see that approach as normal and acceptable, and to see horses' reactions to it as inevitable. When good horsemanship is perceived as the ability to "ride out the bucks" or "show a horse who's boss," it is easy to overlook the quietly competent people who do not provoke unwanted behavior in the first place.

As I worked to improve my leadership skills, I looked for opportunities to spend time with horse people whose horses were not just obedient, but relaxed and confident. I shared ideas with horse friends who were trying to improve their own horsemanship. I thought back to people I knew in the past whom I now recognize as Protector Leaders, and reviewed in my mind how they had handled various situations. I joined an online group of like-minded people who share ideas and problem-solve together. I watched countless videos of people using body language instead of pressure to communicate with their horses. As I watched and listened to Protector Leaders, their approach became my new normal.

No one person knows everything. I have learned useful things from more people than I could possibly count.

In the end, our most important teachers are the horses themselves. Each horse is an expert on himself, and each horse will tell us his own truth if we listen. When in doubt, I ask my horses. Theirs is the final word.

## Safety

All ideas I present are offered with the assumption that you already have safe horse-handling skills. One of the most important of those skills is the ability to read a horse's body language and assess his emotional state so you can be aware when trouble is brewing. As you plan your work with horses, please give very careful consideration to your own skills, experience, and safety relative to the behavior of every horse you handle.

When I describe working with horses whose behavior was potentially dangerous, please consider that I am a certified riding instructor with many years of experience working with a variety of different horses, including re-schooling horses with problem behaviors. Protector Leadership provides guidelines that help prevent and resolve problems; it does not magically turn dangerous horses into safe ones. You must always be mindful that horses are powerful animals, easily frightened, and that even the kindest, best trained horses make mistakes and bad judgment calls, just as we do.

## Things to Try

At the end of each chapter are suggested "Things to Try" with your own horse, or any horse available to you. These are *experiments*, not training exercises. Only two rules apply: First, of course, stay safe. Second, do not measure your success by how "obedient" your horse is. There are no right or wrong answers in this context. Instead, focus on *understanding* your horse's responses. If you have more than one horse to engage, so much the better. Notice individual variations in their responses.

## Summary

Horses look for leaders they trust to protect them because security is more important to them than who is in charge. Many unnecessary problems and disappointments stem from overlooking horses' need for security, while focusing instead on what we want them to do. The amount of pressure often used for training, cues, and corrections is a common source of trouble.

You can offer the security horses need by being a protector/leader instead of an authority/leader. Then, horses readily accept your direction and your rules. You get better cooperation, faster learning, and more reliability. This has worked for horse people of every riding style and skill level for many centuries. Research validates that a "protector" approach to leadership is compatible with horses' natural social order. Authoritarian leadership is not.

### THINGS TO TRY

- Write down three things you like about your relationship with your horse and might want to build on.
- Write down three things you would like to change in your relationship with your horse.
- As you read on, watch for ideas on how to make those changes.
- Recheck those lists a few months from now, and notice your progress.

## chapter 2
# Earning Trust

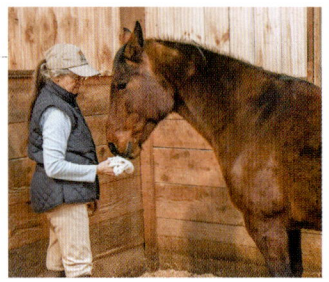

> "Horses are never misled like humans into believing that they are completely safe from all danger. They always seek someone to whom they can turn in a strange or threatening situation...a horse seeks freedom from fear and stress above all else...."
>
> —Magali Delgado and Frédéric Pignon *(Gallop to Freedom)*

Establishing yourself as a leader who can be trusted starts with the message your body language sends when you first approach a horse. A person concerned with authority announces, "I am in charge, and I expect to be obeyed." If a horse is already behaving respectfully, making an issue of authority is pointless, and may actually confuse him. You can always add later if needed, "And by the way, I am the leader here." But if you come on too strong, you do not get a second chance to make a reassuring first impression.

A person offering protection says first, "I'm safe. You can trust me to look out for you." This is so important because it is not good enough for *you* to think the horse is safe. He needs to *feel* safe. With a horse who is already comfortable around people, a reassuring introduction is deceptively simple, yet powerful. You show the same respect for the horse's personal space that you expect him to show for yours.

### First and Lasting Impressions

You have probably seen people walk up to a strange horse and grab the lead line, expecting the horse to follow. Or take up the reins and stick a foot in the stirrup

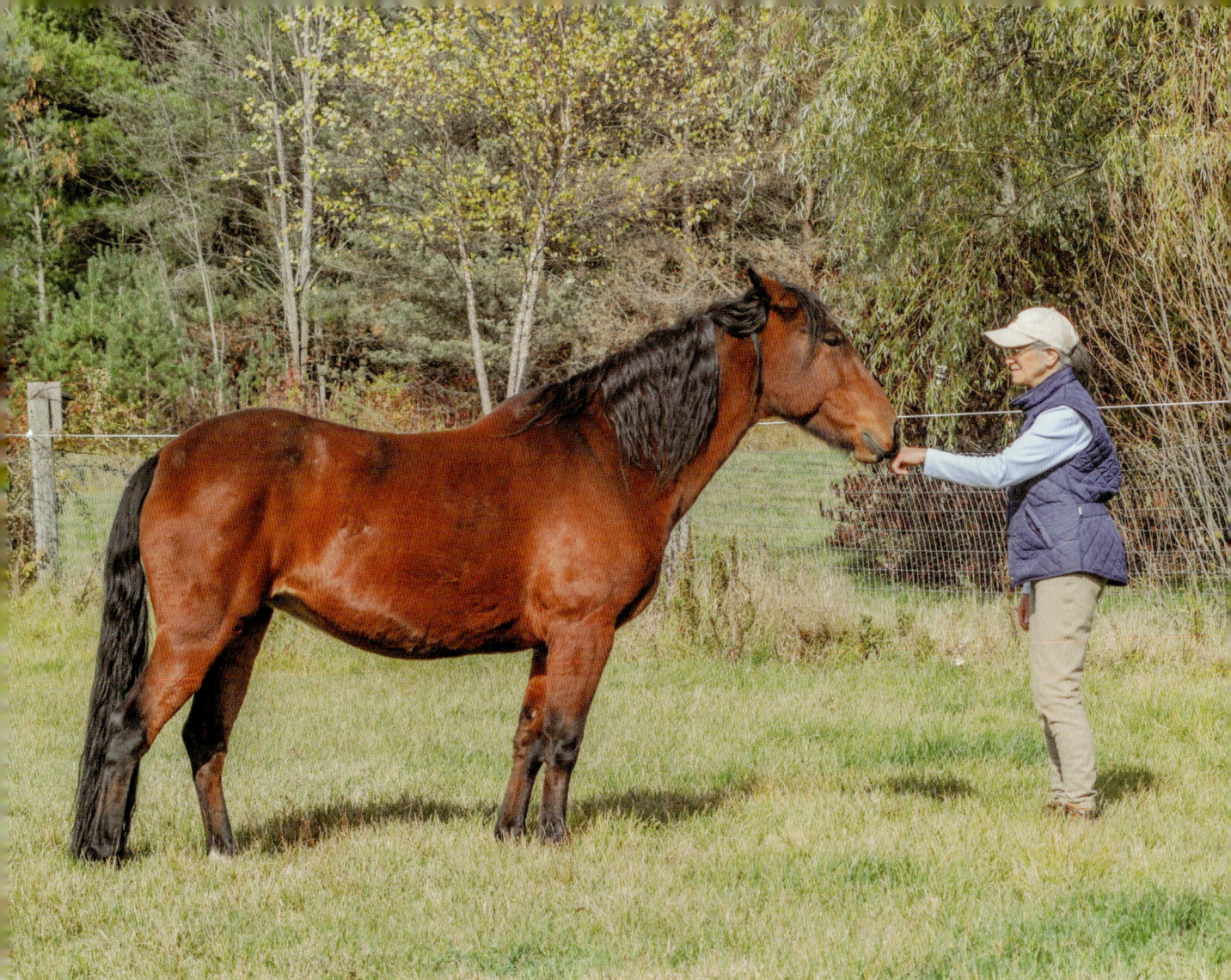

without so much as greeting the horse. Although many horses learn to tolerate this behavior, it is a disrespectful invasion of their personal space. It can make horses uncomfortable just as you might be uncomfortable having a stranger get too close.

It takes only seconds to pause a few feet away, speak to the horse, and wait for him to acknowledge your presence by glancing or flicking an ear your way. You have just announced your intention to treat him respectfully. You have also given yourself a chance to assess his emotional state. If he looks relaxed and friendly, you offer a hand for sniffing, and carry on (fig. 2.1).

When the horse looks tense or anxious, you can take extra time to talk quietly, extend your hand slowly, and assess his response. If a horse backs up nervously at your approach, reaching for him announces loud and clear that you are not to be trusted. To invite trust, you must let the horse come to you. That gives him a choice instead of making him

2.1 Brandy and I demonstrate an unthreatening way to introduce yourself before entering a horse's personal space. This gentle nose touch, which Sharon Wilsie teaches in *Horse Speak,* reflects a greeting between two horses who are friends.

PART ONE: HORSES WANT A LEADER THEY TRUST — 17

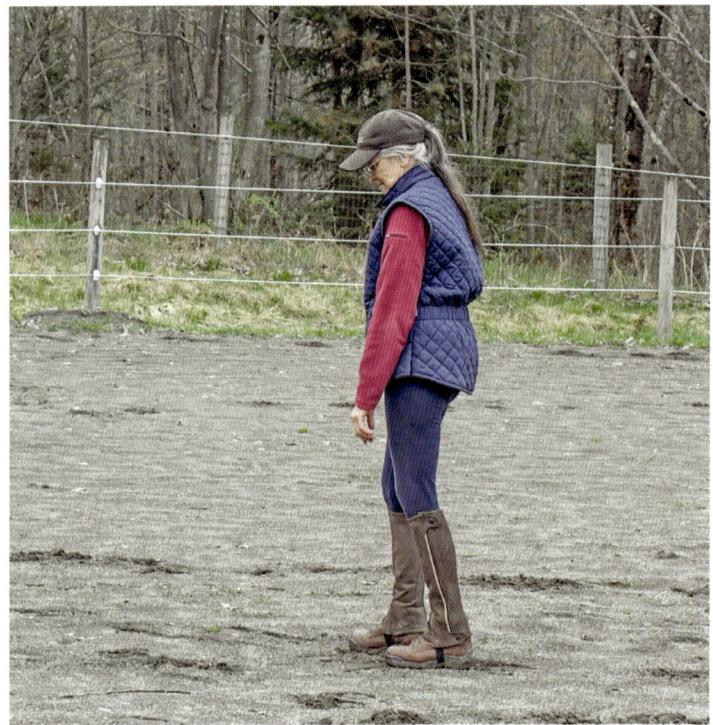

2.2 Approaching an anxious horse applies pressure that makes him more anxious. My unthreatening posture as I take a tiny step backward is what invited Brandy to approach me instead.

feel trapped. If he is reluctant, you can encourage him by turning so you are not facing him directly.

Making a habit of greeting a horse before you enter his personal space is also a good safety precaution in case he is dozing or distracted. You simply speak to him as you approach, or pause just outside his personal space zone, watching for an acknowledgement before you move in. Speaking to horses makes sense because they identify you by your voice as well as scent and appearance, and because a friendly tone reinforces your intent.

I have noticed that people often look confused when I introduce myself to their horses, but dog people are never surprised when we introduce ourselves to their dogs. In fact, dog people are inclined to *assume* we will greet their dogs first!

## Catching the Uncatchable Horse

You might be tempted to skip this section if your horse is already easy to catch, but consider this: good horsemanship includes preparing for the unexpected, such as a gate left open, a rider down, or a loose horse frantic in a situation where he is in the most danger. Our impulse is to rush toward him in a desperate attempt to grab reins or halter, the action most certain to scare him off. Horses who are frightened or excited for any reason need a delicate approach.

The day we met Brandy, her increasingly desperate charge around the arena clearly showed fear, heightened by Donna's attempts to approach her. I did what I have always done with horses who do not want to be caught. I invited her to "catch" me instead. This approach is the best starting place even with horses who appear stubborn because such "bad behavior" often masks anxiety.

I strolled toward the center of the ring with a casual slouch, head down, unthreatening (fig. 2.2). When Brandy looked at me, I backed away, thus rewarding her for looking at me. When she stopped looking at me, I got her attention by moseying obliquely into her line of sight, weaving little serpentines. When she looked at me again, I stopped. When she began to slow down, I stepped back.

When Brandy looked like she was *thinking* about stepping toward me, I took another step backward. After a few more laps, she actually did step toward me. I took a bigger step back.

It is an intricate dance, each step meant to reassure the horse that I will not chase, harass, or scare her. The more skittish the horse, the slower my approach. Each time she looks at me or moves my way, I reward her by stopping or backing up. If she moves away, I resume moving, careful to keep my angle of approach in front of her, to avoid chasing her.

When Brandy walked toward me, I backed up slowly, letting her catch up to me. Then I stood still, hands down, just talking quietly to her for a moment. Since reaching toward a horse from the front is more threatening, I executed a slow about face so I was standing next to her, facing the same way. Slowly I reached up and scratched her shoulder. It had taken her about 10 minutes to catch me.

At this point, if I wanted to halter the horse, I would slowly reach the lead line *under* her neck with my left hand, reaching over the crest to grasp the line with my right. This is less threatening than placing a rope over the neck. Having already faced the same direction as the horse, I am in position to slowly slip the halter on. If she is already wearing a halter, I work my hand up to it.

Every move is gentle, in slow motion. I breathe deeply.

Instead of haltering Brandy, I just visited with her for a few quiet minutes, then walked back to the gate where Donna and my husband waited. Brandy followed me. She parked herself within arm's reach of me, and stayed there calmly until we left, about half an hour later. While I was not surprised that I had persuaded Brandy to catch me, I was surprised when she followed me and stayed with me. This told me that she *wanted* to trust.

As to whether she could become a reliable riding horse, there was only one way to find out.

## Earning Brandy's Trust

We met Brandy in December but didn't plan to bring her home until spring, when the weather was more conducive to riding and training. That left me time to ponder what to do with her when she got here. I had laid a foundation of trust in our first meeting. I did not want to blow it.

The problem was that I did not know how to train a horse without pressure. I had used *less* pressure with Snickers, but the basic techniques were still the same: direct pressure from halter, lead, bridle, or touch; indirect pressure from my body language. But Snickers basically trusted people. Brandy did not. She was afraid to even be near people. *Any* pressure was going to activate her flight response.

Yes, she would eventually have to cope with pressure, but she needed to trust me first. Then she needed to learn that specific types of pressure were cues for her to perform certain actions, and that she could relieve the pressure by performing those actions so she wouldn't feel trapped. Meanwhile, I needed a way to communicate with her and begin her training without pressure, so we could build a trusting bond. Enlightenment came from an unexpected source.

## A Teacher Appears

Visiting another barn, we met a newly arrived pony who was terrified of people, especially men. Guests were asked not to even approach her stall, and it was obvious why. The mere sight of my husband, peering over her door before he was warned, had her scrambling to the back of her stall, hitting the wall in terror.

> *I needed a way to communicate with her...without pressure, so we could build a trusting bond.*

When I heard a couple months later that a *male* employee of the stable was having great success with her, I asked him for a demonstration. My first question was how did he even get close enough to the pony to get a halter on her? He showed me. He opened Thistle's stall door and stood sideways to her, halter in hand, not looking at her. The first time, he said, he waited half an hour for her to come to him. Today, the little mare hesitated only briefly before approaching him. Slowly, he held out the halter and she stood still as he placed it on her head.

He signaled the pony to walk with him by bending forward at the waist, inviting forward motion. She fell in step beside him like an obedience dog at heel. They went down the barn aisle, out the door, across the driveway, and into the indoor arena. There she continued to copy his every move like a dance partner. Walk, trot, turn, stop. Her head stayed right next to his body. The lead never went tight. Her manners on the lead line were better than many horses ever learn.

The young man unclipped the lead, and Thistle continued to stand by his side as we talked. Suddenly, she took off, cantering around the arena as if he no longer existed.

"What do you do now?" I asked, expecting him to be flustered by this "lapse" in training.

"Nothing," he said calmly. "She'll be back."

She did not come back right away. She was too busy finding things to inspect. Jump standards, poles, plastic flowers and hedges, chairs, mounting blocks. She had her nose into everything. Then she knocked a pole over and scared herself. Spinning around, she made a beeline for her trainer and parked herself at his side for security.

That is when the light bulb went on in my head. *She chose to come back because he gave her the freedom to leave!* No pressure, no demands. He had simply offered her security by making himself her safe haven. Had he tried to teach her by using pressure on the lead line, she would have felt trapped and thought only of escape. Seeing him as her security, Thistle had willingly copied his movements, thus learning those skills with no pressure or stress.

Even when Thistle returned, the trainer did not look at her, pet her, or offer reassuring words. Too much pressure for her at this stage, he said. She just needed him to *be* there and be clear about what they were doing.

A few months later a small adult was riding and schooling the pony.

## Brandy Arrives (May)

The following spring, Brandy's previous trainer trailered her to us. She all but fell off the trailer, dripping with sweat and shaking. It was not a hot day. The trainer offered to demonstrate what he had done with her. The moment he turned to face her and lifted his right hand, she shot to the end of the rope, head high, trotting frantically around him before he even twirled his rope. When he swung his rope in front of her, she did not process it as a signal to change direction. She froze.

Her feet were stuck, he announced, not acceptable. It wasn't clear whether he failed to see her fear or did not consider it important. He swung his rope ever closer until it hit her on the nose. She spun around and raced off in the opposite direction.

This was not training; it was chasing and intimidation. Brandy was moving because he had triggered her flight reflex, not because she had learned anything. My husband and I quickly assured the trainer that we understood just what kind of work he had done with her and showed him which stall to leave her in.

Before he left, I clarified, "I was told that you trail-rode Brandy." No, he replied firmly, he never rode her outside a round pen. When I asked if he knew how she was with children, he was adamant. He would never let children near her. I began to suspect there was a lot more to this little mare's story than I had heard.

## The Velcro Pony

With the help of Thistle's young trainer, I made a plan for building Brandy's trust in me. It wasn't complicated. Hang out near her. Ask nothing of her. No training or "discussion" of leadership except what was required for safety. This sounded pretty radical to me, accustomed as I was to establishing right off the bat that I am in charge and expect to be obeyed. But that approach had already been tried on Brandy with dismal results. There was nothing to lose with a radically different approach.

I started by turning her out in my arena. The first day, it took her 15 minutes to catch me. The next day, she cantered to the gate to meet me! On her third day, I started adding brief pasture turnout to acclimate her to our grass. She continued to meet me at the gate whenever I appeared. This is the bonus of inviting horses to catch you; they become easier to catch each time. That is assuming, of course, that nothing unpleasant happens after you catch them, in which case there is no method that will make them want to be caught.

Horses routinely spend undemanding time just hanging out with each other; it is part of social bonding. We humans tend to show up only when we want horses to do something for us. In our goal-oriented, overscheduled culture, spending even a few minutes just "hanging out" with our horses might seem like a waste of time. It is not. It is an investment in your bond with the horse, not only when you are first getting acquainted, but for your entire partnership.

To avoid putting any pressure on Brandy at this stage, I mostly pretended to pay no attention to her. I dug weeds, trimmed bushes, and scooped manure. By the third day she was following me around. At first, she stood nearby, watching as I worked. Then she began to creep in closer, sometimes poking her nose into the middle of what I was doing. Considering her intent, I realized it was not meant as a disrespectful invasion of my space. She was curious about what I was doing, responding to my tacit invitation to hang out with me, and feeling safe closer to me. Rather than risk frightening her by pushing her away, I just quietly put out an elbow to deflect her if I felt she was too close for safety.

At first, I did not touch or look at her, but I did talk to her as I worked. Although opinion is divided on the value of talking to horses, I have always talked to them, and I had the impression that chatting with Brandy increased her interest in being near me. Sometimes she wandered off, investigating other parts of the arena or sampling weeds, but invariably she came back. Even though I had seen how Thistle stuck to her trainer when she had the choice to leave, I was shocked that it actually worked for me! Brandy soon followed me so consistently that we called her the "Velcro Pony."

Although I did not want to start training right away, Brandy had several unsafe behaviors that I could not ignore. I addressed them in non-punitive ways in the context of the everyday routines when they occurred.

## Leading and Following

Brandy had been taught to walk directly behind her handler when led. This leading position is sometimes described as respectful of the leader's authority, but nothing in herd dynamics supports this claim. Quite the contrary, the rear position is the power or driving position. In any case, I do not want a horse directly behind me because I cannot see her; if I trip or slip I can fall in front of her; and if she spooks I am in her flight path.

I changed Brandy's position by turning slightly toward her, wiggling (not pulling) the lead line to get her attention, and clucking to encourage her to come forward so she walked with her head beside me. This took some gentle nagging because it was contrary to what she had previously been taught.

## Personal Space

The other unsafe behaviors related to personal space.

One occurred when we went through a gate and turned around to close it. Brandy wanted to lift her chin and swing her head above mine as she turned. I did not want her crowding that close, and I especially did not want her flinging her head over mine. To change this, I used the tactic of making the behavior I wanted more attractive than the one I did not want.

Every time we turned and Brandy started to lift her chin, I just *happened* to stretch my free arm straight up in the air so that as she swung her head over mine, she bumped her face into my arm. I did not look at her or say anything when I did it. I was not punishing (hitting) her; she was bumping herself on my arm. This is a critical distinction, and horses get it. She quickly decided to back up so she had room to turn around without whacking her nose on my arm. This corrected the unsafe behavior quickly and without jeopardizing the trust I'd earned.

Our other personal space issue was a bit more complicated. When Brandy hovered close out of interest in what I was doing, I chose to allow it, though other people might not, especially with a larger horse.

When she crowded because she was anxious, that was a different story. There was nothing belligerent or disrespectful about it. She was looking to me for reassurance, like a foal makes body contact with her mother when she's worried. But it was still dangerous.

*I made the behavior I wanted more attractive than the one I did not want.*

Sadly, most people don't recognize this action for the compliment that it is. Instead of trying to escape, the anxious horse is looking to you for protection and reassurance. This is what Protector Leadership is all about! Your big chance to say, "Yes, I'm here to protect you!"

What do most people do instead? The opposite! They push, poke, chase, slap, scold, yank the lead, or anything else unpleasant to "back the horse off," which only makes the horse more frightened and desperate for reassurance. The horse, who meant no disrespect, has no way of knowing what he is being punished for or what the handler wants him to do instead.

The simple, speedy solution that makes everyone safe and happy is to show the horse in a non-punitive way where we *do* want her to be. Without looking at Brandy or speaking to her, I flapped my elbows as if overcome by an urge to do a "chicken wing" exercise (fig. 2.3). When she stepped out of my space, I praised her as if it had been her own excellent idea and put a reassuring hand on her withers, the mutual grooming spot. Then we just stood. If she stood quietly, which she usually did, I rewarded her by easing closer to her so our bodies touched, which was what she wanted in the first place.

If a horse is too tall for elbows to be effective, you can use a raised-arm exercise like windshield wipers that involves motion *inside your personal space bubble*. It simply has to be a consistent neutral motion that is not directed at the horse. Horses are good at judging distance. As long as your maneuver stays right inside your personal space, they figure out exactly how far away it is comfortable to

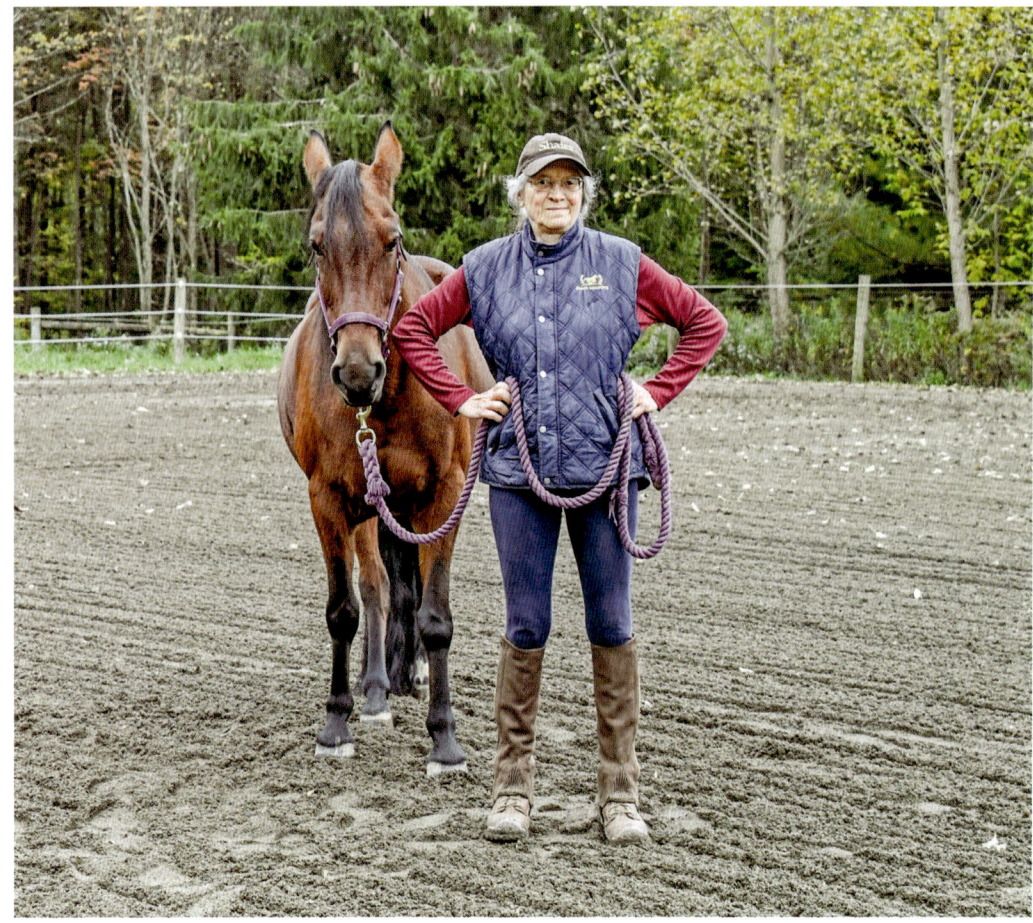

2.3 The chicken-wing exercise discouraged Brandy from crowding my personal space because she quickly discovered it was more comfortable to stay outside elbow range. This is non-punitive because you do not look at the horse, scold, or direct your actions at her.

stand, and they get it more quickly than you could teach them.

The same personal space bubble approach works with horses who crowd for other reasons, including the "schmoozy" characters who want to frisk everyone for treats. In chapter 11 (Rewards Are Positive Feedback—p. 128), I will show how to use treats to keep horses *out* of your personal space. Counterintuitive though it may sound, it works great.

## Saddle Phobia (June)

Brandy was a quick learner and very cooperative, but if I forgot how vulnerable she was to being frightened, she reminded me in a hurry. I normally flip the lead rope over my own horses' necks when I go to halter them. The day I absentmindedly did the same to Brandy, she dodged way beyond the end of the rope—my mistake for taking a liberty she was not ready for. I saw no need to stress her by flinging ropes around to "desensitize" her. Snickers had shown a similar fear of ropes, and it had subsided by itself after a few months of quiet handling and casual rope dangling.

One event did worry me. The first time I walked *past* Brandy's stall carrying a Western saddle, she dove to the far corner in wide-eyed horror. How, I wondered, had anyone ridden her if that was her reaction to the mere sight of a saddle?

My sister came to visit shortly after this, and I wanted her help assessing which of my English saddles might be most comfortable for Brandy when she was ready to ride. A Western saddle was not in the running since most of them are too big for her, and we hoped that an English saddle would look different enough to not be terribly alarming. No such luck.

We could not get near Brandy with an English saddle. Or a bareback pad, or a lunging surcingle, or a saddle pad. No such thing was touching that little mare's body. This definitely did not sync up with the reports that she had already been ridden. Was this a reaction to trauma? Or pain?

My vet could find no evidence of pain in Brandy's back, so I proceeded on the premise that Brandy was reacting to a past trauma. I would restart her saddle training, making the experience as positive and stress-free as possible.

## Remedial Saddle Training (July)

This was my biggest leadership challenge yet. Protector Leaders, *by definition*, do not force horses to do things they are afraid of. If I restrained Brandy with a halter and lead, she would feel trapped, no matter how slowly and gently I worked. I could have given her a choice between being touched and "working," for example, laps in a round pen or on a lunge line, but that is still a form of coercion because the horse cannot escape. Yet Brandy had already made it clear that she

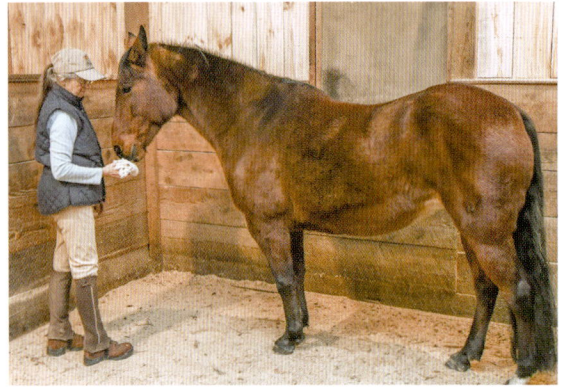

2.4 A  Free to move away from me, Brandy chose to check out the folded towel.

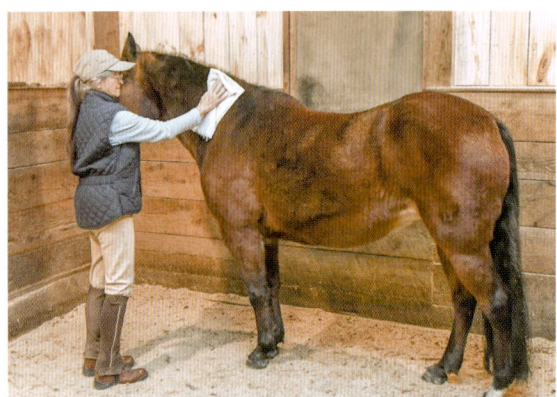

2.4 B  When she was relaxed being "petted" with the tightly folded towel, I partially unfolded it and repeated the process.

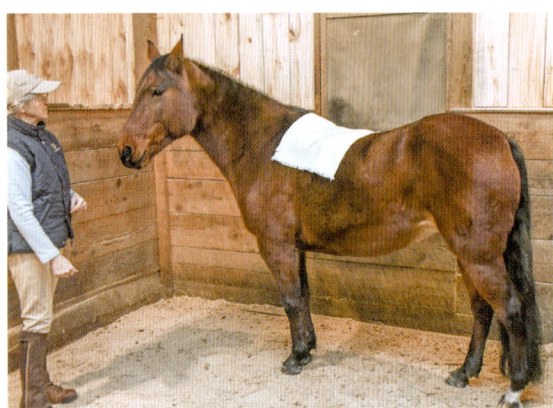

2.4 C  Her left ear says she is noticing the towel, but she is not worried enough to move. Wearing the towel on her back represented trust and progress for Brandy.

would not voluntarily let me put so much as a small towel on her back.

Thistle's trainer had moved and was not available for consultation, so I fell back on one of the most basic of training principles: Start with what I *could* do, and break the problem into the smallest steps necessary to proceed successfully.

Brandy would let me touch her with a small towel if it was folded to the size of a washcloth. That is where we started. In her stall, with her loose so she could walk away any time. Sessions were short. I was not conditioning her to stand still; I was looking for her to understand she was safe enough to relax.

I started by petting Brandy with the folded towel in my hand. When she walked away, I waited. If she did not come back in a minute or so, I asked her to. She always did. Gradually, I unfolded the towel (figs. 2.4 A–C). Then I let it flap around a bit. My criterion for moving to the next step was that she was *relaxed*. Standing still does not prove the horse *feels* safe. It risks anxiety building up until something unpleasant happens.

When Brandy was comfortable with the towel touching her entire body, and having it waved around and draped over her, I repeated everything with a real saddle pad. Then I reviewed that with her loose in my 80- by 200-foot arena (fig. 2.5).

In *Considering the Horse*, Mark Rashid describes leaving horses loose to work on head-shyness and other handling problems. His reasons are the same as mine. A restrained horse feels trapped, making him a danger to

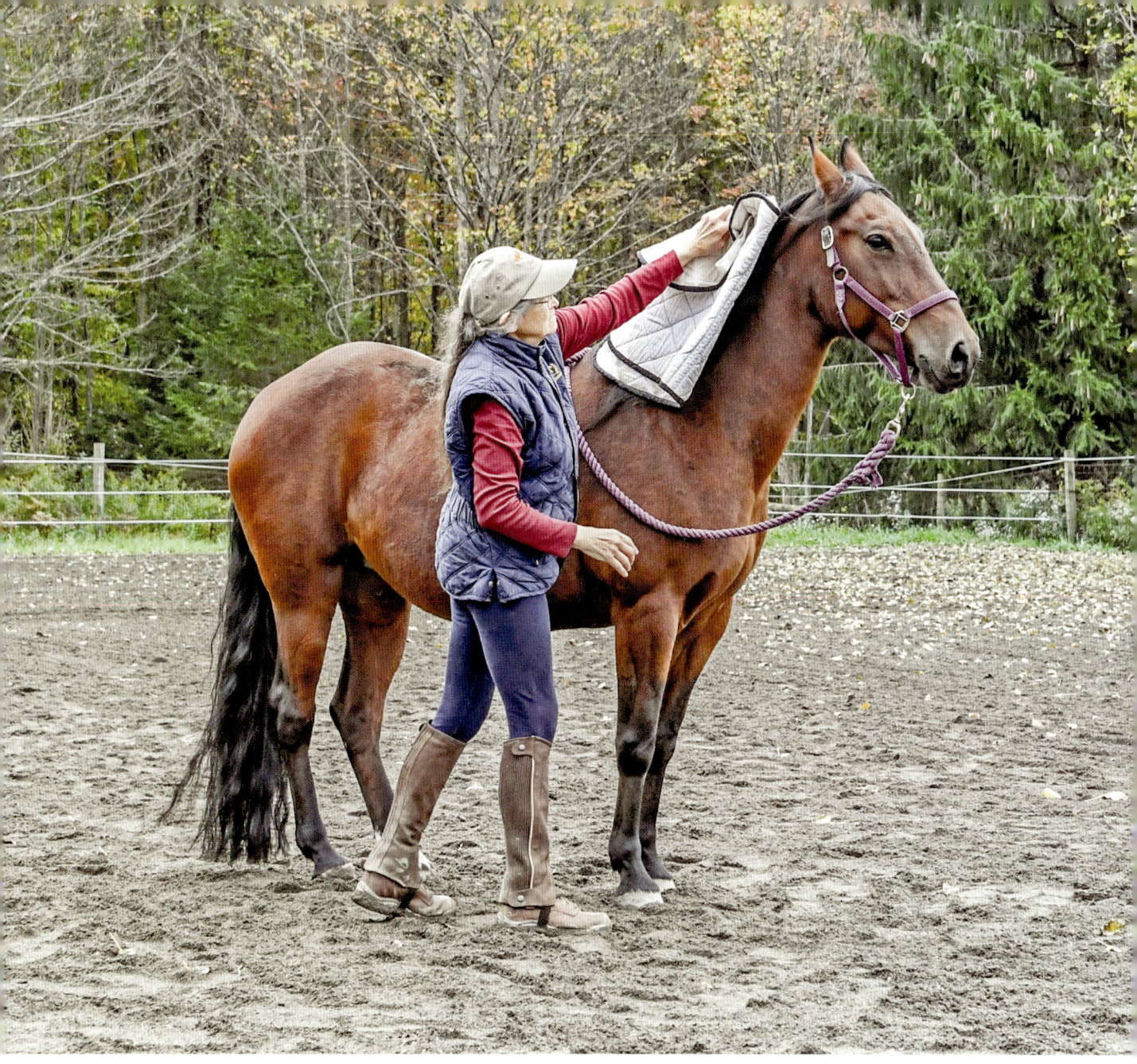

2.5 Brandy's high head shows anxiety about the saddle pad touching her neck, but she is not offering to leave even though I am not holding her lead.

himself and everyone around him. In his words, "The thing that I like most about the method is the genuine lack of desire of the horses to fight. I have now used it on more horses than I care to remember, and in each case, when the pressure became too great, the horse would simply leave. The interesting thing is that they all returned of their own free will or would allow me to approach them."[14]

Mark Rashid's success using this approach with many different horses satisfied me that my success with Brandy was not a fluke.

When I was ready to girth up the bareback pad, I did put a halter and lead

PART ONE: HORSES WANT A LEADER THEY TRUST — 27

on Brandy, so as not to risk her being loose if she panicked with equipment attached. But I left the lead loose, allowing her the freedom to move away from me to the far end of it. By now she seemed to trust that I would not force anything on her, and I was cautiously optimistic about overcoming her fear of saddles.

Brandy, however, had many more surprises in store for us, all of them providing new challenges for my leadership skills.

## Becoming a Protector Leader to My Own Horses

It was more difficult to shift to a Protector Leader relationship with my own horses than it was to establish it from the start with Brandy. Sapphire, Bronzz, and Shiloh had all been with us for over a decade. They were used to my more authoritarian way of relating to them, and I assumed their responses were normal. Nothing had ever happened that required me to rethink how I related to them. If Brandy had not come on the scene, we might have trundled along in the same groove forever.

Subtle contrasts made me wonder. Brandy was the one who consistently met me at the pasture gate, just as Snickers had always done. She was the least likely to misbehave, the most focused and earnest about doing whatever I asked of her. She seemed content to have me just stand next to her doing nothing but being in each other's company.

Slowly, as I learned to be a better Protector Leader, my relationships with my other horses changed, each in a different way. Bronzz greeted me more often with happy ears. He was less fidgety when I worked around him, more focused when I rode him. Shiloh became less tense, less quick to startle.

The biggest change was in Sapphire, who had always been considered the quintessential dominant mare. "Give her an inch, and she'll take three miles," warned her previous owner. I never gave her an inch; I was strict and stern. She constantly "tested" my authority. I never imagined that might be a vicious cycle that I set in motion.

Carefully, I trained myself to relate to her differently. I never lowered my expectations. I was just quieter and more patient about enforcing them. The change in Sapphire's behavior, which I will describe in more detail in chapter 5 (Brandy Changes Our Herd Dynamics—p. 51), was dramatic.

## Summary

Trust is the foundation of Protector Leadership. These are actions that earn trust:

- Greet the horse in a way that shows respect for his personal space.
- Handle the horse in a calm, quiet manner.
- Show the horse what you want instead of punishing what you do *not* want.
- Discourage unwanted behaviors with neutral actions instead of punishment.
- Use relaxation, not actions, as a measure of success.
- Watch for signs of anxiety, and back off as needed. You never know what might have happened in the past to justify the anxiety.
- Avoid using force or making the horse feel trapped in any way.

### THINGS TO TRY

- The next time you meet a new horse, try introducing yourself before entering his personal space. Notice how he responds to you. Try greeting horses you know in the same way. Do you see a difference in the response of the horse who does not know you (and makes no assumptions about your behavior) compared to those who already know you?

- Try inviting horses to catch you. See if those who do not know you show a more obvious positive response than those who may anticipate more "assertive" behavior from you.

- Take time to "hang out" with your horse, in his stall, paddock, or pasture, asking nothing of him. Notice how he responds to your presence, and whether he initiates interaction.

# PART TWO:
# Horses Want Security and Social Bonds

> "When you study a species under natural conditions, the beauty of social order is more apparent....In undisturbed populations of horses with plenty of space, overt, serious aggression is rare. That's because the order has long before been worked out and perhaps even passed from one generation to the next within a herd."
>
> —Sue McDonnell, Ph.D. *(A Practical Field Guide to Horse Behavior)*

Protector Leadership is based on the premise that security and social bonds are more important to horses than rank or dominance. The accuracy of this assumption cannot be evaluated by observing domestic horses, because they do not typically live a natural lifestyle. More often, they live in confined spaces, with people managing their social groups, food supply, reproduction, and raising of the young.

We cannot assume that these conditions create the same social behaviors as those of their wild ancestors, who evolved to live in open spaces, roaming at will, eating marginal vegetation, living in social groups of their own choosing.

Ideally, horse behavior would be studied by observing wild horses in their natural setting, without human influence. Since true wild horses became extinct in 1968 with the demise of the last wild Pzrewalski Horse in Mongolia,[15] "wild" horse behavior is studied by observing feral and free-roaming horses. Feral horses are wild-born descendants of domestic horses. Other free-roaming horses include domestic and semi-domestic herds allowed to run loose with varying degrees of human intervention. Veterinary care might be provided; colts might or might not be gelded. The defining point is that the horses are free to roam at will, responsible for finding their own food, water, and shelter, and establishing their own social groups. As described in chapter 3 (p. 34), these herds are not led by a single individual. Leadership is shared, and is based on social connections, not rank or dominance. Aggression is rare, and the young learn important social skills from older horses.

Chapter 4 (p. 43) shows that social dynamics in domestic horses can be very different from those of free-roaming herds because of significant differences in socialization, diet, and lifestyle. These differences are important to us as leaders because they can be the source of problem behaviors that are easily misinterpreted. Understanding what causes these problem behaviors is the first step in minimizing their negative impact on our relationships with our horses.

Chapter 5 (p. 51) shows how some of these social dynamics played out in my herd, and how Brandy's integration into the group altered interactions dramatically.

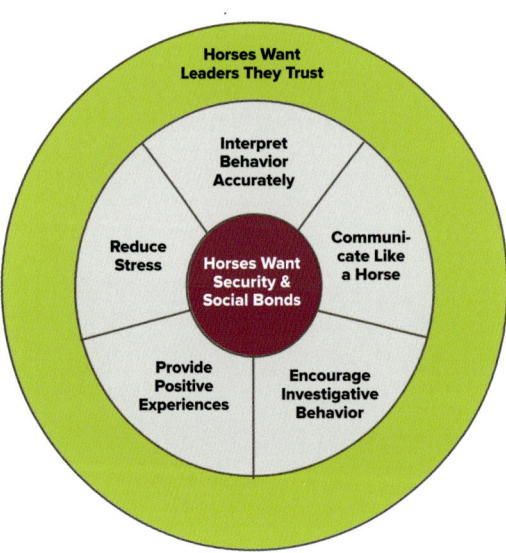

**Part Two Key Points:**
- The behavior of domestic horses is very different from that of horses who are allowed to roam freely.
- Free-roaming herds have complex social networks that provide security through long-term social bonds. Leadership is shared, aggression is rare, and rank is unimportant.
- Domestic horses show more stress-related behaviors and aggression because their living conditions are at odds with how nature meant them to live.

**You will learn how to:**
- Recognize friendly interactions that show healthy social connections between horses.
- Understand behaviors that might be influenced by domestic living conditions.
- Reduce the negative impacts of domestic living conditions.

## chapter 3
# Free-Roaming Herds: Complex Social Networks

> "Under natural conditions, horses rarely have the equivalent of an alpha individual within a band...."
>
> —Sue McDonnell, Ph.D. *(A Practical Field Guide to Horse Behavior)*

Free-roaming herd behavior has been studied in a variety of countries around the world.[16] This diversity is a great bonus since it is only human nature to describe behavior in the context of our cultural and personal belief systems. These observations of horse herd behavior have greater credibility because researchers from different cultures are largely in agreement. Findings vary enough to show that no single study can be taken as the final word on horse behavior, but the big picture shows clear patterns with a complex social structure. This social structure explains a great deal about leadership, friendship, rank, and aggression, all of it relevant to us as leaders.

The ponies shown in this chapter are residents of Assateague Island National Seashore in Maryland. Although they live in close proximity to human visitors, they are feral ponies protected from human contact and interference. Their behavior reflects that of free-roaming horses everywhere. (They are not involved in the annual Chincoteague pony roundup and auction as ponies on the Virginia end of the island are.)

## Lifestyle of Free-Roaming Herds

Mares typically live in "harem bands," consisting of a stallion and two or more mares with their immature offspring (figs. 3.1 A & B). Turnover is low in harem bands. While a filly might join another band as she matures, an adult mare may spend the rest of her life with the same band.

Stallions without mares live in "bachelor bands." As colts mature and leave their natal bands, they might join an existing bachelor band or form their own. There is more turnover in bachelor groups as some stallions leave to form their own harems.

## Social Bonds

Horses form strong social bonds with other individuals in their group. Mares have long-term friendships, usually with other mares of similar age and rank. Stallions also form social bonds. Lower-ranking stallions who remain in their bachelor band may have friendships that last a lifetime. (In the context of herd dynamics, the term "friend" means another individual with whom the horse has a close social bond.)

Actions that create and maintain social bonds include greeting, sniffing, rubbing, and other non-aggressive body contact, resting and grazing near each other, huddling together for warmth in winter and bug protection in summer. Mares may look after each other's foals (figs. 3.2 A–C). Both mares and stallions engage in mutual grooming with friends: two horses face opposite directions and scratch each other's necks and withers with their teeth, sometimes moving on

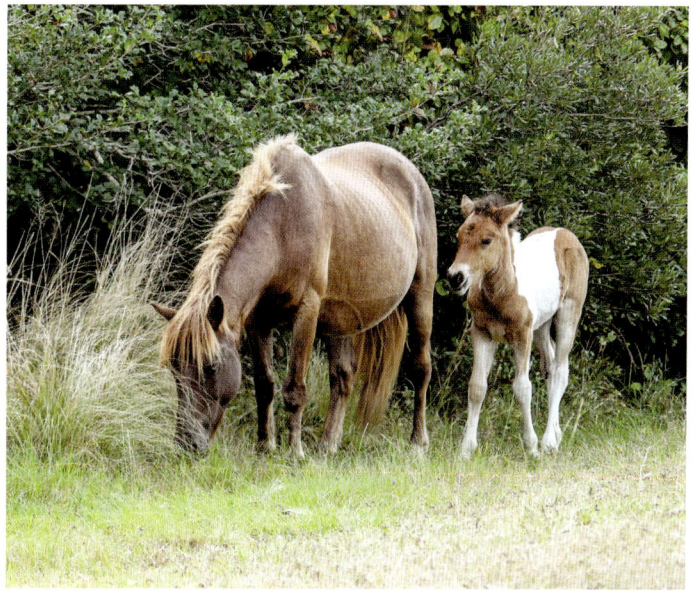

3.1 A  This mare and her filly are part of a feral harem band at Assateague Island National Seashore in Maryland.

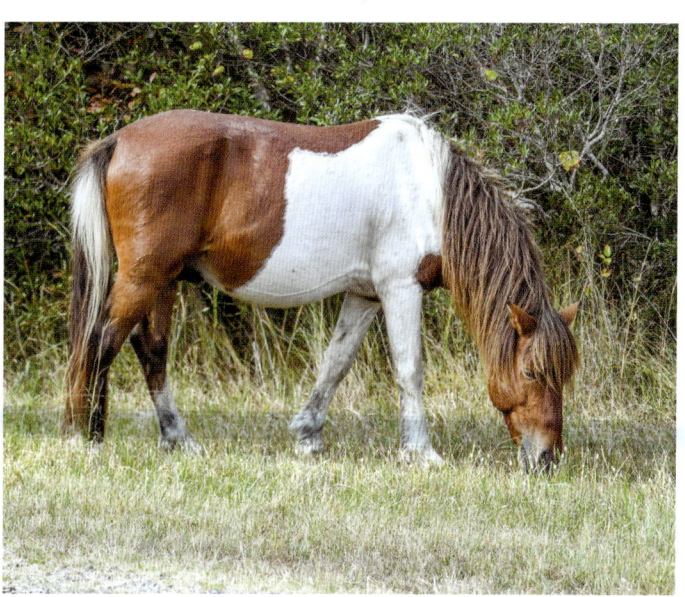

3.1 B  This stallion, the father of the foal in photo A, is grazing nearby.

3.2 A  Social bonding behaviors include friendly greetings.

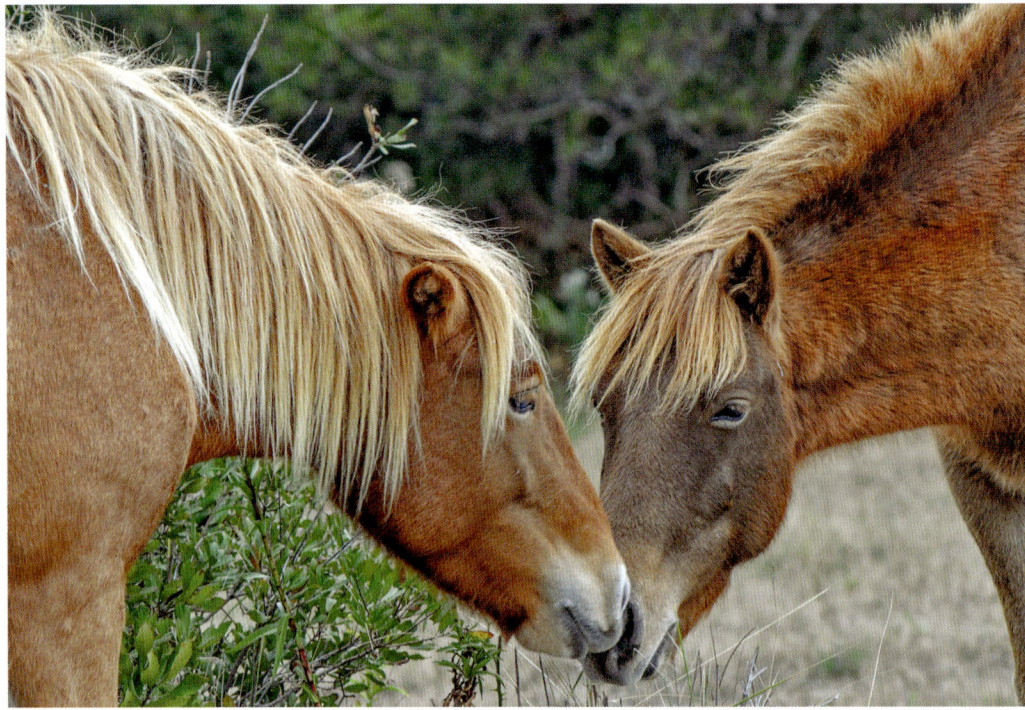

3.2 B  Grazing together and sharing friendly body contact also reinforce social bonds. This is the stallion (pinto) with one of his mares.

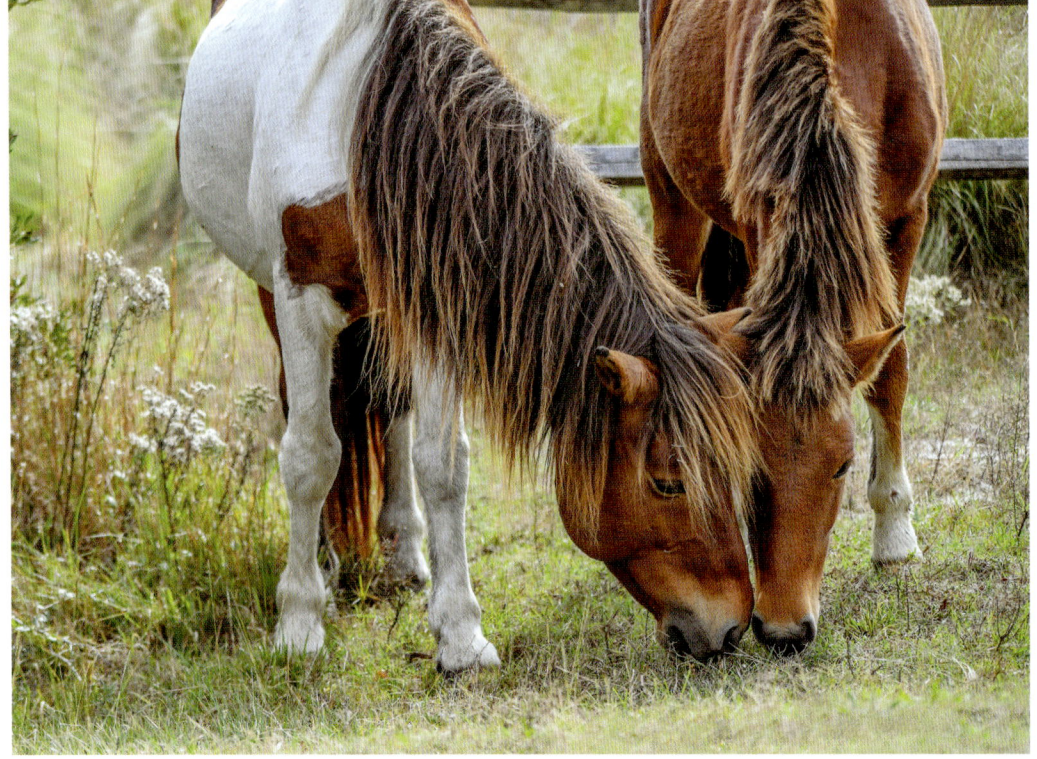

to backs and legs. This activity not only relieves itches, it lowers heart rate and releases endorphins.[17]

## Rank

Rank is most often predetermined by age and does not change. Thus, rank tends to correlate with the life experiences that make older horses more trustworthy as decision-makers.

## Aggression

There is little aggression in free-roaming herds. When it does occur, it is primarily over personal space. The offender is warned off, retreats a satisfactory distance, and the incident is over.[18] In a natural setting, horses do not have to compete for concentrated food sources. If food is scarce, they graze farther apart. When everyone doesn't fit around the water source, then rank determines the order of access, but all get a turn.

Given this well-ordered social system, conflict would make no contribution to the survival of the group or the reproductive success of individual mares. Conflict can be so rare in mare bands that one researcher commented, "Aggressive–submissive behavior was so infrequent during spring that rank determinations could not be made."[19]

We have no pictures of behavior indicating rank or aggression because the photographer saw no such behavior in the harem band.

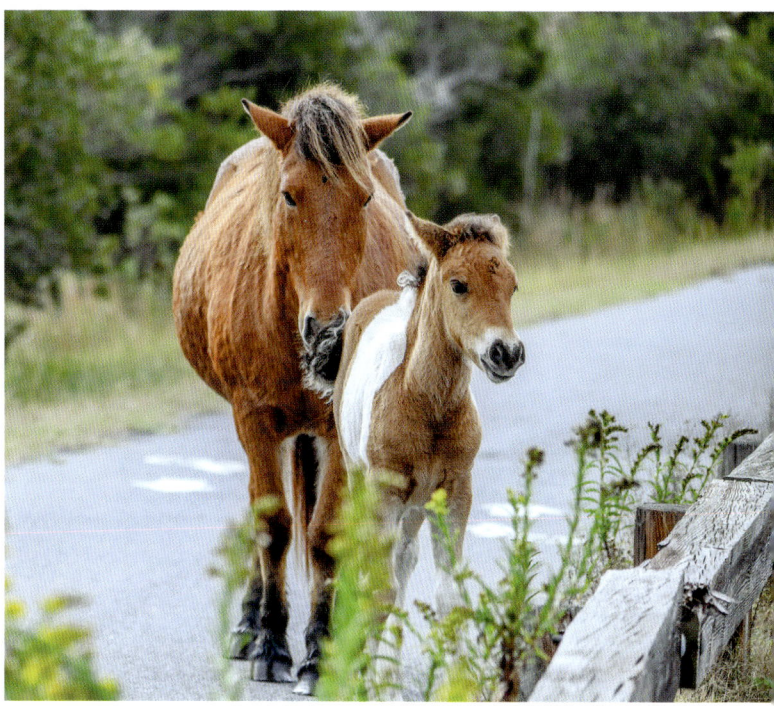

Aggressive behavior is seen more often in bachelor bands, where turnover is greater, and stallions are honing the skills that prepare them to establish and maintain their own harem bands. A certain amount of that "aggression" is mock fighting and, in any case, more time is still spent in the social bonding behaviors than in aggressive acts.[20] [21]

## Mares and Geldings without a Stallion

Observations of free-roaming Icelandic mares and geldings without a stallion are particularly relevant for most domestic situations. As with other free-roaming horses, aggression was low, rank correlated significantly with age, and social bonds were important. Mares and

3.2 C  This mare, who is not the foal's mother, pauses for a gentle body touch greeting as she passes by. Other mares in the band had similar friendly interactions with the foal.

geldings formed separate groups, and adult mares generally outranked adult geldings.

Among mares, social bonds were based on mutual grooming; the closer they were in rank (and thus age), the more they groomed each other. Bonds between geldings were based on mutual grooming and also on play. Fillies and younger geldings gravitated toward the gelding group. "Males played more than the females, had more playing partners and were more popular as playmates." Adult mares did not play.[22]

## Living Conditions and Diet

Free-roaming horses spend about 50 to 80 percent of their time foraging, depending on the availability of food.[23] Locations of food and water determine the distances they travel, which may be many miles a day, mainly at a walk. Diets vary depending on what is available geographically and seasonally, but are normally low in carbohydrates (figs. 3.3 A & B). These characteristics are significant because domestic living conditions tend to alter them drastically and that, as we'll see in the next chapter, can also alter behavior.

## Friends, Leaders, and Social Networking

Forget the old myths of the stallion leading the herd, and more recent images of a wise, dominant mare in charge. In free-roaming horse herds, there is no single leader who is always followed. Any individual can initiate movement. Different horses might tend to take the lead on different occasions. For instance, one might decide most often when to go to a water source for a drink, while another decides when to stop grazing and find shelter. The horse most likely to initiate flight might be one of the more anxious members of the group.[24] [25]

When one horse starts off, everyone else is free to follow or not, regardless of the rank of the departing horse. If no one follows, the would-be leader generally chooses not to continue. Each horse's decision whether to follow or not is influenced by the horses nearest her, who would typically be those with whom she has the closest social bonds—that is, her friends.

It works like this: One horse gives subtle physical cues that she is about to move. Her closest friends are the most likely to follow, then *their* friends join in until the whole herd is moving. Thus, the horse with the strongest social network is most likely to be followed. Dominant horses are *not* the ones most likely to be followed, suggesting they do not have as many friends.[26]

The stallion rarely initiates movement and is not apt to be followed if he does. His job is rear guard while the herd is moving. He monitors surroundings and hurries stragglers along.[27] [28]

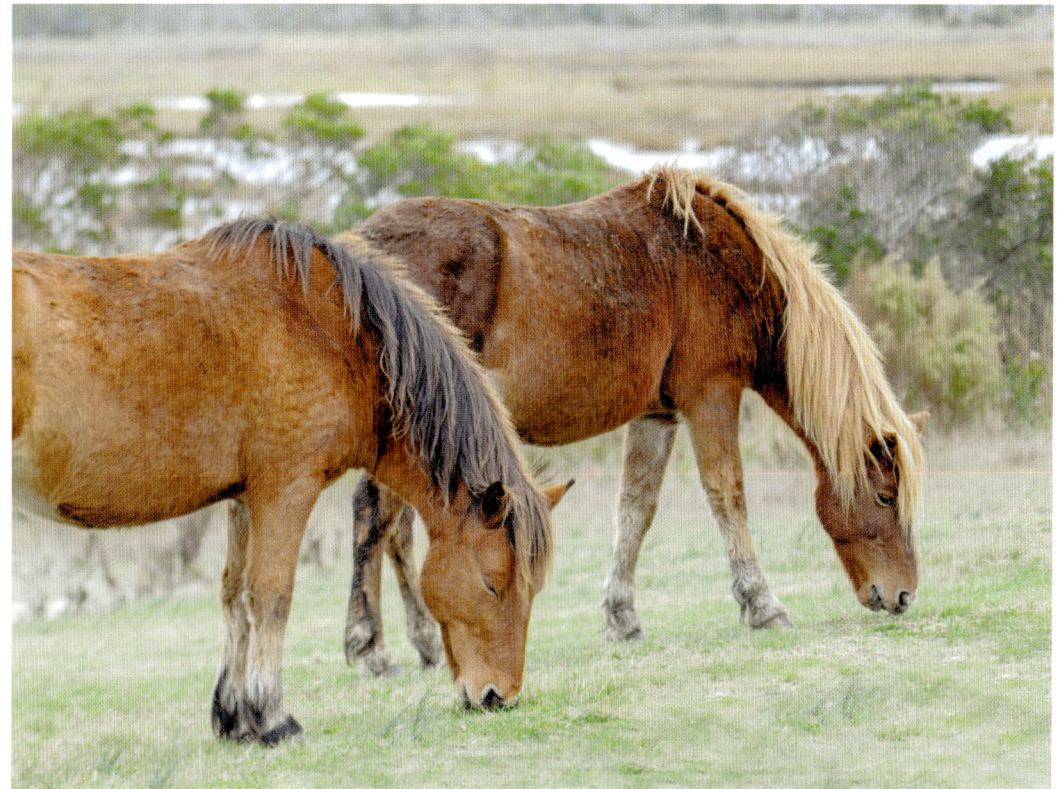

3.3 A  Contrary to popular images of wild gallops, feral horses spend most of their time walking and eating marginal vegetation.

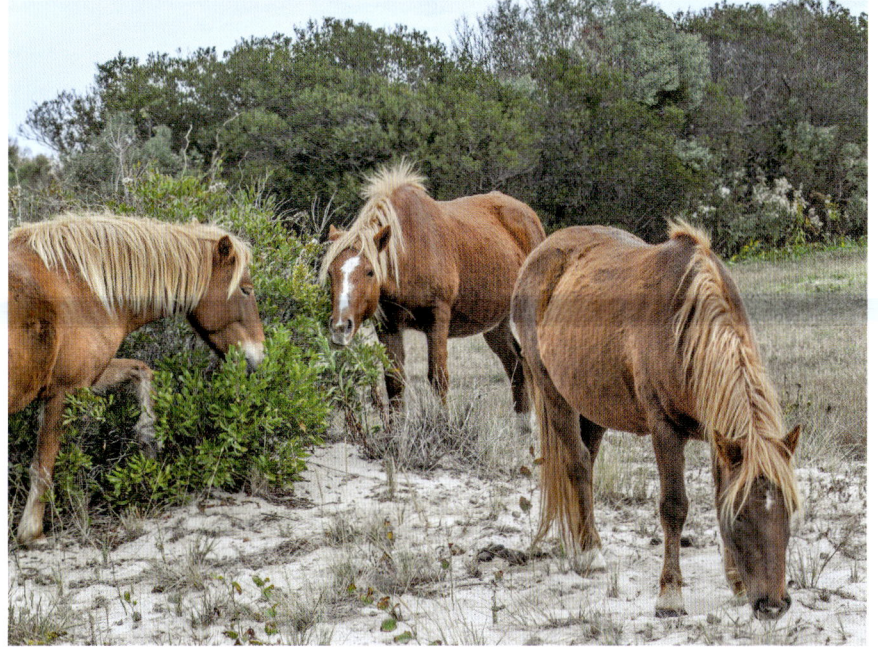

3.3 B  The diet of these Assateague ponies includes marsh and sand dune grasses, rosehips, and bayberry twigs, which the two on the left are nibbling.

Note that leadership refers to following, and no one is required to follow anyone else. A horse might warn another out of his personal space, and a stallion might herd his mares away from an intruder, but these are chasing maneuvers.

## The Education of a Free-Roaming Foal

Free-roaming foals grow up playing with other youngsters and exploring the world, indulging their curiosity under the watchful eyes of parents and other herd adults. The stallion actively participates in parenting the foal. As Dr. Sue McDonnell describes his role, "This includes playing with the foals and yearlings, staying with the young play groups when they wander or play short distances from the mares, and retrieving them from straying off too far from the herd."[29]

The social behaviors horses need to know to get along in a group are not instinctive; youngsters must learn them from older horses. They learn the social bonding behaviors such as mutual grooming that help them form attachments with age-mates. Aggressive behaviors are a package deal; it is not enough to know how to threaten and fight. It is critical to know how and when to avoid a fight, to appease an attacker or signal submission; and for an aggressor to recognize these signals and break off an attack. It is also important to understand the rules of mock fighting.

Foals learn from parents and other older herd members as they copy practical skills like what plants to eat or not eat (figs. 3.4 A & B), and what types of things or situations they should be fearful of, and which are safe. This ability to learn by copying trusted individuals is something you can put to good use, as you will see in chapter 10 (Friendly Body Language—p. 113).

Weaning is a gradual process that starts between six and twelve months, and can take up to two or three years. A photo in Dr. McDonnell's *Understanding Horse Behavior* shows a two-year-old mare nursing from her mother while her own foal nurses from her. Throughout the weaning process, the young horse has the security of familiar companions, the diversion of playtime with other youngsters, and the freedom to continue exploring the world.

The cowboy author, Will James (1892–1942), was an exceptionally astute observer of horses, and his lifestyle provided on-going opportunities to observe free-roaming herds. In his classic *Smoky the Cowhorse* he describes herd dynamics and the education of a foal from Smoky's point of view as he grows up on the range.[30] Although this is typically classified as a children's book, it is actually an insightful portrayal of life from a horse's point of view. Will James' observations of horse behavior are remarkably similar to those of modern researchers.

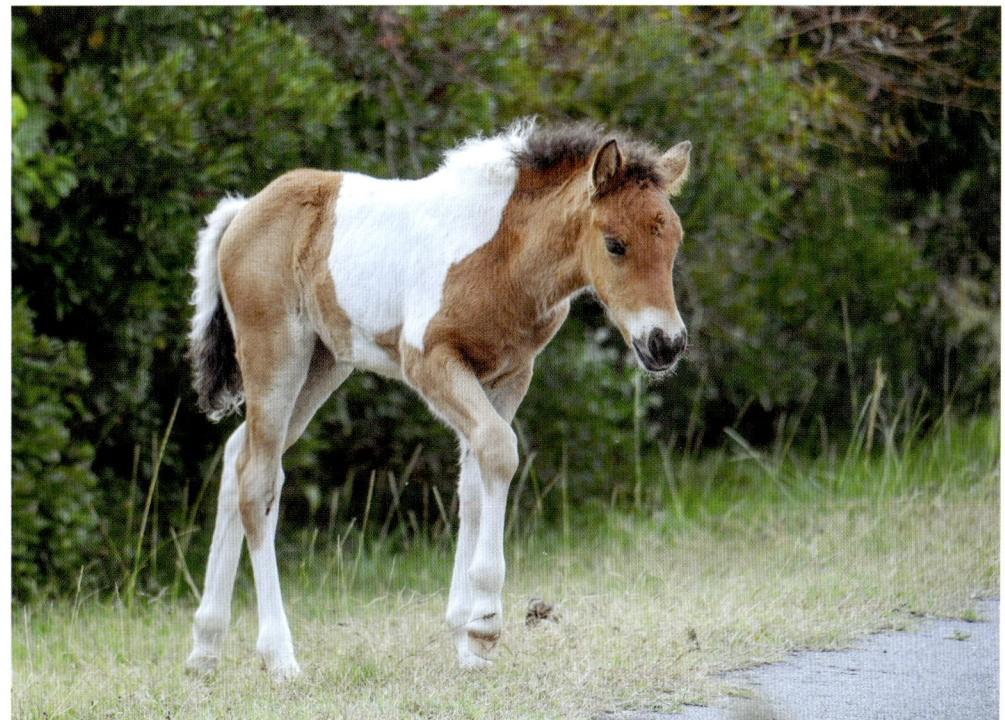

3.4 A  This foal is free to explore her surroundings.

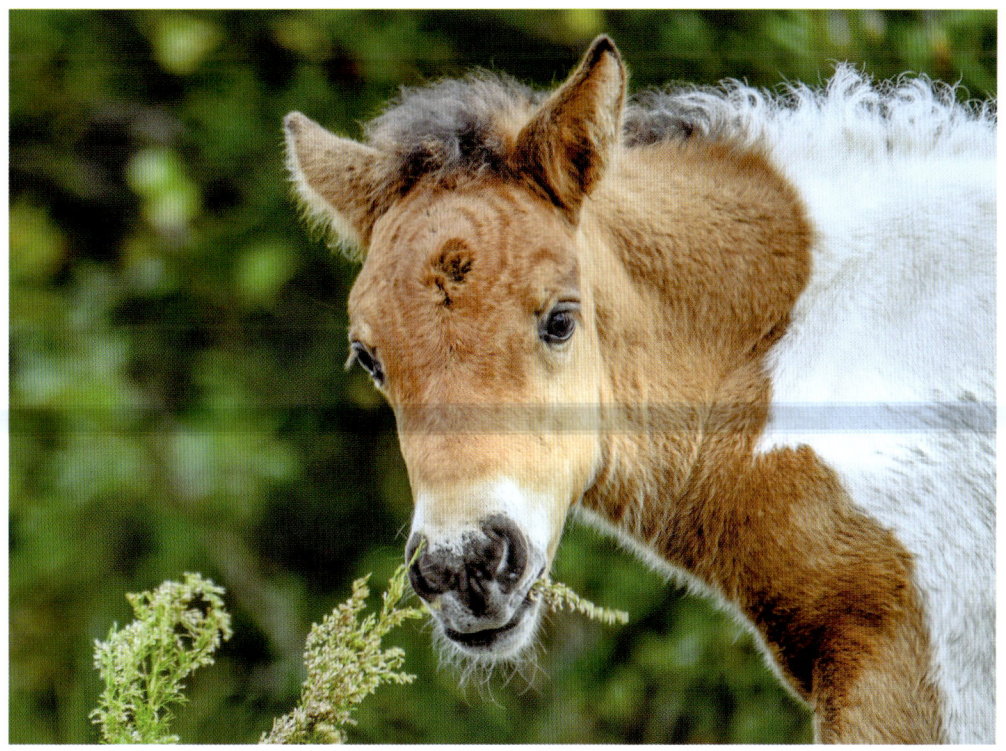

3.4 B  Here she is testing edible possibilities. Her family is just out of sight in the background.

## Protector Leadership Validated

Studies of free-roaming herds provide scientific validation for the principles of Protector Leadership: social bonds are more important than rank, and horses follow leaders they trust and with whom they have a social bond. Nothing in free-roaming herd behavior suggests that authoritarian leadership would make sense to a horse. Quite the contrary. Since security means being close to one's friends, who do not force one to do anything, it is only logical that bossy horses and people would be avoided if possible.

## ❧ Summary

Free-roaming horse herds have a complex social structure built on strong long-term bonds between individuals. Rank is most often determined by age and does not change. Aggression is rare except among stallions defending their mares. Leadership is shared, with any member of a band free to initiate movement, and no one is required to follow. Individuals are most likely to follow those with whom they have close bonds.

Youngsters have great freedom to play, socialize, and explore the world. Both genders participate in raising them, protecting them, and teaching them essential social skills. Weaning is late and gradual.

The photographs of the feral Assateague ponies in this chapter show behaviors of a cohesive, well-socialized group, just as researchers typically describe in free-roaming horses.

### THINGS TO TRY

- ▶ Observe a group of two or more horses turned out together. Watch for behaviors that show social connections such as sniffing, rubbing, mutual grooming, and other non-aggressive body contact; sharing a hay pile, spending time together as they rest or graze; following another horse's lead as he or she moves to a different place.

- ▶ Watch which horses play with each other. Do youngsters and geldings play more than mares?

- ▶ Can you see a *network* of social connections, separate from a dominance hierarchy?

- ▶ If there are foals to watch, what social and exploring behavior do you see?

*chapter 4*
# Domestic Horses: Social Networks Disrupted

> "The label of alpha animal within a group of domestic horses is usually based on the individual's ability to control a limited resource, say a feed bunk or a row of grain buckets along a fence. We all know horses that can control such a focused resource, or create havoc trying. But this is a fairly unnatural condition created by our husbandry practice. Under natural conditions, it is rare to see overt aggression or a single individual controlling a limited resource."
>
> —Sue McDonnell, Ph.D. *(A Practical Field Guide to Horse Behavior)*

Domestic herd behavior has also been widely studied. A review of over 20 studies of free-roaming and domestic herd behavior, conducted over three decades, shows how the behavior of domestic horses can differ significantly from that of free-roaming ones.[31]

## Lifestyle of Domestic Herds

Domestic herd structure is artificial because it is determined by people, not by the horses themselves. Mares and geldings may be mixed together, unlike free-roaming horses who separate themselves by gender. Young horses are typically separated from adults, instead of growing up under the supervision of well-socialized older horses.

Turnover is usually higher than in free-roaming bands. I cannot find statistics on the average number of owners a horse has in a lifetime, but for our crew the number is at least three-and-a-half and everyone I have asked thinks that's low. Sapphire had at least four owners, Bronzz two, Shiloh five, Brandy at least three. That does not count additional moves made when an owner changed stables or sent a horse off for training. Even if a horse doesn't move, odds are that herd mates will come and go. Since free-roaming mares can live their entire adult lives in the same band, it has been suggested that moves might be even more traumatic for mares than for geldings.

## Social Bonds

The security of long-term social bonds is the exception for domestic horses. Many grow up without learning the social bonding skills to make positive connections with other horses, or to temper their own aggression or deflect that of others. The result is more aggressive behaviors, fewer social bonding behaviors. Even when they manage to make friends, those bonds are frequently severed because one horse is sold, moved, or switched to a different turnout arrangement.

Isolation often prevents horses from making social connections at all. Peering through bars at other horses is not social contact, and turnout in separate paddocks is a poor substitute for the physical closeness that provides security. The severity of the impact is shown in the fact that horses kept in stalls with little or no access to other horses are more likely to be aggressive toward humans.[32]

## Rank and Aggression

Rank is not typically determined by age, as in free-roaming bands. It is determined more often by "aggressiveness, temperament, or social experience".[33] [34]

Domestic living conditions often include the three factors most likely to cause aggression among horses:

• **Confined spaces** increase the likelihood that personal space will be invaded, a common cause of aggression.

• **Having food supplied** brings horses into close proximity, and invites guarding of resources. It is possibly the most significant source of aggression among domestic horses.

• **Artificial social groups with high turnover** means that rank must be re-established with each change in group membership.

It is no surprise, then, that domestic horses spend more time in aggressive behavior and less time in social bonding behavior than their free-roaming cousins. These higher levels of aggression explain why people unfamiliar with free-roaming herd behavior mistakenly believe that rank is important to horses and that aggression is a normal part of herd behavior. This makes it easy to overlook the importance of social bonds.

Other aspects of domestic living also contribute to stress, and potentially to aggression:

- **Being confined is abnormal for horses.** The less turnout time and space a horse has, the more likely he is to have behavior problems. When turnout is not possible, appropriate daily exercise is important for mental and physical health.

- **Lack of opportunity to use curiosity and explore their surroundings** makes horses more fearful and less adaptable to new situations.[35][36] Fearful horses are clearly a common problem. Consider the prevalence of calming supplements for horses; the anxious horses and riders one sees at many events, and the great interest in "de-spooking," "desensitizing," or "bomb-proofing." How many horses are sold or relegated to pasture-ornament status because their owners are afraid to ride them? Horses' reactions to anxiety-producing situations are intensified when they are already stressed by their living situations and/or inappropriate diets.

- **Diets high in carbohydrates and/or low in forage** can contribute to stress-related behaviors and excitability. They are a risk factor for ulcers, which are found in 30% to 90% of domestic horses depending on the population studied. Such diets make horses more prone to aggression toward people, possibly as a result of gastric pain.[37] Ulcers are rare or non-existent in free-roaming horses.

## Leaders, Friends, and Social Networking

The shared leadership of free-roaming herds is based on a complex social network where horses decide whether to follow another horse based on their social bonds. Without these bonds, the system of leadership that is most natural for horses is not possible.

Instead, a domestic social system may be a pecking order with rank determined by aggression. The highest-ranking horse may not be a leader any of the others would choose to follow, but a bully who has achieved rank through aggression while other horses do their best to appease or stay out of the way.

## The Education of a Domestic Foal

Domestic foals lead very restricted lives compared to free-roaming foals. At best they are turned out with other foals and their mothers. Social interaction with different age groups is the exception. Many spend large portions of time in stalls or small paddocks with little opportunity to play, to socialize with anyone other than their mothers, or to exercise their bodies or their curiosity.

Foals are typically weaned abruptly

around four to seven months of age. This is a highly stressful event, as one might expect compared to the long, gradual weaning of free-roaming horses.

Weanlings are sometimes placed together in pairs or groups for company, but stressed-out peers are a poor substitute for a reassuring adult presence. Maternal deprivation stress is expressed in a variety of behaviors: increased vocalizing, raised cortisol levels (a common measure of stress), decreased time spent eating (resulting in weight loss), attempts to nurse from each other, and increased aggression toward each other.[38]

To avoid injuries, weanlings may be placed alone in box stalls, a recipe for mental and physical health problems. Now, in addition to maternal deprivation stress, they suffer from the stress of social isolation. This leads to significantly more time spent in abnormal behaviors such as licking or chewing the stall wall, kicking the wall, pawing, and bouts of bucking and rearing. Stalled weanlings also spent more time lying down than paddock-kept counterparts (20 percent compared to 5 percent), which researchers suggested might explain their decreased bone density.[39]

*It's no coincidence that stereotypies tend to emerge within a month of weaning.*

Considering the stress-related behaviors exhibited by isolated weanlings, you might question how much "bad" stallion behavior is provoked by the long-term isolation that is so often a stallion's lot in domestic life.

Yearlings and two-year-olds are often turned out in same-age, same-sex groups to limit injuries from older, larger horses. While this sounds prudent, it is rather like leaving a group of young children to fend for themselves with no adults to set limits or teach appropriate behavior.

## Stress-Related Behaviors

*Stereotypies* are repetitive behaviors that occur only in domestic and captive horses. They include cribbing, stall- or fence-walking, weaving, pawing, digging, pacing, circling, wall-kicking, and self-mutilation through biting. Commonly referred to as "vices," they actually correlate to stress-related behaviors in people. They are more prevalent when weanlings are stall-kept, do not have access to grazing, or are fed large amounts of concentrates.[40] It is no coincidence that stereotypies tend to emerge within a month of weaning.

Stereotypies may appear pointless to us, but they are not pointless from the horse's perspective. They release the endorphins a horse would get if he engaged in social-bonding behaviors, such as mutual grooming, with herd mates. The release of endorphins makes the behavior self-rewarding.[41] It also creates structural changes in the brain related to learning and habit formation, thus making it difficult to "cure" horses of stereotypies.[42]

While horses do learn some behaviors from other horses, research suggests that stereotypies are not among them. Though it is possible that a predisposition is inherited,[43] the behaviors are triggered by stress. When multiple horses in a barn engage in them, it is more likely because they have all been subjected to stressful conditions, if not currently, then in the past. The particular stereotypy a horse develops may be related to the need for which it is compensating. Oral stereotypies such as cribbing relate to lack of chewing time; three meals a day does not make up for the time (as much as 17 hours a day) that horses would naturally spend foraging. Oral stereotypies may also increase saliva flow and reduce acid in the gastric tract.[44] Weaving and stall-walking seem related to lack of opportunity for natural movement, that is, the many miles horses' wild ancestors would have walked every day.[45]

Studies of brain development show that when the young of a species live with ongoing stress, the fight/flight pathways develop more strongly. In contrast, young who grow up with appropriate socialization and opportunity to explore develop stronger cognitive/learning "brain circuits."[46] A study of stereotypies and learning did indeed show that the horses with stereotypies were less able to learn the task used in the test: opening the lid of a chest with their nose. Those who did learn took longer than the horses without stereotypies.[47]

In dogs, another social species, lack of socialization is recognized as a cause of fear-related aggression (fear-biting). An early environment that lacks interest and stimulation fails to build confidence and learning ability. That's why service dogs are not raised in kennels. They go to puppy-raisers who form positive bonds with them, and introduce them to the real world in ways that promote confidence.

## The Importance of Early Learning

Foals who lack opportunity to explore real-life situations with calm adult influence are primed to be more fearful as adults. This was demonstrated in a study comparing the fear levels of two groups of foals.

The "Demo Group" saw their mothers responding calmly to potentially scary situations: walking over a tarp, passing colorful objects, being wiped with a plastic bag, and having an umbrella held over their body. They had 10-minute sessions once a week for eight weeks. The mares had previously been accustomed to these activities, so they modeled their own lack of fear. The foals were free to explore and play with the equipment.

The foals in the "Control Group" had no such experiences.

Both groups of foals were given standardized fear tests at eight weeks of age. *All* of the foals in the Control Group

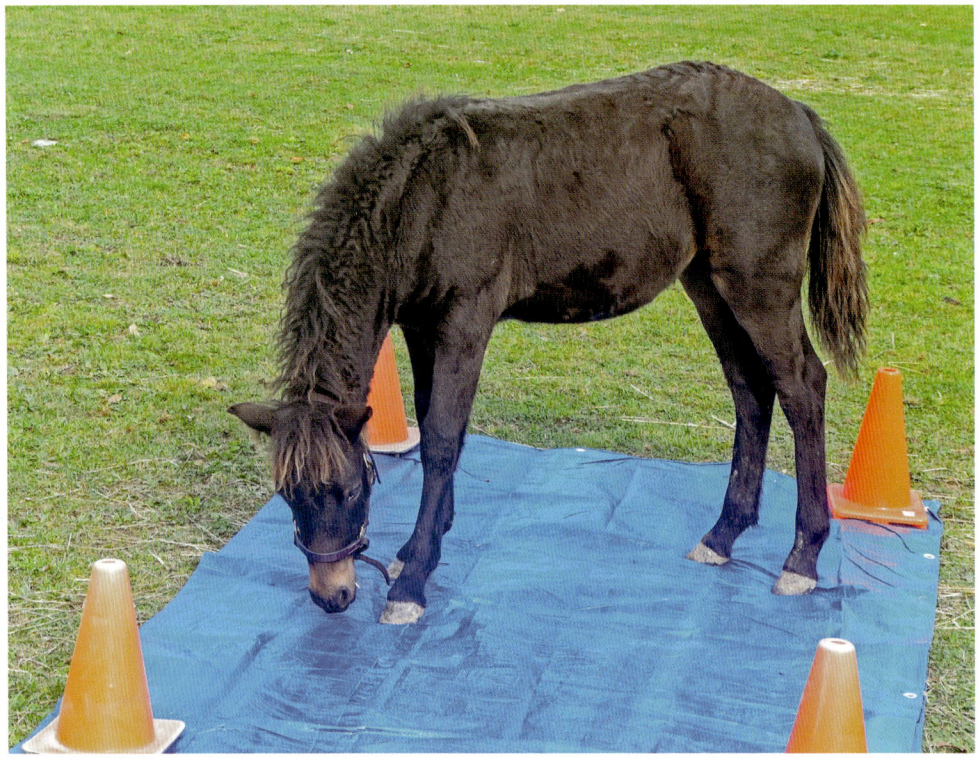

4.1 A  After seeing his mother blithely stroll across the tarp, Tiger went to explore it on his own.

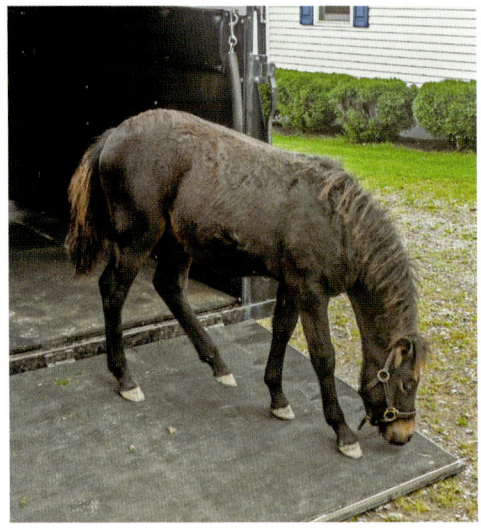

4.1 B  Having the same opportunity to watch his mother go in the trailer, and then explore it himself, Tiger taught himself to load calmly. His first trailer ride, to our place with his mother, was a stress-free adventure.

showed more fear than *any* of the foals in the Demo Group. Both groups were retested three months later with no further "training." The Demo foals remained less fearful, not only in the type of situations they had already experienced, but in all tests of fear.

I saw the value of this calm adult modeling after my friend Melody brought me her pregnant Dartmoor pony, Love, for agility and (light) riding training. Love became confident with a variety of equipment while she was with me. When her son, Tiger, was five months old, we put some obstacles in the pasture that they shared with other members of their small herd. Confidence built in one setting carries over to others (figs. 4.1 A & B).

## ❧ Summary

Free-roaming horses spend most of their time strolling and grazing on low carbohydrate forage, in the company of friends and herd mates. While their living conditions may be harsh, this is the life nature prepared them to live. They have the security of long-term companions and the freedom to make choices.

Domestic horses frequently face challenges not encountered by their free-roaming counterparts or their wild ancestors. Inadequate socialization can result in a lack

### 4.2 HERD CHARACTERISTICS

| Characteristics | Free-Roaming | Domestic |
| --- | --- | --- |
| **Herd Structure** | Determined by horses, social groups separated by gender, low turnover | Determined by people, genders may be mixed, high turnover |
| **Social Bonds** | Strong, long-term | Limited, disrupted |
| **Social Skills Required to Establish and Maintain Bonds** | Learned from older herd members | May not be learned due to lack of appropriate adult interaction |
| **Rank** | Determined by age, not a source of conflict | Determined by temperament, social experience, aggression |
| **Aggression** | Rare | Common |
| **Living Conditions** | Open spaces, lots of walking, opportunities to explore | Confined spaces, limited opportunities to move or explore |
| **Diet** | Marginal forage, grazing at will, resources spread out | High-carbohydrate food, schedules set by people, fed in confined spaces |
| **Leadership** | Shared, based on social bonds, following is voluntary | May be replaced by dominance related to resource guarding |
| **Growing Up** | Social interaction with all age groups, unlimited opportunities to move, play, and explore, gradual weaning | Limited social interaction and learning, limited opportunities to move, play, explore, early abrupt weaning |

PART TWO: HORSES WANT SECURITY AND SOCIAL BONDS

of skills needed to get along safely with other horses. It can also mean failure to learn rules that help them get along with people, such as being aware when they are invading someone else's personal space. Lack of opportunity to explore and learn about the world creates more fearfulness. Limited opportunity to move around, exercise, and build social bonds, compounded by domestic feeding programs all contribute to stress (fig. 4.2).

This stress frequently provokes unwanted behaviors that add to the challenges of leadership. Anything you can do to provide outdoor time with space to move, appropriate diet, and compatible long-term companions improves horses' quality of life, and thus the quality of their interactions with you. Where that is not possible, you can recognize that resulting behaviors are consequences of their living conditions, not the horses' fault, and possibly not correctable with training.

Ahead you will find out how Protector Leadership can help you meet the challenges created by domestic living.

## THINGS TO TRY

- ▶ If you assume that horses' interactions are mainly about rank, you can overlook other influences on their behavior. Try watching a group of horses relating their behavior instead to their living conditions, personalities, and stress: Which horses are comfortable with which other horses? Which ones might be stressed? Who guards food? Who is anxious about getting enough food, or about invasions of his personal space?

- ▶ Consider how far their living conditions deviate from horses' natural lifestyle. Problems are least likely when horses have:

  - Maximum turnout time (24/7 is ideal).

  - Compatible companions with minimum turnover in the group.

  - Room to move, run, and get out of each other's space.

  - Maximum forage, minimum concentrates that their health allows.

  - Hay piles spaced far apart to minimize conflict.

## chapter 5
# Brandy's New Herd

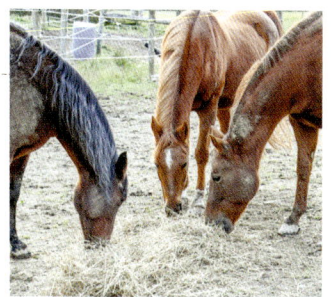

> "A great deal of their behavior concerns communication among herd mates and the establishment and maintenance of a social hierarchy that enables peaceful, ongoing interaction."
>
> —Sue McDonnell, Ph.D. *(A Practical Field Guide to Horse Behavior)*
>
> "The only way to have a friend is to be one." —Ralph Waldo Emerson

The dynamics in our little herd have changed dramatically since Brandy first arrived six years ago. She was the catalyst, and each of the changes she prompted illustrate some dimension of herd dynamics. Positive changes in herd dynamics have corresponded to positive changes in our horses' relationships with us.

## Our Semi-Dysfunctional Herd

For many years, I had assumed that the behavior of our three horses (Sapphire, Bronzz, and Shiloh) reflected normal herd dynamics. This was based on my faulty assumptions about a linear hierarchy, competition for rank, and the most dominant horse naturally being in charge.

Sapphire, my husband's Palomino, was the oldest and clearly in charge, claiming first dibs at hay piles, water tanks, and gateways. If she said "move," which she often did for no apparent reason, the other two scrambled. In retrospect, I recognize this as the resource guarding that Dr. McDonnell describes at the beginning of chapter 4 (see p. 43).

Bronzz, my chestnut Arabian gelding, was second in age and rank. Shiloh, a chestnut Quarter Horse type, was youngest and lowest in rank. Bronzz often lunged at Shiloh with pinned ears and bared teeth, making her dodge out of his way. When the horses filed into the barn at mealtimes, it was always in rank order. I sent them out in reverse order so no one had to scoot past a higher-ranking horse. There was never the slightest doubt about rankings.

I supposed this was normal because nobody was getting hurt, and it wasn't all chase and scramble. The trio huddled together in a corner of the turnout shed when wind or flies bothered them, Sapphire always in the middle. They lined up together at the paddock fence to stare across the back yard and into the house when they wanted me to come out and serve meals or open a pasture gate. Sapphire and Shiloh even groomed each other, though only when Bronzz was not with them.

Sapphire's dominant attitude with other horses seemed to match her pushy manner with people. Two previous owners indicated that she had been the head honcho in every group she was turned out with, and that she also intimidated people everywhere she had lived. I was very assertive with her, cutting her no slack.

Yet there were things that did not add up. She behaved best for my husband, the person who was least strict with her. She carried him around our rugged state forest trails for over a decade, never letting him fall off or get hurt. She was attentive and careful when we lead-lined children on her. Her farrier manners were impeccable, and she was a model patient when she was injured. Why did she give me such a hard time?

## Snickers

When Snickers first arrived, Sapphire reacted as she did toward most horses who visited our farm. She took every opportunity to charge at him with pinned ears and bared teeth, screaming and striking. Only stall doors and fences kept them both safe. Snickers mostly ignored her.

Over the next couple months she stopped reacting, and sometimes even grazed near him in their adjacent pastures. Snickers was clearly unhappy pastured alone, so we tried turning all four horses out together. Amazingly, there seemed to be no issues between Sapphire and Snickers. However, kick-fests between Snickers and Bronzz escalated, with Bronzz getting the brunt of the scrapes.

We separated the boys rather than risk a serious injury, but it looked like Snickers and Sapphire might be a successful pasture match. At 30, she was missing a few teeth, and starting to lose weight. With insulin-resistant Bronzz and overweight Shiloh both on limited, muzzled

> *She behaved best for my husband, the person who was least strict with her.*

pasture time, Sapphire could get more grass with Snickers to keep her company.

For two days all was well—or so we thought. On the third day I arrived at my optician's office to be met with an urgent message. Sapphire was badly injured… the vet was on her way…I needed to come home fast.

Who knew that one bare pony hoof could cut a hole that deep in a horse's backside? But we got off easy. Nothing critical was damaged, the vet assured us. It was just a sewing job, albeit a time-consuming one. Though the wound took a year to heal, it never slowed Sapphire down. Who was the problem this time? Hard to say. Maybe Sapphire bullied Snickers too far, but on the other hand, he later got into pasture fights in his new home, too.

## Brandy Changes Herd Dynamics

Sapphire reacted to Brandy's arrival with her usual aggression, instantly squelching any fantasies we might have entertained of turning them out together.

Meanwhile, Brandy's positive response to my new leadership approach convinced me to change the way I related to Sapphire. Instead of correcting her sternly when she did things I didn't like, I quietly redirected her to do what I *did* want, then waited for her response. Instead of pinning her ears at me, she calmly did as I asked. The more gently I handled her, the more cooperative she was, and the clearer it became that she was actually very sensitive and easily distressed. We began to wonder. Could it be that her aggressive reactions to people were coming from anxiety, like dogs who are fear-biters? From her point of view, her "aggression" was self-defense.

We started to re-think the source of Sapphire's aggression with other horses. Several owners ago, she lived at a boarding stable where 20 horses vied for hay served outside, and the whole herd charged into their stalls in the barn at grain time. No wonder she was aggressive around food and wanted everyone out of her personal space at mealtimes.

Bronzz never worried about food. There was no competition for food where he grew up. Hay was served generously in stalls; turnout was a large pasture, no hay. On the other hand, he was very disrespectful of other horses' personal space, and constantly crowded Sapphire—just the thing that stressed her most at mealtimes. Under the circumstances, it is much to her credit that she never kicked him.

Shiloh frets incessantly about food, always nickering for more, and obsessively cleaning up any morsel left behind by anyone else. She never challenges anyone for food, but it is not hard to guess where her anxiety came from. At 16 months old she was sold to a dealer, then went to another dealer, then to a novice owner, and then went to a large boarding stable, all before she turned three. Yet Shiloh does respect personal space of higher-ranking horses, so perhaps she and Sapphire would have become friends without Bronzz in the mix.

Ironically, only Brandy who lived on her own and needed to be "rescued" showed no anxiety about food, was always respectful of other horse's personal space, and was comfortable with them in her personal space.

## A Friendship Develops

The fall that Sapphire was 33, her weight dropped alarmingly. She needed maximum grazing time. Meanwhile, Brandy was in her third year with us, and we had seen a major shift in Sapphire's behavior

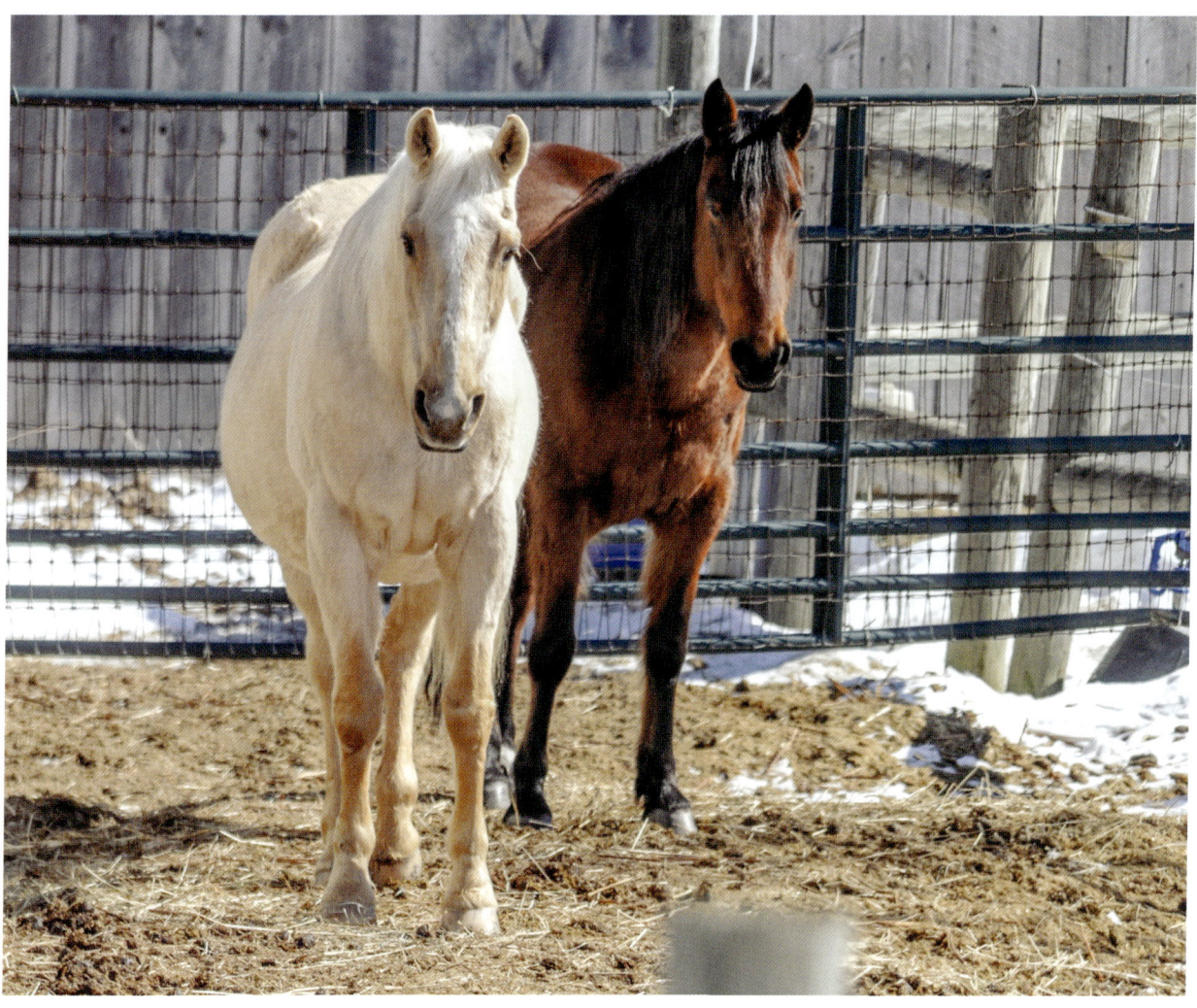

5.1 By late winter, Sapphire and Brandy had become friends and routinely hung out together.

toward her. There were friendly overtures over fences, and they were calm in adjacent stalls. With much trepidation, we turned them out together. Recognizing that confined spaces and introduced food are two of the biggest causes of aggression, we put the mares in a large pasture with no hay. In case we needed to chase them into separate pastures, I lounged against a fence post with a lunge whip, while my husband took gate duty.

The mares ate grass. Brandy gravitated toward Sapphire, but when Sapphire laid her ears back, Brandy calmly moseyed off. My husband and I got bored and also moseyed off.

As we watched the mares over the next weeks, we saw a pattern. Brandy would ease closer to Sapphire as they grazed. When Sapphire pinned her ears, Brandy calmly angled away. Gradually, Sapphire let Brandy ease closer and closer. After a few uneventful weeks, we risked placing hay piles in the paddock, far apart. Brandy continued to respect Sapphire's very large personal space bubble around food, and all stayed peaceful.

Over the winter, the mares became friends, and it was impossible to tell who had the higher rank (fig. 5.1). They hung out together, groomed each other, shared the same hay pile, and kept careful track of each other when they were separated (fig. 5.2). Neither warned the other out of her space, or cared who went through gates first.

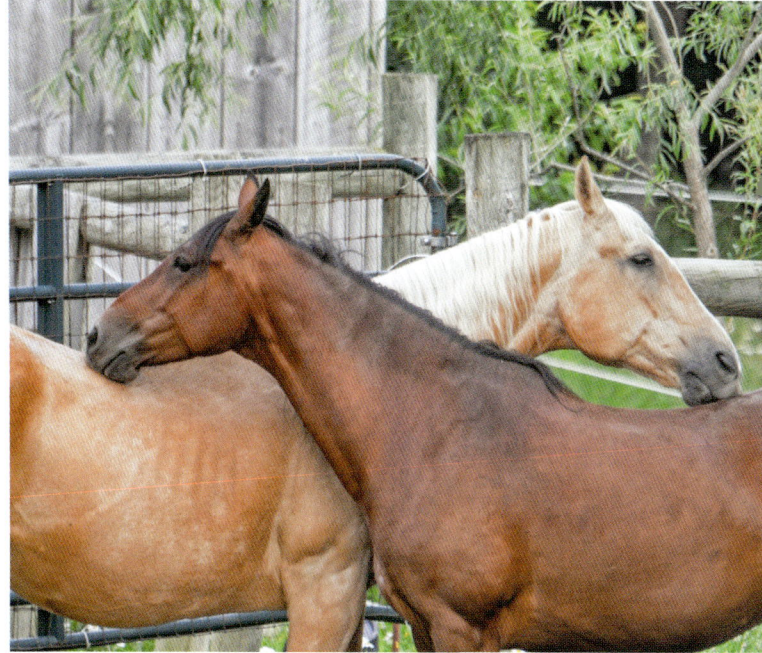

5.2 The mares often engaged in mutual grooming: nuzzling and nibbling each other's withers, shoulders, and backs.

There was just one incident that showed Brandy looked to Sapphire for guidance when she was unsure about a situation. This is documented in photographs in the first chapter on Investigative Behavior (see p. 143).

Sapphire's manner with people changed. She was calm and mellow with everyone, practically cuddly. I commented to my husband that Sapphire's personality had changed since she was pastured with Brandy, and he replied sadly that it had not changed; her real personality had finally had a chance to come out. I'm afraid he is right. It was more apparent than ever that Sapphire was very sensitive and easily upset. In retrospect, her "bullying" seems like the behavior of an anxious individual trying to wrest some control over her environment.

I'm not sure what it was about being pastured with Brandy that made the difference for Sapphire. Brandy's respect for her personal space? The lack of gelding interference? Or perhaps it was that having lived "wild," Brandy projected an air of savvy caution that reassured Sapphire she could go off-duty and trust Brandy to be on guard. One thing I am sure of. Brandy never cared about rank. She cared about being friends, and she set about winning Sapphire over by being *her* friend. She waited patiently for Sapphire to become comfortable with more physical closeness, and ultimately with mutual grooming and sharing hay piles.

It was a relationship that developed slowly, a relationship of trust and comfort in each other's company.

## Horses Grieve

Sapphire and Brandy had been together for eight months when Sapphire had a stroke. The coordination in her hind end was compromised, making her unsteady on her feet, a danger to herself and everyone around her. Since she showed no sign of distress, we waited nearly two weeks in case there was some recovery. There wasn't. During that time, with Sapphire's mobility severely impaired, Brandy's behavior toward her never altered. She remained a calm, undemanding companion.

None of the horses called or looked for Sapphire after she was gone, but I think that was because we let each of them see her after the vet left, and before she was buried. Each horse reacted differently, but the one thing they all did was sniff her nostrils, and that apparently told them what they needed to know. That night at turnout time, I led each of them into the pasture where Sapphire was now buried, so they could see she was no longer there. Brandy pawed at the grave.

For the next 10 days all three horses were unusually subdued. No one whinnied hello when I came to the barn or tried to engage me in games. They seemed to want me to be with them, but they did not want to be touched or asked to do anything.

Then two of our young grandchildren arrived for a two-week visit, and the timing could not have been more perfect. All of us, horses and humans, were ready for cheerful, young energy. Horses were hugged, petted, brushed, hoof-picked, pampered, and played with. They craned their necks over stall doors to watch kids play in the barn aisle, and receive endless bouquets of loose hay served up by small hands.

## Brandy and Shiloh

My husband and I had already concluded that Brandy was meant to stay with us, so we soon started the next phase of herd integration: Brandy and Shiloh together. We had no qualms about Brandy, having seen the patience and finesse with which she won Sapphire over. It was Shiloh we worried about.

When Shiloh first arrived here as a two-year-old, she slid right into the bottom rank without a fuss. It was a different story a few years later when we agreed to board a friend's young Arabian mare. Trusting Shiloh's social skills, we turned the two young mares out together. Shiloh charged at the other mare and kicked her, then attempted to corner her in the turnout shed. As soon as we had the mares safely separated by a gate, Shiloh jogged over to stand beside me, head down, shaking in terror. Whatever prompted her aggression, there was clearly fear behind it. Our friend found a safer place to board her mare.

When Brandy arrived, Shiloh reacted as she had to the Arabian mare. She lunged at her with bared teeth every time Brandy walked past her stall. When we put them in adjacent stalls, Shiloh kicked her wall incessantly. Brandy steered clear of Shiloh but never responded aggressively. Over time, Shiloh's reaction had faded to the "grumpy" ears that seem to signify her anxiety.

We watched Brandy and Shiloh like hawks at first. Brandy did the same thing she'd done with Sapphire, edging closer until Shiloh put her ears back, then veering off. After a few uneventful weeks, we left them out together overnight. Brandy kept a cautious distance from Shiloh, but neither had scrapes or scratches.

We had two alarming incidents in which Shiloh charged aggressively at Brandy, with no apparent provocation from Brandy. Both incidents occurred when my husband was in the paddock with the girls, dispensing treats. With our new understanding of herd dynamics, we realized that this was a human-created problem. Shiloh was guarding a valuable resource: Jerry and the treats he served up. Since Shiloh had become Jerry's mount after Sapphire retired, she perhaps felt a special claim on him and the goodies. Jerry agreed to serve treats only to Shiloh and only in her stall. End of problem.

*Whatever prompted her aggression, there was clearly fear behind it.*

We gave the mares two months together, hoping that a friendship would develop. It didn't. Satisfied with peaceful coexistence, we put Bronzz in the mix.

## Brandy and Bronzz

I was sure Bronzz would be no problem with Brandy, which just shows that the only guarantee with horses is that they will surprise you. Although Bronzz had gotten into kicking matches with other geldings, as he had with Snickers, he had never offered to kick a mare. We had never seen Brandy kick anyone. Should be fine, right?

Bronzz did his pinned-ear lunge at Brandy as he'd always done with Shiloh, but Brandy did not scoot away. She swung her butt at him in warning. He tried herding her, all but pushing her with his chest. She kicked the air in his direction, high and swift, but he did not get the message. When he continued to push her, she whipped around and hit him square in the ribs with both hind feet, catching him three times before he backed off. He tried again a few days later and got slammed in the chest. After that, all Brandy had to do was swing her butt toward him when he got pushy.

Now here is the intriguing twist. Brandy only threatens to kick if he lunges at her. If she approaches Bronzz's hay pile, and he asks her "nicely" to leave (ears back, nose flick, and feet still), she often walks away. She appears to be rewarding him for appropriate behavior!

## A Year Later: The Circular Hierarchy

Bronzz deferred to Brandy, who deferred to Shiloh, who still deferred to Bronzz. Dr. McDonnell says this "triangle" is not unusual in free-roaming horses. Friends who watch pasture politics on their own farms have also observed it.

Rankings were not rigid as they were in Sapphire's day. Brandy did not care who got which hay pile, drank first, or went through gateways first. Her priority was having a friend to hang out with. Bronzz seemed happy to fill that role and respect her rules in the bargain. They grazed together, shared hay piles, and took turns standing guard when one of them would lie down to rest.

Shiloh mostly stayed on the periphery, but Brandy continued to make friendly overtures. She offered gentle nose touches when they were in adjacent stalls and went to stand beside Shiloh if Shiloh stayed off by herself too long. Shiloh stood guard when Bronzz and Brandy would lie down to rest at the same time.

A mundane incident one day showed how Bronzz viewed Brandy as his protector. Hearing an unusually loud banging and clanging at the intersection below our farm, all three horses galloped to their pasture fence to stare in alarm. Suddenly Bronzz glanced around and noticed that Brandy had stopped behind him. Swiftly, he backed up until she was in front of him. The leader is the protector.

## Three Years Later: Circular Hierarchy or Family Group?

Our herd dynamics are increasingly harmonious. Bronzz has not only stopped lunging at Brandy, he no longer lunges at Shiloh. He asks her to move politely, with a nose flick. Since we never saw Shiloh react differently to his chasing, it appears that he learned this more appropriate behavior from Brandy, and now applies it with Shiloh, too.

Shiloh and Brandy often share a hay pile. When Shiloh's ears say she does not want to share, Brandy quietly moseys off, yet Shiloh always lets Brandy come in the barn ahead of her at mealtimes. I'm not

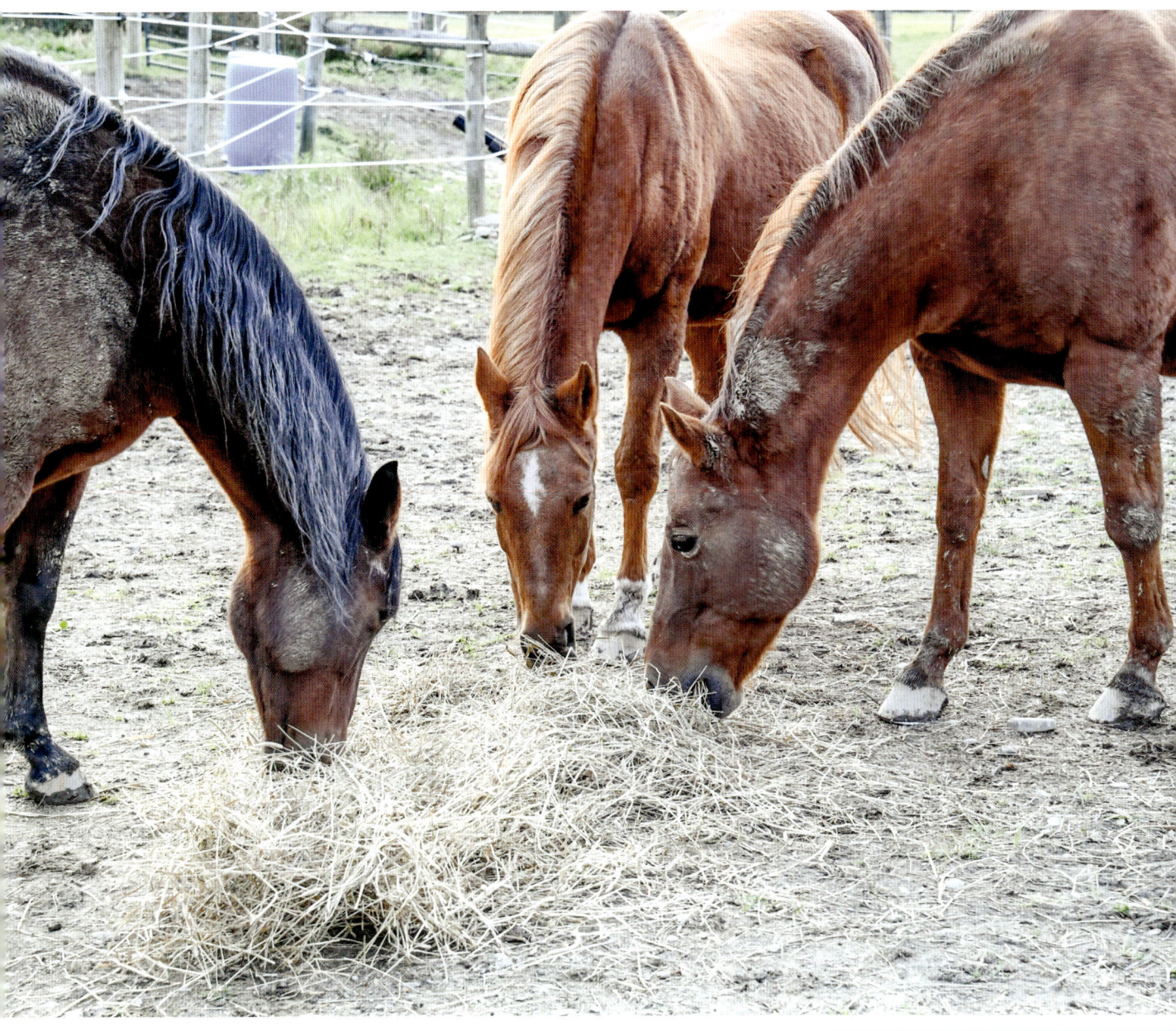

5.3 Even though we put out multiple hay piles, all three horses sometimes choose to share the same one.

sure which of them has the higher rank, and I'm not sure they care.

I used to think that the only "relationship" horses had to work out was the pecking order, and when the dust settled from any disputes, the relationship was established. My horses have shown me over and over that establishing rank is just the beginning and, ultimately, perhaps not that important. If horses are lucky enough to be turned out with compatible companions, and allowed to stay together over time, their relationships continue to grow (fig. 5.3).

## Changes in Relationships with Us

We saw a change in both Bronzz and Shiloh when they began living with Brandy. They are more relaxed and more tuned in to whatever we ask them to do.

In the past, Bronzz's ears were often back in a "grumpy" expression and, despite his excellent people manners, he always seemed a little bit on edge. Now he greets everyone with happy ears, ready for whatever we have planned.

Shiloh had a "wary" look, backing away or flinching from even normal, *un*threatening actions. We had discussed the issue with our vet and tried various

**5.4** Sapphire always stood guard when other horses rested, yet did not lie down to rest herself.

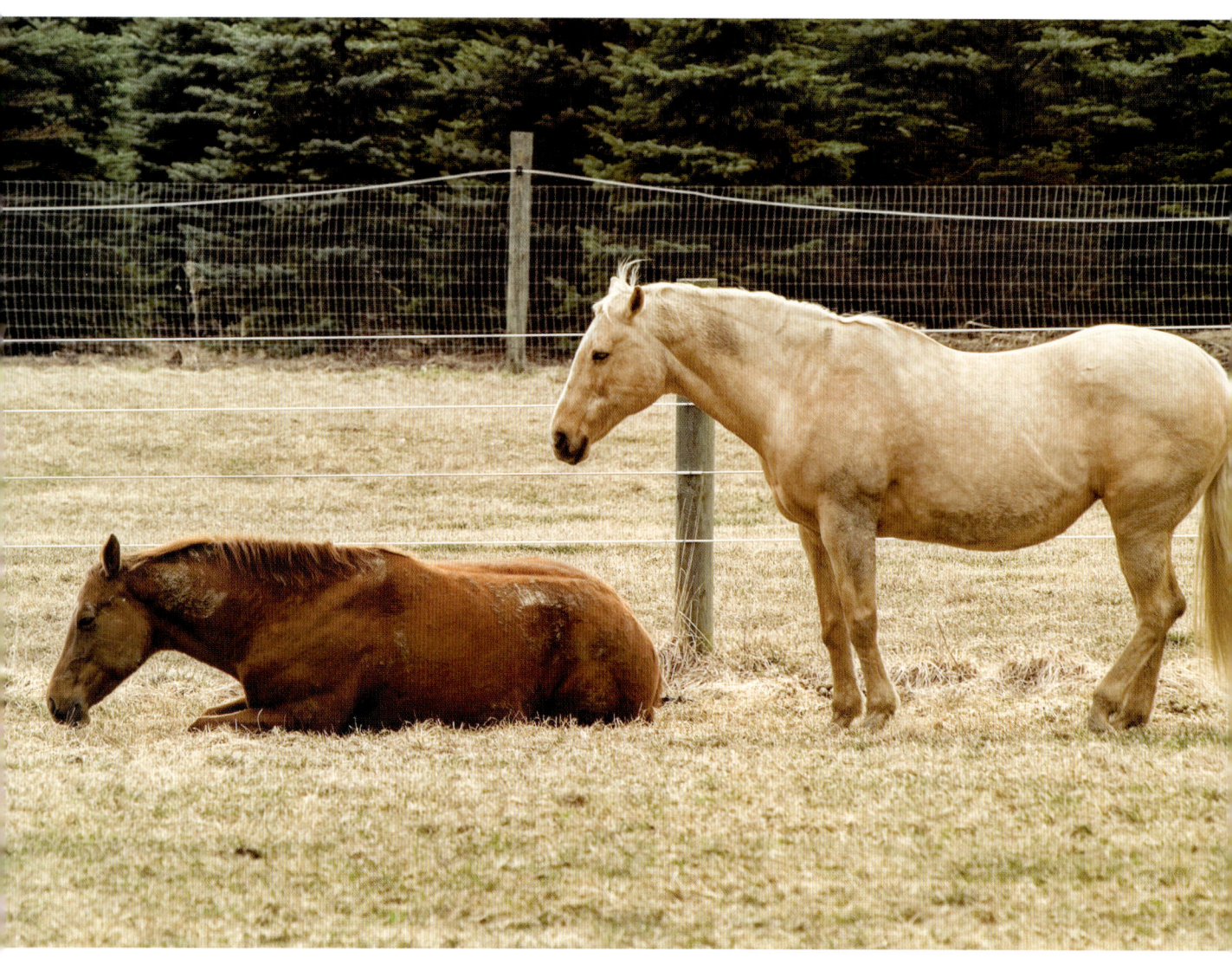

supplements in hopes of calming her. None of them helped. She is calmer now. I think that results from a combination of calmer herd dynamics, and my gentler way of interacting with her.

## Sapphire's Point of View

Considering the old dynamics from Sapphire's perspective, she had several significant causes of anxiety. First, at least one previous living situation had taught her to fight for her share of food, and Bronzz added to her mealtime stress by constantly invading her space. Second, for most of her time with us, I was her main caretaker and an authoritarian leader.

Finally, whether she actually wanted to be leader or not, the position came naturally to her as the oldest, a mare, and the horse who had been with us the longest. She was always the one on guard and seemed to feel a burden of responsibility (fig. 5.4). We never saw her lie down to rest. She developed sores on the fronts of her fetlocks, which I have since learned is a sign of sleep deprivation.

Had I understood Protector Leadership sooner, I would have handled her much differently, relieving some of her anxiety, and perhaps her need to be on duty all the time. Serving her hay separately from the other horses (but within sight) might have eased her fears of not getting her share.

## ◆ Summary

People often see bonds between horses as a bad thing, fearing that horses will be too herd bound to focus on them. Separating friends is not the solution. When horses get along without hurting each other, there is much to be said for quitting while you're ahead. If you rearrange turnout companions often enough, odds are that sooner or later there will be two horses who really do not get along. I know a stable where turnout arrangements are deliberately changed on a regular basis to discourage bonding. They have an unusually high incidence of serious (even fatal) injuries inflicted by pasture mates.

Breaking up a friendship will not improve your relationship with a horse any more than you can improve your relationship with a human friend by coming between her and her other friends. That is not just unkind, it can blow up in your face.

Instead of interfering, consider the positive. A friendship is a sign of the horses' good mental health and social skills, and of your good planning (or luck) in putting them together. The security that friendship provides makes a horse feel safer and, therefore, calmer and better able to focus. If your horse resists leaving four-legged companions to be with you, then you need to focus on becoming another friend who makes him feel safe and secure.

I have told Brandy's "herd story" here from arrival to present because it is relevant to the topic of herd behavior and the connection between our horses' relationships with us and their relationships with each other. The rest of Brandy's story, including her training, saddle phobia, and new career, will resume in chapter 8 (p. 90).

### THINGS TO TRY

- Observe a group of horses and notice if there is a connection between the way the horses behave with each other and the way they behave with people.

- Consider the horses' behavior in the context of whatever you know of their history: how well-socialized they might have been, how often they were sold, moved, or switched to turnout with a new group, what their turnout and feeding arrangements might have been in previous homes.

- Is there a correlation between their interactions with people and the amount of grain and/or turnout they get?

# PART THREE:
# Interpret Behavior Accurately

"Deeper bonds of friendship will blossom as you show your horse you are willing to listen and learn his language instead of just expecting him to respond to yours."

—Sharon Wilsie *(Horse Speak)*

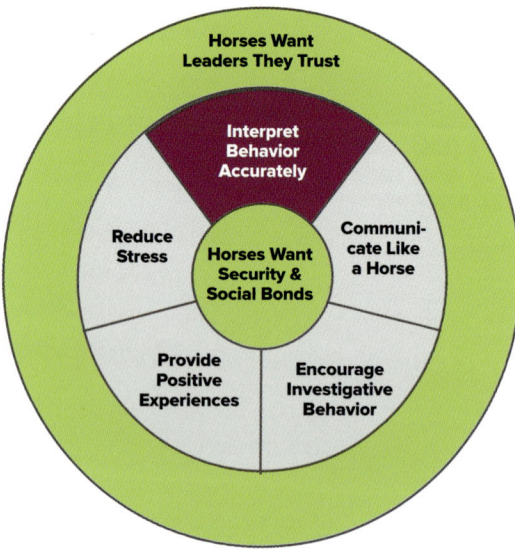

Horses' behavior is their only means of communicating with you. It's how they tell you if they are comfortable, tuned in, and confident; whether they are in pain, confused, or anxiously wishing they could be anywhere else. Their body language is an important predictor of behavior to come, allowing you to address small problems before they become big ones. It also shows you opportunities to build on positive interactions.

However, body language provides useful information only if you interpret it accurately. You must notice what a horse is doing, *and* ask yourself what he is trying to tell you. You must also consider each horse's unique personality, and his way of expressing himself and relating to the world.

The most important part of listening to horses is the willingness to actively tune in to the messages behind the behaviors. In my experience, people who watch horses respectfully, including novices, tend to be astute in their observations. Yet I have seen very technically skilled riders and even famous clinicians who failed to recognize these messages so completely that they were shocked by behavior that a horse warned of well in advance. In fact, they had no idea that a horse had actually been very tolerant of a stressful situation long before "misbehaving."

Unwanted behavior is often *mis*interpreted when people project human motives onto horses, such as believing that horses want to be dominant, disrespectful, lazy, resistant, or take advantage, for example. Blaming the horse encourages a negative response from the person, usually making a bad situation worse. It also focuses attention on "fixing" the behavior. Much time is wasted trying to train away behaviors without addressing the underlying problems that caused them in the first place.

Horses don't want to misbehave. They want the security that comes from harmony in their social group. Their very subtle body language helps them maintain that harmony with each other in a well-socialized group. When we tune in, it can help maintain harmony in our relationships with them, too.

This part is devoted to interpreting communication that is commonly seen as "misbehavior." Some of these actions are actually positive signs that a horse accepts your leadership and is thinking like a partner (see chapter 6—p. 66). Other behaviors tell you something is seriously wrong (see chapter 7—p. 77). Chapter 8 describes some problem behaviors we encountered with Brandy, Bronzz, and Shiloh, and how sorting out the reasons behind their behavior helped resolve them (p. 90).

**Part Three Key Points:**
- Horses' body language or behavior is their main means of communicating with us.
- Behavior problems are a common sign of confusion or distress, but they are frequently misinterpreted as disobedience or lack of respect.
- Trying to solve behavior problems without addressing their cause can make matters worse.

**You will learn how to:**
- Interpret unwanted behavior so you can identify and address underlying causes.
- Recognize "misbehavior" that is actually a positive sign that your horse is thinking like a partner.

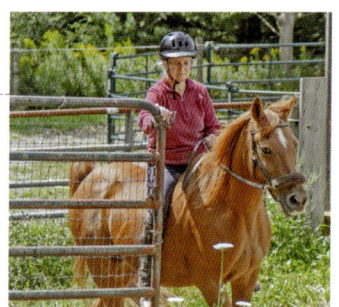

## chapter 6
# Positive Behaviors Misinterpreted

> "Since the horse cannot speak the rider must endeavor to guess his thoughts and to interpret his reactions and draw conclusions from his behavior."
>
> —Alois Podhajsky *(My Horses, My Teachers)*

Horses want to be partners, not obedient servants. Partners think. This means they do not always do exactly what you ask (or think you're asking). Or they sometimes do things you have not asked for. This can be a good sign that they are thinking like a partner, trying to communicate with you, keep you safe, or show signs of trust and attachment.

These actions can be misconstrued as disobedience. They might even be punished. It is like being with someone who ignores what we say, and places a negative interpretation on everything we do. When we do this to our horses, we overlook important information, and turn ourselves into a source of anxiety instead of security.

This chapter describes six actions of horses who are acting like partners. Protector Leaders recognize these actions as compliments that show we have a good relationship.

### Initiating an Action in an Attempt to Communicate with You

For many years I thought of horses' behavior mainly in terms of their responses to what I wanted them to do. I overlooked the fact that horses do not just *react* to what we do. They also *initiate* communication with a goal in mind, a strategy to achieve that goal, and the ability to come up with a new strategy if the initial one fails.

In one study, a bucket of delectable goodies (apples, carrots, or oats) was placed beyond each horse's reach. The horses experimented with different methods of getting the attention of a human standing nearby, and directing her attention to the bucket. When the human was facing them, horses tended to seek eye contact, then look at the bucket. When that didn't work, horses tried more creative strategies to get the person's attention, and direct it toward the goody-bucket. Some were subtle; others used whole body motions.[48] [49]

Sometimes my horses' meanings are clear to me. Brandy gazes longingly at the grass on the other side of the gate. "Please open the gate." Shiloh tips over the water tank. "Empty. Need a refill." Sapphire once met me at the pasture gate, and stuck her forehead right in front of my eyes so I could not miss the burdocks that completely snarled her forelock. "See this mess? Fix it!" Bronzz limped up to me and held his lame foreleg out to me. "It hurts."

Other times I am really slow. Shiloh often lifted a hind leg while we were grooming her. Assuming this was a disrespectful gesture, I scolded her sternly. One day, I noticed that her ears were not pinned, and her leg was waving *under* her belly, not at me. When she put her foot down, I very cautiously reached under her belly and worked my way back. When

> **Actions of the Horse Acting Like a Partner**
>
> 1. Initiating an action in an attempt to communicate with you.
> 2. Pausing or experimenting to figure out what you want.
> 3. Anticipating what you are going to ask.
> 4. Volunteering an action that has been rewarded in the past.
> 5. Disobeying for what the horse believes to be a good reason.
> 6. Showing signs of trust and attachment.

I reached her udder, great gobs of crusty mare goop came off in my hand. Shiloh sighed with relief. This is a perfect example of misinterpreting Shiloh's meaning because I was focused on her waving leg without noticing that the rest of her body language was not threatening. And because I was too busy assuming she was being disrespectful to notice that she was desperately asking for help!

So, why didn't she find a more polite way to call attention to her plight? She had tried. She had danced around in her stall, lifting her leg and swinging her face at her flank. She'd rubbed her tailbone bald. To my embarrassment, I never connected those actions to her udder. When she lifted her leg, all but pointing at her udder, I had scolded her. Many horses give up trying to communicate with people. To Shiloh's credit, not mine, she persevered until I finally caught on.

Now, if Shiloh needs to remind me to take care of her udder, she shifts so a hip is in front of me. This could look like a threatening gesture to someone who does not know her, but I know she is just "showing" me the body part that needs help. If I don't "listen," then she lifts her leg.

Horses have a concept of what we do and do not know, and this influences their communication. This is a sign of the social intelligence that makes for sophisticated communication in horse herds.

In another study, food was hidden in a bucket that only the horse's caretaker could reach. Each horse saw the item being hidden, but in some instances, the caretaker was not present when a second person hid the food, so presumably the caretaker did not know about it. When the caretaker apparently did not know about the hidden goody, horses worked harder to get her attention and direct it to the bucket.[50]

This means horses understand that they might have information that we do not. This is especially relevant when horses spook or act suspicious of a situation. If we act like nothing's there, as I was taught long ago, we suggest that we haven't noticed a potential problem. In this case, a horse might escalate the behavior in an attempt to direct our attention to it. We have more credibility as a leader if we let the horse know we *do* notice the situation. I look ostentatiously at whatever the horse is worried about and announce with great authority, "Yup, I see that. It's a whatever. No problem." Assuming, of course, that I know for a fact there is no danger. When the horse is still not satisfied, further investigation might be needed, as described in Part Five (Investigative Behavior—p. 139).

Sapphire once gave a dramatic demonstration of pointing out a danger that proved to be real. She and Jerry were in the lead on a lazy summer trail ride when she suddenly took a flying leap, whipped around, and stood snorting and glaring at the trail. Since Sapphire was typically the last horse to spook, we all searched until we found the cause: a ground-hog hole nearly hidden in the weeds at the edge of the trail.

One way to interpret the meaning of a horse's behavior is to notice what it accomplishes. As a result of Sapphire's warning, which the other horses probably deciphered before we humans did, no one stepped in the hole.

How often is this sort of behavior misunderstood when the cause is not obvious to people? "Stupid horse, he spooked at nothing." Yet it is nearly impossible to prove that a horse has spooked at "nothing." They hear and smell things we do not. Their vision is specially adapted so that, in addition to splendid peripheral

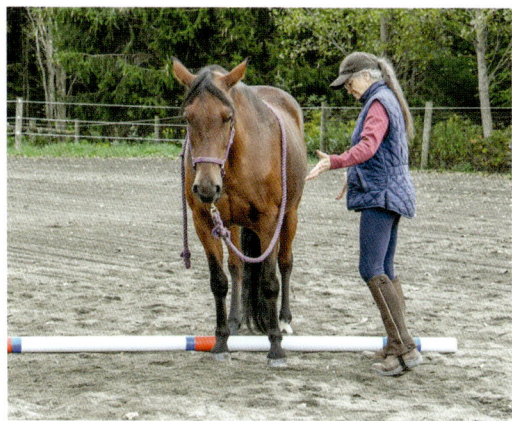

6.1 A  When I ask Brandy to side-pass along a pole, she pauses to think about what I mean.

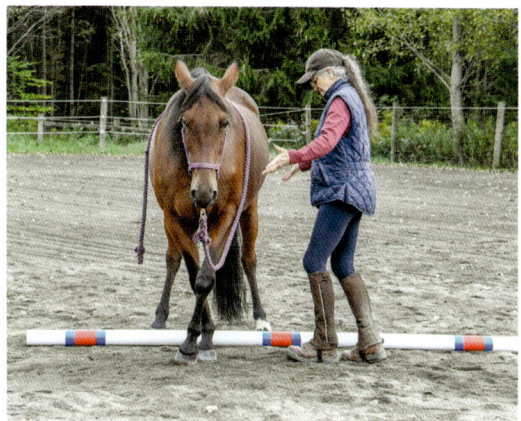

6.1 B  After pondering the options, she responds correctly.

vision, they are not deceived by color camouflage as we are. (More details on this in chapter 12, How Horses Explore the World—p. 141.)

## Pausing or Experimenting to Figure Out What You Want

Horses are not born knowing what different cues mean. When they first encounter a new cue, or a rider who gives cues differently, they need to decipher what is wanted. This process might involve trial and error as the horse tries out different options. Or it might start with a pause as the horse, apparently doing nothing, is really considering the options.

The first time I asked Shiloh to side-pass under saddle, she was confused because the cues were different than when I was on the ground. She tried going forward then back, moving her haunches then her shoulders. I just waited, gently holding the cue, until she tried moving shoulders and hips at the same time. Although ragged, it was the right idea, so I instantly released the cue and praised her lavishly.

Experimenting is a compliment that says our horses trust us not to punish them for honest mistakes. Shiloh would not experiment when she first came to us. It took her a long time to trust that she was safe making mistakes.

Unlike Shiloh who now readily experiments, Brandy often does nothing right away when presented with an unfamiliar cue. This was disconcerting at first, because it felt like she was ignoring me. I was so used to expecting an instant response, even if it was a wrong one that even 10 seconds felt like a long time to wait. Apparently Brandy is actually thinking through her options (figs. 6.1 A & B). If I just wait, her first try is usually close to what I want. With practice and confidence, her responses get quicker.

## Anticipating What You Are Going to Ask

When I want to ride through a gate, I do not need to maneuver Bronzz into position to open it. He automatically lines himself up so my right hand is at the gate latch. I did not plan this; it evolved because we opened a gate on every ride, either to go into the arena or out of the paddock to the woods. I praised him when he first lined up on his own, and he generalized it to any gate we encounter.

Bronzz also learned the maneuvers needed to close gates with minimal cues from me, allowing us to easily close even heavy gates that swing uphill (fig. 6.2).

This kind of initiative shows that a horse is tuned in, understands his job, and is performing it willingly.

Sometimes a horse is tuned in to such subtle nuances of your body language that he responds to cues you are not aware of giving. If I am thinking about trotting, and my horse starts to trot, he is probably responding to a minute shift of weight or tightening of a muscle. It is only fair to give horses the benefit of any doubt because they are usually more aware of your body language than you are.

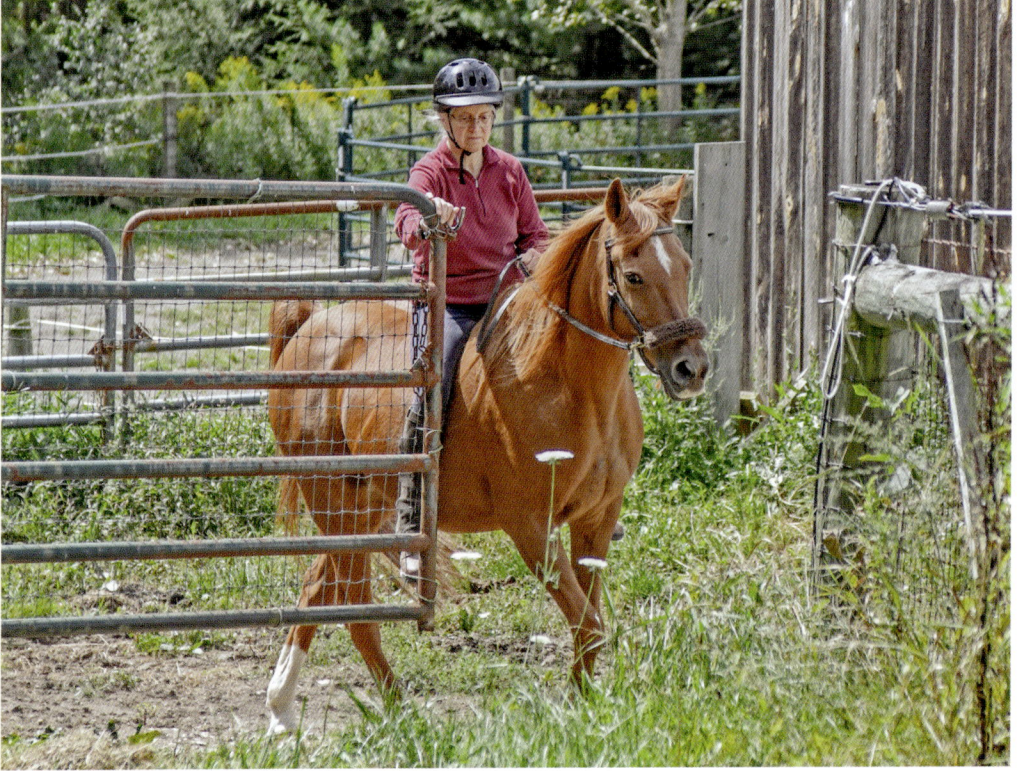

6.2 With one eye on the gate, Bronzz walks an arc, staying just close enough for me to reach the gate.

Convenient forms of anticipation are often taken for granted. A horse lowers his head when you pick up his halter. At hoof-picking time, he has each hoof off the ground when you get to it instead of waiting to be asked.

Anticipation is not necessarily appreciated when a horse's job involves precision responses to a rider's cues. In that case, you can discourage it with clear cues for the action you want instead. Horses are quite capable of understanding that initiative may be appreciated in some circumstances and not others. For instance, yes for gates or hoof-picking, but not in a show ring.

Horses may also anticipate when learning a new skill for which they have not yet coordinated cues, timing, balance, and execution. For example, a green horse learning to canter might break into a canter when he *thinks* (correctly or incorrectly) that his rider is getting ready to ask him. He should be praised for his willingness. When he is confident about cantering, secure in his balance, and clear on cues, then you can gently remind him to wait for the appropriate cue.

Anticipation should never be punished because the action is offered in good faith, and not intended as disobedience. I once knew a nice lady whose talented dressage horse worked hard to please her. When he was learning flying changes, he started to offer them before she gave the cue. Her instructor insisted that she punish him for anticipating the cue. The horse took the correction so much to heart that he never did another flying change under saddle for the rest of his long life.

## Volunteering an Action That Has Been Rewarded in the Past

In this instance, you are confident that you have *not* asked for this action, and did not intend to; the horse is acting on his own initiative. A horse may do this to earn praise, or to "negotiate" a different activity than the one you're asking for. The crucial point is that he is volunteering an action that has received a positive response in the past. This is a huge compliment to you and your relationship. He is trusting that you will not punish him for making a suggestion of his own. Horses who have been taught to do only as they are told, and punished for any deviations, do not take such initiative.

As soon as Snickers learned how to do turns-on-the-forehand (a pivot around the front feet), he began to offer them whenever we halted. I laughed, and let him practice because a horse who is trying to score himself an "atta-boy" and a withers scratch obviously is not out to cause trouble. When he had the maneuver down pat, and the little dance got tiresome, I either ignored it or asked him to do something else.

Horses may offer a substitute

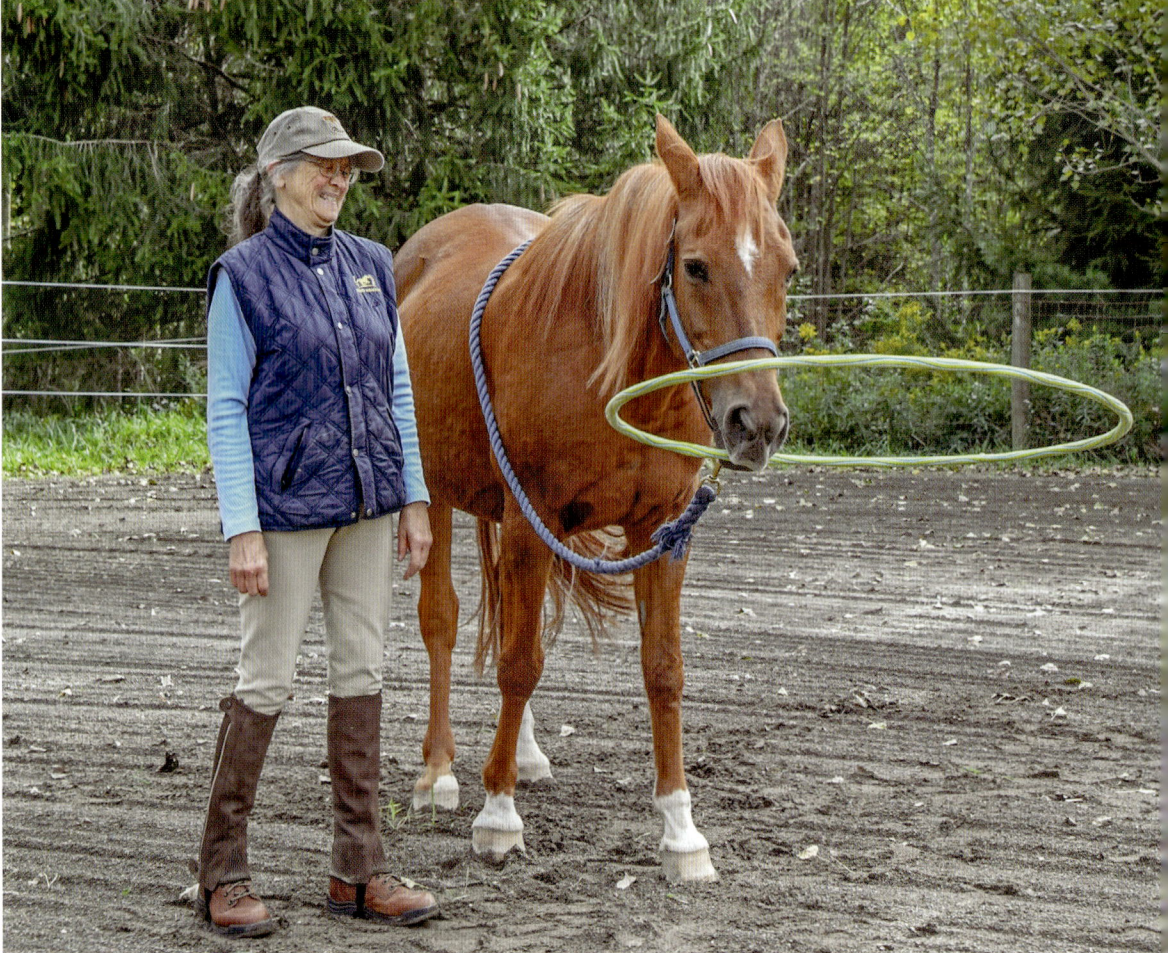

6.3 Bronzz picks up the hula hoop, apparently hoping I will be amused enough to forget that I just asked him to stand in it.

behavior when you ask for something they find difficult, confusing, or just less interesting. Bronzz's favorite lateral move is haunches-in (traveling with the hind feet slightly inside the track of the front feet). It is easy for him, and he sometimes offers it when I ask for shoulder-in, which he finds more difficult. When we do agility courses, he'd rather pick up a hula hoop than stand in it (fig. 6.3).

Although you do not normally want to let horses change your agenda, you can notice what they like to do, and ask for it as a reward after they do something else well.

## Disobeying for What the Horse Believes to Be a Good Reason

We have a state forest adjacent to our farm. Bronzz and Sapphire learned the trails on our end of it the first year we lived here. One day both of them flatly refused to cross a culvert they'd crossed before without hesitation. Bronzz went as rigid as a statue. Sapphire went into reverse, her pretty palomino neck arched, nostrils flared.

My husband and I agreed this was not disobedience; it was a warning. Even though the culvert looked fine to us, the horses did not trust it. They readily agreed to an alternative that was much more work: bushwhack through underbrush, scoot down a muddy creek bank, clamber across rocks, climb up the other bank, and squeeze through a maze of saplings.

Their suspicions were validated a couple weeks later when we got a phone call from a friend who rides the same trails. Erosion around the culvert had created dangerous sinkholes that were now obvious.

Refusing to obey a command for a *valid reason* is called "Intelligent Disobedience." Service dogs are *taught* to do this. It is what stops a guide dog from leading his handler into traffic. For a horse, warning us of possible danger is part of being a responsible herd member or **partner.**

Horses see, hear, smell, and feel (through their hooves) things that we cannot. Faulty or misunderstood cues from a rider often require a horse to guess what to do. Unexpected circumstances may require a horse to react faster than we can. Horses who have been punished for using their own judgment can actually be more dangerous. My worst fall occurred when a horse obeyed my faulty command, and we landed on *top* of a jump. Had he refused, I would have been spared a serious injury. That was when I recognized the danger of demanding absolute obedience.

Intelligent Disobedience is at work when horses slow down for insecure footing, refuse to go forward onto footing that looks unreliable, refuse jumps because their rider is poorly balanced, or opt to detour around situations that look risky (fig. 6.4). No prey animal wants to risk falling or getting trapped, and his caution protects us, too.

Slowing down with riders who are wobbly or anxious is a job requirement for horses used for lessons, public trail rides, or therapeutic riding. If they did not ignore or "disobey" unintentional leg motions and shifts of weight, they'd terrify their riders with all sorts of unexpected moves.

Some people fear that letting horses "get away with disobeying" undermines future **obedience. My** experience is exactly the opposite. When we fail to trust our horses' good judgment, we lose credibility. I once overruled Sapphire's objections, insisting we cross a flooded creek in a February thaw. I did not realize the danger until I felt Sapphire bracing her body against the current as she picked her way

PART THREE: INTERPRET BEHAVIOR ACCURATELY — 73

6.4 Bronzz looks over the tangle of branches in front of us and turns his head to show that we should go around it. He would not step into this treacherous mess even if I asked him to.

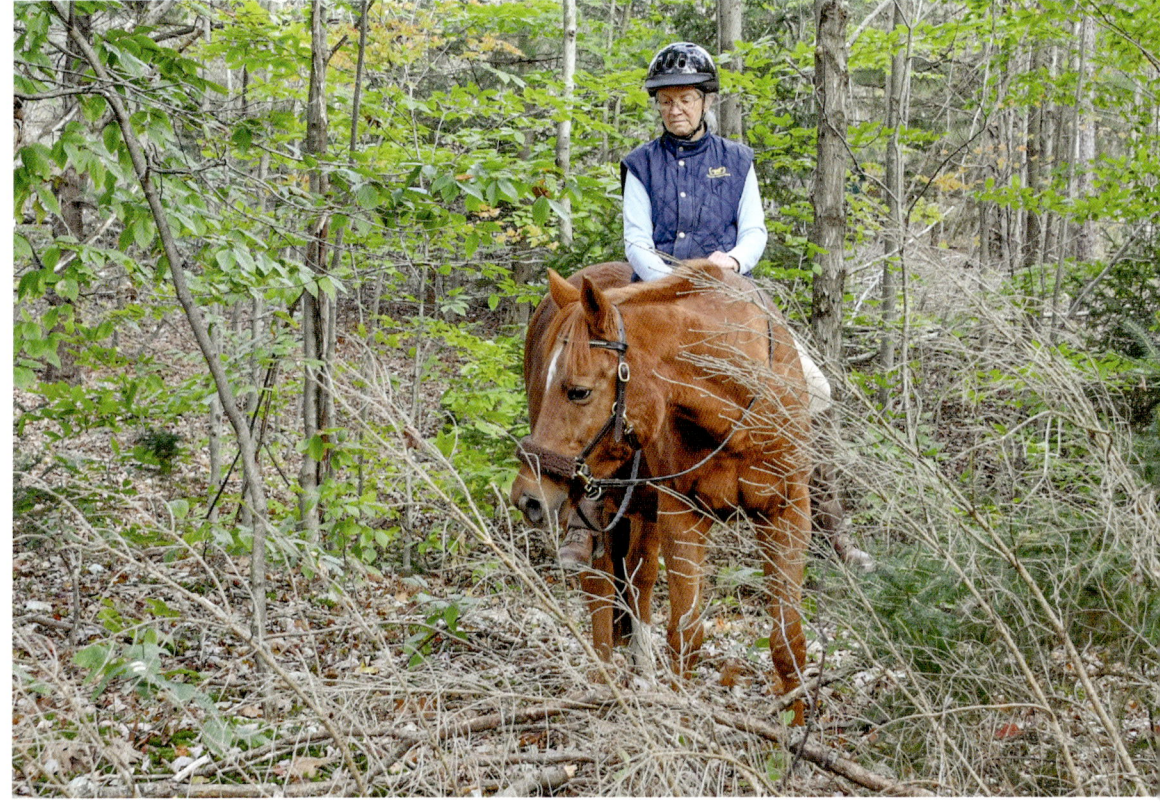

across slippery rocks. I peeked down to see icy chocolate-colored water swirling around my waterproof boots and thought, "If she slips, I'm going to drown." After that she refused to get anywhere near the creek when it was high.

When you trust your horse, he is more likely to trust you when you do need to overrule him. If you suspect a horse could be right about danger, you retain your position as decision-maker by deciding on Plan B after the horse has warned you that Plan A might be risky.

## Showing Signs of Trust and Attachment

Your horse's attachment to you is significant, and not only for sentimental reasons. Horses who are attached to their trainer have a stronger sense of security, and, therefore, are calmer, more focused, and able to learn. Horses who lack this security are more likely to be fearful and distracted. Thus, attachment impacts the success of training, independent of the techniques used.[51]

People may not doubt that their dogs love them, yet few notice that their horses are attached to them. The idea is even scoffed at by many, and surely it is easier to sell a horse if we don't believe the horse cares. But many do care…and deeply.

We saw it the day Sapphire was delivered to us. Her teenage owner was committed to showing in Western Pleasure. Sapphire despised ring work and repetition, but was reliable on trails. A career change made good sense. When Melissa brought Sapphire to us, Sapphire appeared to think they were on a routine clinic or lesson expedition. She dove happily into the clover-laced grass in the little pasture where we turned her out, until she saw Melissa's truck and trailer disappearing down the road without her. Then she ran to the edge of the pasture screaming that heart-rending, "Don't leave me!" whinny.

It was months before we felt that Sapphire was getting attached to us; it was very clear a year later when we left her overnight at the equine hospital at Cornell in preparation for a lameness exam. Her desperate screams rang in our ears as we left, and met us when we arrived the next morning. The moment she saw us, she quieted, and became a model patient.

Possibly Sapphire got unusually attached to people, but I do not think so. I think she was just quicker to suspect she was being left behind permanently, and more eloquent about showing her distress.

Signs of attachment can be so mundane that they are misinterpreted or overlooked altogether. Welcoming us with a nicker, or leaving a hay pile to greet us. Relaxing contentedly when we groom, talk to them, scratch itchy spots, or just hang out. Not walking off immediately when we turn them out. Tuning in to us even when we're not asking for anything.

I have seen this tuning in when I ride a student's horse to demonstrate something. Even as the horse is politely doing as I ask, he keeps an eye and ear on his owner, and gravitates to her the minute I dismount. Few owners notice this or appreciate its significance until I point it out.

Attention-seeking is another sign of attachment. Brandy comes to nuzzle me in the paddock. Bronzz plays silly games like sneaking out of his stall when my back is turned; picking up the wrong foot at hoof-cleaning time; or lifting anything he can fit his mouth around, including pitchforks, wheelbarrow handle, or the cats' water bowl, undaunted by the mess.

Changes in behavior when we've been away are another clue. While Bronzz was still living with his breeder, Fritz, I went away for two weeks. The day I returned, Bronzz did not come to the pasture gate as usual when he heard my car. Instead, he walked to the far corner of his pasture and stood there with his butt toward me, acting like he couldn't hear me calling him. As I prepared to hike out and fetch him, Fritz translated jokingly, "Bronzz says you hurt his feelings by going away, and now he's going to hurt yours."

Sapphire's reaction was just the

opposite. She met us at the gate with happy nickers, and knocked herself out to please us for the next two days.

The most disconcerting sign of attachment is a horse "clinging" to us when he is scared. If a horse has not learned to stay out of our personal space, it can feel like he is trying to run us over. He is really acting like a scared foal who wants to press himself to his mother's side. Since no one wants a half-ton panic attack plastered to her side, it is hard to see this behavior as a positive sign that he is looking for our leadership. A horse who respects personal space can look to us for reassurance and guidance without becoming a danger.

## Summary

The behaviors described in this chapter are the purposeful actions of thinking partners. They show that horses have confidence in you as a leader. Protector Leaders appreciate and build on them.

1. Horses *initiate* communication with you.
2. Horses trust that when something new is asked of them, they can safely *pause* to think through their options or *experiment* to decipher the right answer because they will not be punished for honest mistakes.
3. Being tuned in to what you are doing, they may *anticipate* what you are likely to ask of them next, and offer it before you ask.
4. They *volunteer* behaviors that have pleased you in the past.
5. They exercise *Intelligent Disobedience* instead of obeying commands that could place them or their people in danger.
6. They show signs of *attachment* to their people.

### THINGS TO TRY

▶ Think of positive behaviors you've observed that show your horse is thinking like a partner; if your responses have not encouraged these behaviors, what could you change?

▶ Watch for behaviors that might be misconstrued as disobedience, but are really expressions of your horse's unique personality. Consider positive ways to respond to these behaviors.

## chapter 7
# Interpreting the Causes of Unwanted Behavior

> "Behaviors such as rearing, which often lead to horses being described as 'bad' or 'dangerous,' are in fact a result of the horse coping with stress in the only way it knows how....By the same token, 'stubborn' and 'unwilling' horses have frozen up and withdrawn as a means of minimizing the stress being placed on them."
>
> —Dr. Carrie Ijichi *("Researchers Develop Subjective Equine Personality Test")*

Horses want security, not conflict. Behavior problems are a sign that something is wrong, and often appear after subtle early warning signs have been overlooked. If a horse becomes distressed enough, his behavior escalates to a level we cannot ignore. Labeling behavior in a negative way (bad, pushy, flighty, disrespectful, stupid, stubborn, ornery, vindictive, and more) puts the focus on changing the behavior instead of addressing the cause. Meanwhile, negative interactions undermine our horses' trust in us.

The real cause of a problem, however, is not always obvious. Any behavior has multiple possible causes, and horses' coping behaviors differ based on their individual personalities.[52] Fortunately, when we encounter behavior we do not want, there is a limited set of likely causes. The following list is a composite drawn from a variety of sources. This chapter describes the dynamics around these causes. Pain and anxiety rate the most attention because of the frequency with which they occur.

When I asked my veterinarian what percentage of behavior problems were caused by pain, her immediate response was, "The vast majority." She explained that includes not only current pain, but memory of past pain, and anticipation of pain. Other equine veterinarians and chiropractors I have queried said the same thing. Behaviorist, Dr. Sue McDonnell, describes undetected pain as "...one of the biggest persisting threats to domestic horses' welfare."[53]

Statistics back them up. Pain is the first cause that should be ruled out when problem behaviors occur, especially aggression.

The prevalence of anxiety-related problems is reflected in the many calming supplements advertised for horses, and the popularity of books and articles on rider anxiety. Anxious horses make people anxious, and rightfully so. An anxious horse is focused on monitoring his own safety, and primed to react to anything he sees as suspicious, making himself a potential danger to rider or handler.

Although some horses are inherently anxiety-prone, much anxiety is the result of situations that are stressful to a horse, or that he anticipates will be stressful. Problem behaviors might result from a single, specific cause, or from a series of smaller stresses that add up to more than the horse can cope with in the moment. This is akin to what happens to us when we're having a bad day, everything seems to be going wrong, and a perfectly reasonable request from someone else suddenly feels like too much, and the other person has no idea why we've lost patience.

I have saved anxiety for last because, as you read through the first nine topics, you will notice that most of these scenarios can cause or contribute to anxiety. This shows what a pervasive problem it is.

Whatever the cause of a problem behavior, we humans are usually a big part of it. Once we understand what is going on, we can be part of the solution instead. Future chapters describe how Protector Leadership skills can help.

Keep in mind that a horse's behavior might reflect treatment from previous owners, handlers, or riders, and you are dealing with the fallout. In this case, this is your opportunity to show the horse that you are offering the security he is looking for. Even if you never fully overcome the effects of his past, you can change

### Causes of Problem Behavior

1. Pain
2. Insecure balance
3. Confusion and misunderstandings
4. Inconsistent expectations
5. Punishment
6. Boredom or fatigue
7. Living conditions and diet
8. Pressure the horse cannot relieve
9. Stressful situations
10. Anxiety

his behavior for the better. Good leadership has turned more than one "difficult" horse into a legendary partner, including Alexander the Great's Bucephalus, Kim Walnes' Gray Goose, and Frederic Pignon's Templado, to name just a few.

Always keep your own safety in mind. If you suspect a horse's behavior could endanger you, get more experienced help. If you *are* the more experienced help, consult and strategize with other people who take a positive, non-punitive, approach to horsemanship.

## Pain

The statistics on pain are shocking. Back pain impacts anywhere from 27 percent to 100 percent of ridden horses, depending on the study population, yet three out of four horses with back pain are not recognized by their caretakers as having pain.[54] A study by the Animal Health Trust in the U.K. found evidence that "nearly half of the sports horse population in normal work may be lame, but the lameness is not recognized by owners or trainers." [55] [56]

How can this be? Many horses work in spite of pain, and pain is often overlooked because horses hide it so well. This had survival value for their ancestors as prey animals because any sign of pain or weakness would be a red flag signaling predators, "Easy pickings over here!" This stoicism is a liability for domestic horses because signs of pain are often mistaken for "bad behavior" or training problems.

### Common Signs of Pain

- **Avoidance or resistance** include resisting being caught, grooming, saddling, or mounting; reluctance to go forward, bucking, refusing jumps. The horse is trying to avoid the situation or activity associated with pain.

- **Compensatory behaviors** are things like poor transitions, changing gaits, wrong leads, a favorite diagonal. The horse is trying to work in spite of pain or stiffness.

- **Tension** or **stiffness** can show up in tight or rigid muscles, wringing tail, bracing against reins, difficulty bending. Tension may also show in subtle ways, such as a horse's expression.

- **Posture** is a red flag when you see a high head, low back, and inverted neck.[57] Legs might slant toward each other, or a hind leg might trail out the back (fig. 7.1). Even if a horse's behavior is acceptable, this posture tells you his body is not comfortable.[58] [59]

- **Anxiety** can come from any stressful situation. That includes pain or anticipation of pain just as it does in people; it is a physiological response.

The Animal Health Trust study mentioned above lists these behaviors as early warning signs of pain:

"…Ears back, mouth opening, tongue out, change in eye posture and expression, going above the bit, head tossing, tilting the head, unwillingness to go, crookedness, hurrying, changing gait spontaneously, poor quality canter, resisting, and stumbling and toe dragging."[61] [62]

## Pain Is Often Caused by What People Do—Or Fail to Do

- **Riders** who are poorly balanced tend to hang on reins and bounce on backs, making horses sore, tense, and braced in self-defense.[63] Any rider who uses stronger cues than necessary can create discomfort.

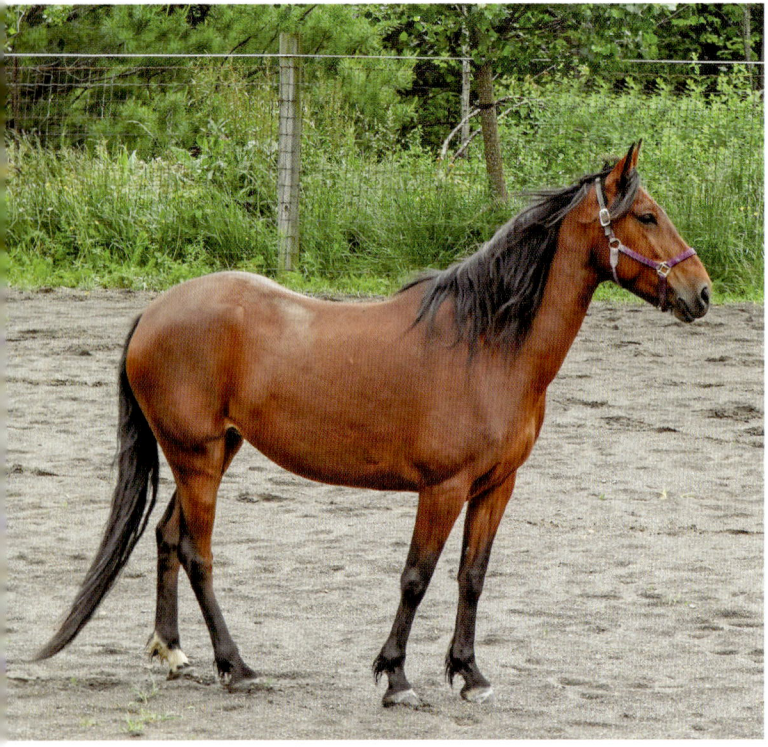

7.1 At age six, Brandy's "goat on a rock" posture showed pain: high head, low back, inverted neck, legs slanting toward each other.

- **Depression, changes in temperament, or any behavior not typical for a given horse**. Being aware of what's normal for a horse helps us spot these changes.

- **Aggression** is a well-recognized reaction to acute pain. That is why we muzzle an injured dog, no matter how sweet he normally is. In horses, *chronic* pain is also associated with aggression. *Any horse who shows aggression should be carefully evaluated for pain.*[60]

- **Lameness** can prompt behavior changes before a horse is obviously lame.

- **Equipment** can cause discomfort when it is poorly designed, poorly fitted, improperly used, or simply not right for that particular horse. For example, Western, dressage, and treeless saddles are often too long for short-backed horses, placing the rider's weight behind the last rib, where the spine has no support. Bits are uncomfortable when a rider has heavy hands, but alternatives such as hackamores or bitless bridles simply shift the pressure to a new place, such as the poll or the bridge of the horse's nose. These are both sensitive areas without the pliability of the mouth. Restrictive equipment such as draw reins or side reins can cause pain when used to force a horse into an unnatural posture.[64]

- **Good hoof balance** is crucial for overall comfort and long-term soundness.[65] If you doubt this, imagine putting a shim in one side of your own shoes. Sooner or later, some part of your body will feel the pain of having to compensate, whether it is your foot, ankle, knee, hip, or back. In horses, long toes with low heels are a particularly common problem that stresses tendons and ligaments, alters posture and gaits, and can cause back pain (fig 7.2). Just imagine wearing shoes that are too long for you, and low in the heel.

- **Dental and TMJ (temporomandibular joint) problems** can cause pain in many parts of the body, as anyone with a TMJ problem herself will understand. A comfortable bite and healthy TMJ are supported by lots of head-down chewing time that domestic horses frequently do not get.[66]

## Insecure Balance

Balance is critical for a prey animal. He might run or fight in spite of pain, but falling leaves him most vulnerable, so anything that makes him feel less than confident of his balance is a source of anxiety. This is a commonly overlooked cause of unwanted behavior.

We do many things that challenge

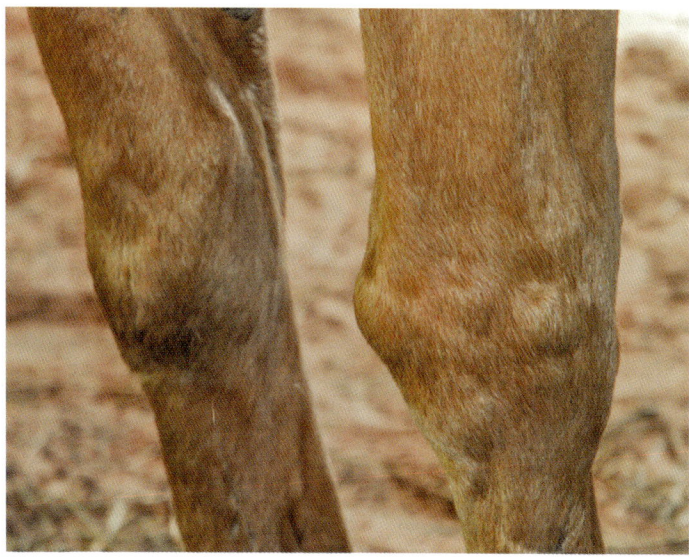

7.2 Sapphire's arthritic knees forced her retirement from riding. Years of long toes/low heels likely hastened the progression of damage.

a horse's balance, starting the first time we ask a youngster to pick up a foot and stand on three legs. Carrying a rider might look easy, but that too is a learned skill, as I discovered the first time I mounted an untrained two-year old Thoroughbred. The trainer I was assisting assured me that the colt was not going to buck as I feared because he would be too busy keeping his balance. Finding this unbelievable, I leaned to the side to test it. Sure enough, the big fellow tottered sideways.

Even a trained horse's balance is challenged (fig. 7.3) when he must cope with a poorly balanced rider, difficult terrain, insecure footing, tight turns, or being forced to carry himself in an unnatural posture.

Good balance is dictated by gravity and equine biomechanics. Head and neck movement is part of a horse's natural

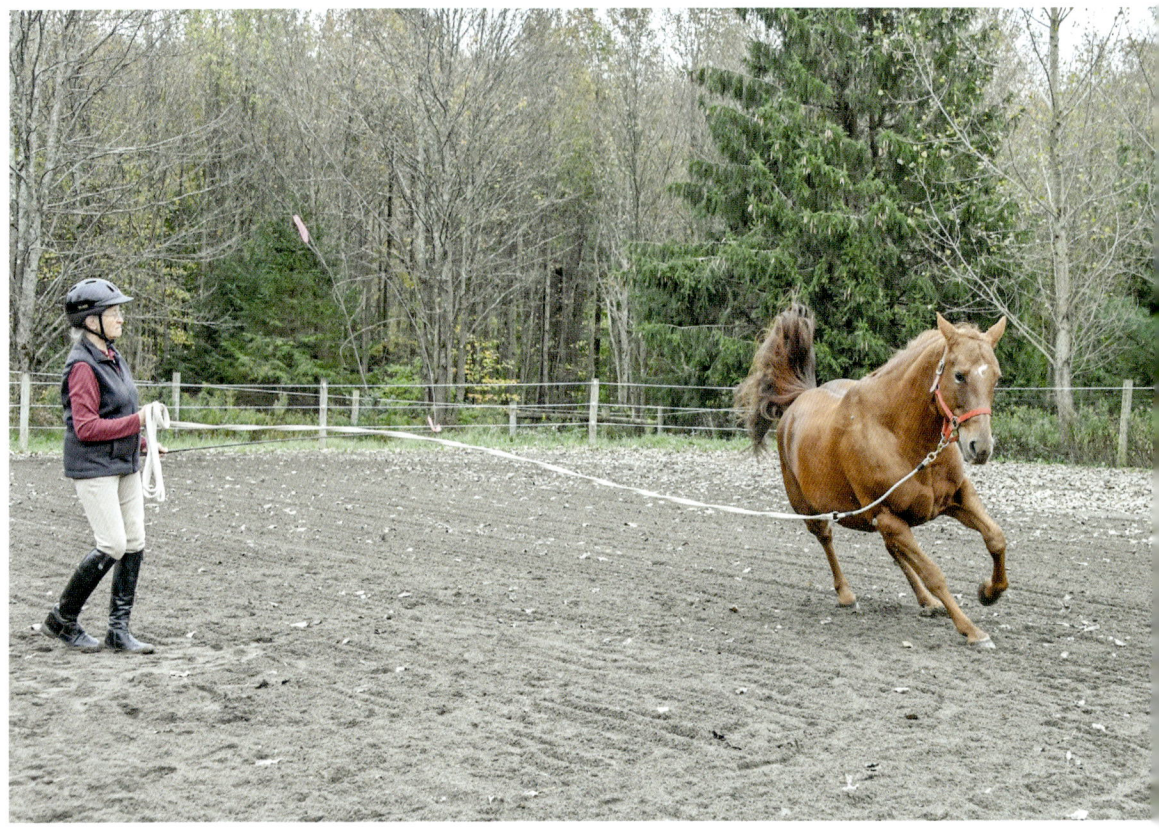

7.3 Shiloh is off balance, my fault for startling her with a twirl of my lunge whip. If I did not immediately slow her down, I could expect her to either buck or charge forward and pull the lunge line from my hand. The angle of her body and legs shows why lungeing on a too-small circle is hard on a horse's joints.

balance in every stride. Restricting this movement compromises balance. That is why, when a horse trips, you let the reins slip through your fingers so he can use his head to help regain his balance.

Training that dictates how a horse should carry his head can compromise balance. This happens when a horse is taught to carry his head too low for his conformation, thus making him heavy on the forehand. It is also an issue when a horse is required to tuck his nose behind the vertical. Instead of learning to balance, horses must compensate for being off-balance, resulting in stiffness, pain, and orthopedic problems. If you doubt that restricting a horse's head movement is a problem, try tucking your own chin to your chest, and then go do something athletic. Also notice what that does to your breathing and your ability to see where you're going (figs. 7.4 A & B).

A horse's reaction to balance problems is often illogical from a human point of view, as Susan Harris describes in *Horse Gaits, Balance, and Movement*. Some horses slow down or stop, as you might expect. Losing balance is scary, however, and their instinct to escape scary situations prompts many horses to speed up or even buck.[67]

You may see the "speed up when off balance" dynamic, for example, in a horse who rushes jumps. A rider holding him back interferes further with his balance, which increases his anxiety and makes the rushing worse.

## Confusion and Misunderstandings

When a horse does not understand a cue, he must guess what to do. This is a common occurrence. Perhaps the horse has not been taught the meaning of a cue, a cue is not given clearly, is accompanied by a conflicting cue, or is different than the cue the horse was previously taught. It is never fair to assume a horse knows anything just because someone says so; horses are often sold with claims that their training is more extensive than it really is. Meanwhile, people are frequently less clear than they think they are. Blaming the horse for the human's mistake creates anxiety and undermines trust, just as it does in people.

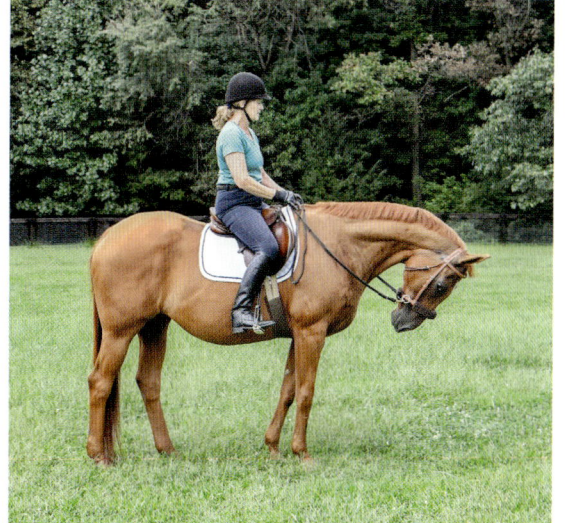

7.4 A  Gracie came to my sister Dani with a habit of tucking her nose behind the vertical. She still does so occasionally despite careful remedial training and a customized bridle without a bit. Notice the tension in her neck, the constriction at her throat, and the restriction of her visual field.

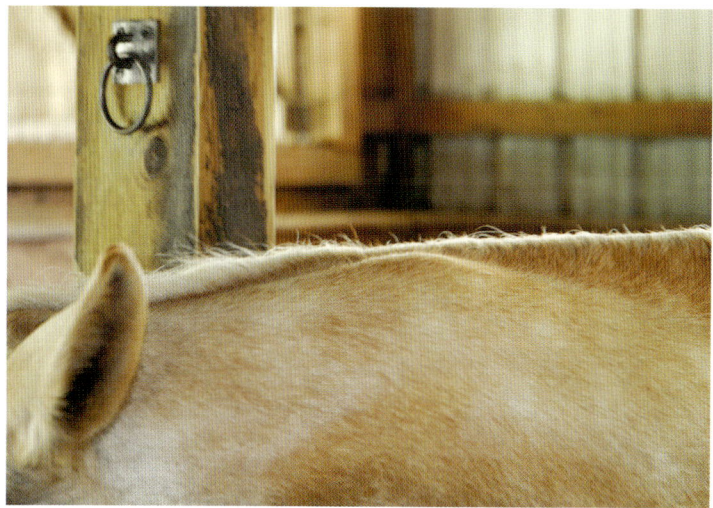

7.4 B  The bulge in Sapphire's neck shows a long-term consequence of over-flexing a horse's neck. Since we never rode her that way, this damage was done early in her life.

## Inconsistent Expectations

Inconsistent expectations also leave horses guessing. Is this the day I can dance around and pull on the lead line, or the day I'll get jerked and scolded? Can I trot to catch up to the horse in front of me or will my rider yank my reins and yell at me? When my rider asks for a canter, does she really mean it, or if I pretend not to notice, will she give up?

Such inconsistencies are a recipe for anxiety, resentment, and even aggression, especially if the horse is punished for gambling that today is his lucky day. A leader who cannot maintain consistent expectations and fair consequences does not inspire trust or confidence.

## Punishment

Few horse trainers list punishment as a *cause* of problem behaviors, but equine behaviorists such as Dr. Sue McDonnell most certainly do, and so does the American Veterinary Society of Animal Behavior (AVSAB). Punishment does not address underlying causes of problem behaviors or show the horse what you want instead. It can backfire for several reasons.

- **Punishment causes negative associations** with people and/or the activity involved. Confusion, resentment, and anxiety are likely if the behavior being punished was allowed or rewarded, however inadvertently, in the past.

- **Intermittent punishment actually strengthens the unwanted behavior** when horses gamble that they will not be punished *this* time.

- **Even mild punishment can cause fear** in some horses, and this fear can be generalized to other situations. If the behavior being punished was caused by fear, then punishment increases the fear and the likelihood of fear-related aggression.

While punishment may suppress fearful and aggressive behaviors, it can also suppress the *warning* signs of aggression. In that case, a horse overwhelmed by fear can become aggressive without warning, the equivalent of fear-biting in dogs.[68][69]

When a horse does something dangerous, a swift and stern reaction may be called for, but your reaction must be fair, predictable, and make sense to the horse. See chapter 9 (Power and Pitfalls of Pressure—p. 102) for non-punitive body language that lets horses know they have stepped out of line.

## Fatigue and Boredom

Horses cannot focus or perform their best when they are tired, any more than we can. They also have the same sorts of reactions to boredom that we do: tune out, go on strike, or create their own diversions.

Much training is based on repetition in the mistaken belief that repetition is the only way horses learn. Not so. They also learn by observing, experimenting, exploring the world, and generalizing what they already know to future situations. They actually learn faster and work more reliably when you encourage them to use these innate ways of learning, as described in future chapters.

Although repetition is needed to develop smooth responses to cues, and the muscle memory to carry out actions correctly, this does not require boring drills. Practice can be incorporated into a variety of activities that hold a horse's

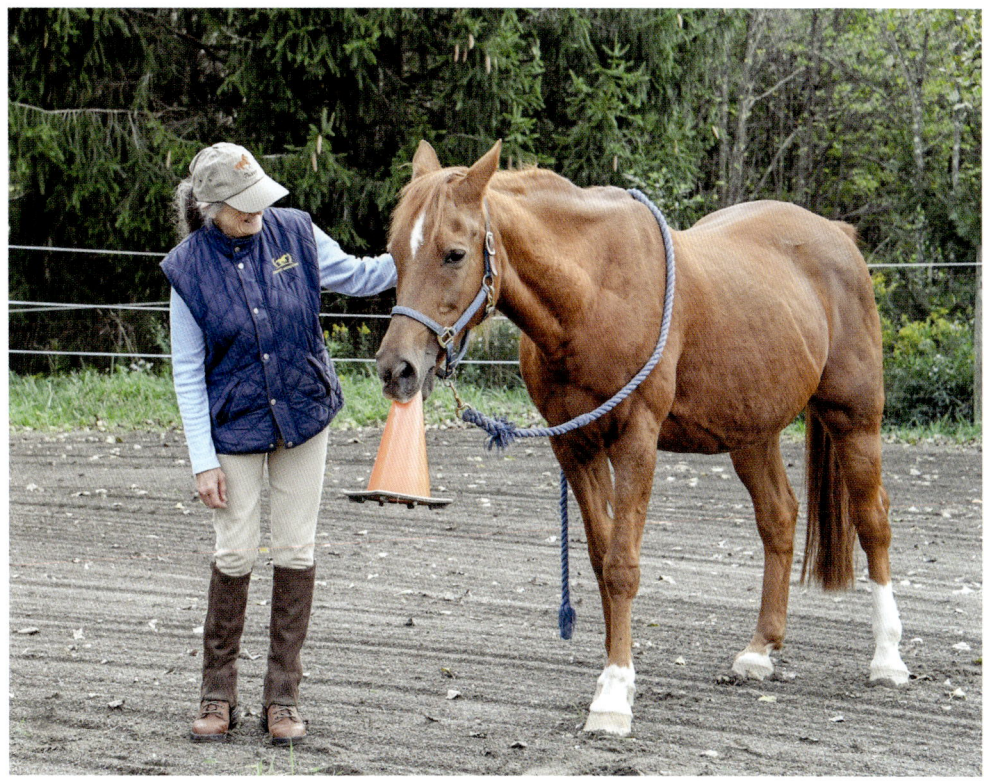

7.5 Bored with weaving through cones, Bronzz picks one up instead.

interest and keep him thinking.

Too much repetition can hide problems, especially when the symptom involves a lot of energy. If a horse is rushing, pulling, tossing his head, prancing, or bucking, for example, these symptoms may be reduced or even go away when the horse is fatigued by enough repetitions. This does not mean he has learned anything or that the problem is solved. He is just tired.

Horses have varying degrees of tolerance for boredom and individual ways of telling you they are bored. Brandy tunes me out, getting slow and sloppy, or just walks away if she is at liberty. Bronzz is more likely to initiate a lateral move I have not asked for or pick up the nearest object he can get his mouth on. People are rarely amused when bored horses get creative, and I think that's a shame. It gives us glimpses into their personality, and can be quite entertaining (fig 7.5).

## Living Conditions and Diet

In the "olden" days, when horses worked long hours, it was customary for them to be tied in straight stalls to eat and rest. A "loose box" was a luxury by comparison. Today, when horses generally spend few hours working, confinement to a stall is a recipe for health and behavior problems no matter how luxurious the accommodations might look to people.

When horses worked long hours, a measure of oats at the end of the day provided valuable calories and nutrition. "Nutrition" programs designed by modern feed companies are designed to sell more feed. Any concentrates beyond what's needed to maintain body condition just fuel a confined horse's frustration.

As described in chapter 4 (p. 43), the further a horse's living conditions deviate from moving, socializing, and eating forage, the more likely behavior problems are. Training does not change that. Calming supplements make sense if they address a nutritional deficiency that causes anxiety. But if anxiety is provoked by external situations, then supplements at best treat symptoms, not the root causes.

*The further a horse's living conditions deviate from moving, socializing, and eating forage, the more likely behavior problems are.*

## Pressure the Horse Cannot Relieve

Pressure is a basic part of our communication with horses. From the ground we exert pressure when we move a horse by touch or with a remote gesture using hand, body, rope, or whip. When riding, we use pressure through our legs, seat, weight, reins, whips, and spurs. All equipment places some type of pressure on the horse; that is how it works. Alternatives such as bitless bridles or rope halters just shift the pressure to different locations, which may or may not make any individual horse more comfortable or responsive.

Theoretically, pressure is gentle, the horse recognizes it as a cue and responds accordingly, we release the pressure, and all is well. Much can go wrong between theory and practice. If our meaning is not clear to the horse, or he is uncomfortable doing what we've asked, he cannot relieve the pressure. Then the pressure becomes a source of anxiety, and we are the cause.

Problems associated with pressure are compounded by the fact that most of us were taught to *increase* pressure when a horse fails to comply. Use more leg or pull the reins harder. As pressure increases, a horse can feel trapped and increasingly anxious until he is desperate to escape. Depending on his personality and background, he might try to physically escape the situation, threaten the person putting the pressure on him, or disengage emotionally and ignore the person.

The amount of pressure required to cause anxiety varies with individual horses, but in general is far less than you might think. This was demonstrated in a study where two groups of ponies were taught to back up on a verbal command. One group was trained with reward (food), and the other with pressure (a whip waved in front of them, *not* touching them). Monitors showed that the whip trained ponies were stressed not only during their training sessions but in anticipation of them. They also learned more slowly, performed less reliably and, when turned loose, avoided their trainer and other people as well.[70]

## Stressful Situations

Stress can be ongoing if a horse's living situation does not meet his needs (see chapter 4—p. 43), or he has pain or other medical problems. Vision loss, for example, can lead to bolting, spooking, bucking, balking, or refusing jumps.[71] Stress can also be ongoing if a horse has the wrong human partner or the wrong job (more on this in chapter 18—224). Anxious horses who do well with one person might be stressed when handled or ridden by multiple people. Ongoing stress can leave a horse in a perpetual state of anxiety.

Occasional stress is inevitable, whether it is a veterinary visit, trailer ride, changes in owner, separation from equine companions, or busy events such as shows or group rides. Future chapters describe ways to help horses cope with stress better so they are less fearful of stressful situations and of the world in general.

## Anxiety

As the previous topics in this chapter show, many things can trigger anxiety. Behaviors that tip you off to anxiety can be summed up in four words: **Fight, Flight, Fidget,** or **Freeze.**

- **Fight** includes any aggression, from mild threats to overt attacks. From the horse's point of view, it is self-defense.

- **Flight** shows up in escape attempts such as spooking, bolting, backing, turning away, or refusing jumps.

- **Fidget** is excess motion such as dancing around, tail swishing, head tossing, pawing, or startle-like reactions to cues.

- **Freeze** means a horse goes rigid and refuses to move (fig 7.6). It may be mistaken for stubbornness or resistance, especially since applying pressure increases the anxiety.

Additional signs of anxiety include loose stools, which suggest immediate fear; and stereotypies and ulcers, both of which indicate historical and perhaps ongoing anxiety.

- **"Hidden Anxiety"** can explain some dramatic behavior that seems to come out of nowhere. Horses might be obedient in spite of anxiety if they are cooperative or eager to please, afraid of the

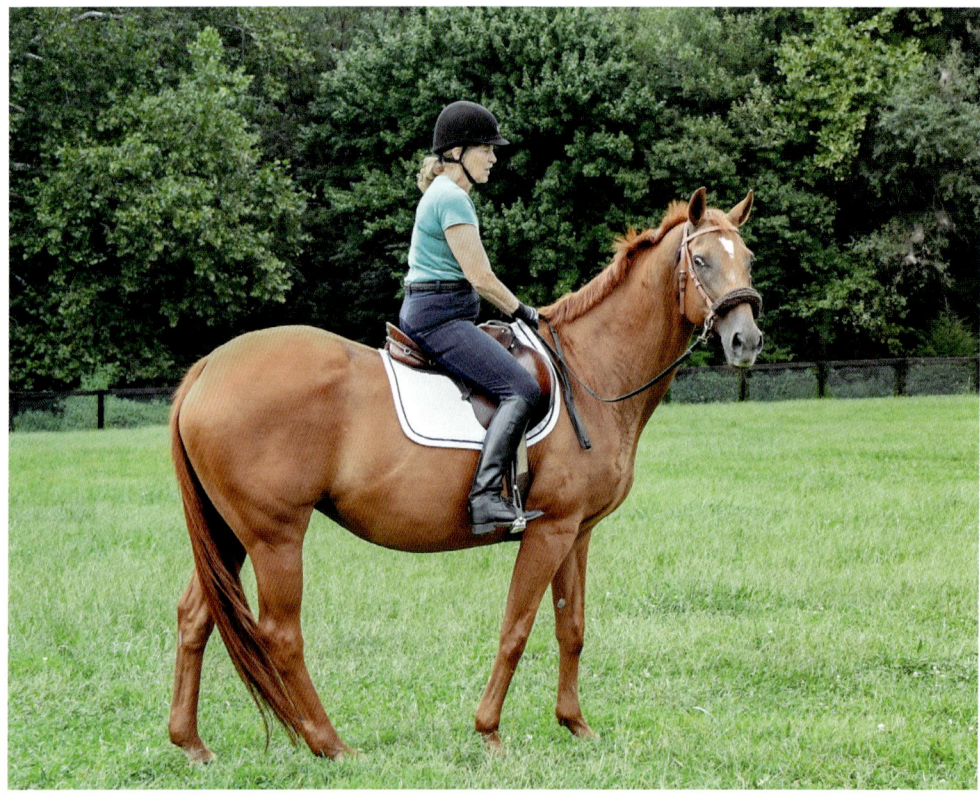

**7.6** Gracie freezes in alarm at a strange sight in her pasture. Since Dani did *not* apply pressure, Gracie quickly scoped out tripod, camera, and partially hidden human behind it. Then she calmly walked on.

consequences of non-compliance, or so food motivated that they will do almost anything to score a treat. If the buildup of anxiety goes unnoticed until a horse is overwhelmed and can no longer control himself, the result can be an explosion that leaves everyone wondering, "Where on earth did that come from?"

Our Shiloh fits the category of highly treat-motivated. The first time I started to blanket her, I cued her to stand still, which she did, anticipating a treat. As I lifted the blanket, however, I saw that while her feet were still, her body was practically vibrating with tension.

Had I looked only at Shiloh's obediently still feet and proceeded to throw the blanket over her back, she would probably have panicked. The result would have been ugly and entirely my fault. Fortunately, I spotted her distress in time to back off and introduce the blanket slowly.

Hidden Anxiety explains some situations where a rider is anxious and cannot explain why. She senses her horse's tension but because he is not *doing* anything wrong, she discounts her own uneasiness. If you find yourself in this kind of situation, please take your own anxiety seriously before you get hurt.

## ⚞ Summary

Horses want to be physically comfortable and emotionally secure. Some discomfort and stress are inevitable in life, but when it is severe or consistent, it interferes with a horse's welfare, behavior, and performance, and jeopardizes your safety. Understanding the underlying causes of these problems points you to solutions.

- **Physical Issues—Pain, Living Conditions, Diet**

Solutions involve addressing causes of pain, and providing living conditions and diet that support good mental and physical health.

- **Training Issues—Insecure Balance, Boredom, Fatigue, Punishment**

Solutions require training that helps a horse learn good balance, riding that does not interfere with it, and planning rides to avoid undue fatigue or boredom. Punishment is not training and should be used only in exceptional situations.

- **Communication and Confidence Issues—Confusion and Misunderstanding, Inconsistent Expectations, Pressure Horse Cannot Relieve, Stressful Situations, Anxiety**

These issues are best addressed with improved communication, life experiences that build horses' confidence in themselves, and leadership they trust. Parts Four through Seven describe how you can use Protector Leadership skills to accomplish this.

---

### THINGS TO TRY

▶ Check out a book, article, or website that describes equine body language and how to interpret different behaviors. The most scientific is *A Practical Field Guide to Horse Behavior* (Eclipse Press, 2003) by Sue McDonnell, Ph.D. with over 300 pages cataloging specific behaviors and the reasons for them, illustrated with sketches and photographs. Sharon Wilsie's *Horse Speak* looks at body language in the context of two-way communication between our horses and ourselves.

▶ Look for an explanation for a behavior that has puzzled you, or a new interpretation for a behavior that might mean something different than you thought it did.

## chapter 8
## Brandy and Friends: "Bad" Behavior Reinterpreted

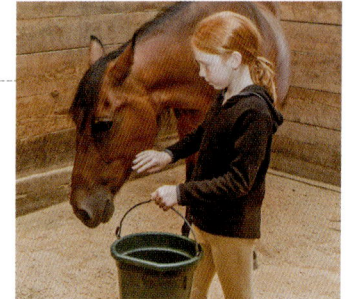

> "How can we possibly think we have a good relationship with a horse if we cannot 'listen' to him or notice when he is depressed or anxious? When a person is unwell, he can try to explain it in words; a horse tries to tell you with all sorts of body language because he cannot speak. It is up to us to learn how to 'read' him."
>
> —Frédéric Pignon *(Building a Life Together)*

Brandy's story continues later in this chapter, but first I will relate my early years with Bronzz and Shiloh. Their stories illustrate with embarrassing clarity how I misinterpreted their "problem behaviors," and made matters worse by trying to "train" them away. Once I finally understood the reason behind each behavior, solutions became obvious.

### Bronzz: Spooking and Bucking

Bronzz sailed through his early training with a cheerful, can-do attitude, and it is now clear to me why that was: trust and communication.

I bought him as a three-year-old from the breeder who had raised and cared for him his whole life. Fritz was, I now realize, a Protector Leader. Bronzz trusted him absolutely and readily extended that trust to me. It was the foundation of our long and happy partnership. On my own, I might have destroyed that trust, but Fritz graciously mentored me through the early stages of Bronzz's training. His gentle feedback stopped me many times from "correcting" Bronzz for honest mistakes or, worse, mistakes that were my own fault.

The training Bronzz already had included clear body language communication. As a foal at his mama's side, he had been taught to lead by watching his Protector Leader's body language. This not only started his training with less pressure, it instilled in him the valuable habit of tuning in to his leader at all times. Thus all of his training and handling required less pressure.

The two behavior problems I had with Bronzz surfaced after I moved him as a four-year-old to a boarding stable closer to home and no longer had Fritz's astute guidance.

The first problem was spooking. The boarding stable was on a busy road. Bronzz, accustomed to living on a quiet dead-end road, found everything new and spook-worthy, so we routinely had the flamboyant flying leaps for which Arabians are infamous. I trained him to turn and face scary things. Though this curtailed his tendency to bolt, it added a mid-air turn to his spooks. It was this "spooking problem" that led me to discover the power of Investigative Behavior to reduce anxiety and spooking, as described in Part Five (see p. 139).

Bronzz's other big problem showed up when I asked him to canter. He bucked. Nothing I could think of persuaded him to canter instead of bucking. I sent him to a trainer. The bucking got worse.

Then I did what I should have done first. I asked my vet. As he ran his fingers down Bronzz's back, Bronzz all but sat down in pain. "There's your buck," said the vet succinctly. He prescribed three weeks rest, a chiropractic adjustment, and a new saddle. The trainer's saddle apparently had hurt Bronzz even more than mine did.

Though I followed my vet's instructions, the bucking soon resumed. The new saddle had made him sore all over again. Even when he was not bucking, his discomfort showed in his high head/low back posture.

Finally, I got it. His bucking was not a training issue. Neither was his tendency to hollow his back and go above the bit. These were pain issues. I focused on relieving the pain (chiropractic, massage, and exercises), and finding a saddle that fit him.

Generous friends and acquaintances loaned me saddles to try, and I spent a fortune shipping trial saddles back and forth. We tried English, Western, flex tree, treeless, saddles specially designed for short-backed horses, hard-to-fit horses, and Arabians (an odd concept since Arabian backs come in many different shapes). Three professional saddle fitters struck out, the large, high-end dressage saddles they sold being poorly designed for small, short-backed horses.

We tried so many saddles I learned

to tell by Bronzz's reaction whether they hurt his back (bucking) or his shoulders (short stride, prancing, and jigging).

Bronzz ultimately settled on a modestly priced synthetic Western trail saddle, and a pad with custom-shaped inserts of memory foam and carpet felt. For a few years he also tolerated an older all-purpose English saddle, but then pain-related behavior resurfaced. Now we use only his Western saddle, which the sports medicine vet said distributes the weight more comfortably for him.

### Bronzz's Behavior Reinterpreted

Bronzz's problem behaviors, caused by *anxiety* (spooking) and *saddle-fit pain* (bucking), are commonplace. Sadly, when they are not resolved, a rider's anxiety may limit what she feels safe doing with that horse. Having addressed the root causes, I have been able to enjoy a great variety of adventures with Bronzz.

### Shiloh: Lazy with Bad Attitude

Shiloh came to us as a two-year-old. Her dog-eared vaccination record, which had miraculously followed her around, showed that she had already been sold four times.

Her previous owner had purchased Shiloh with the belief that she was "fully trained and ready for a novice to ride." The woman reported that while she had managed to wrestle (her word) a saddle and bridle on Shiloh a few times, and climb on her back, she could not get her to go anywhere.

Shiloh, in fact, seemed to have had no training at all. With five owners in quick succession, she had no reason to trust anyone, either. Left to her own devices, she apparently figured out life like this:

1. People give me treats if I nuzzle their faces or frisk pockets. I nip only if they forget what that means.

2. Wherever I want to go, people get out of my way.

3. No one can pick up my foot if I lean on it.

4. Most people can't halter me if I stick my nose in the air and wave it around.

5. If someone does get a halter on me, I decide where we're going.

6. When people bother me, I swing my butt at them. If they still don't behave, I wedge them against a wall.

I was not worried about the skills Shiloh lacked. What bothered me were her pinned ears and the "stubborn resistance" that I interpreted as a disrespectful challenge to my authority. I had recently attended a variety of training demonstrations, and been caught up in the popular misconception that horses want to be dominant. I was determined to show Shiloh that *I* was the one in charge.

Round pen work, I thought, would teach her to be more respectful. I failed to see the flaw in this logic at the time. Respect is a feeling. It cannot be taught. Like trust, it has to be earned, and I did not earn it. I made matters worse. When I saw the pinned ears that I interpreted as "bad attitude," I increased the pressure by sending her around the round pen for extra laps.

I realize now that Shiloh's "attitude" signaled anxiety and confusion. Too many requests were pressure that she did not know how to relieve. In the past, her threatening behavior had probably been successful in persuading people to stop doing whatever made her uncomfortable, and thus had inadvertently been rewarded. Instead of protecting Shiloh from anxiety and confusion, I was a *source* of it. As I got stricter, Shiloh got more anxious ("grumpier")—a vicious cycle that for some people and horses spirals out of control.

I began to rethink Shiloh's "bad attitude" when I started riding her. She did not *feel* stubborn; she felt like a horse in pain. I asked my veterinarian. She was not in pain, he said. She was a lazy Quarter Horse who had my number. Fortunately, I was finally beginning to trust what Shiloh was telling me.

Three vets, many months, and much testing later, we had a diagnosis: Lyme disease. By then, Shiloh's hind end was so stiff her hind toes dragged when she walked. The first round of doxycycline brought marked improvement.

When I started riding her again, I attributed the wobble I felt in her hind end to joint damage from Lyme, which has left her permanently stiff. Our farrier spotted the issue this time. Shiloh stood base narrow on little feet that nature never meant to support such massive hindquarters. The outsides of her hooves were collapsing under the weight.

Shiloh is a sad example of problems created by poor breeding. Unlike humans, nature breeds solely for function. A horse with Shiloh's hoof problems would not survive in the wild. If you doubt the impact of selective breeding on hooves, just consider how much hoof type varies by breed. Our farrier's assessment is blunt: "Mankind has destroyed horses' hooves."

Custom-made shoes with lateral extensions (wings on the outside) for support now widen Shiloh's stance, reduce the wobble, and keep her hooves intact.

Someone riding Shiloh now without knowing her history might describe her refusal to trot a small circle or step over a log as stubborn or disrespectful. We have learned to trust that Shiloh knows her own limitations, and that "resistance" means she is uncomfortable doing what's being asked of her.

> *I realize now that Shiloh's "attitude" signaled anxiety and confusion.*

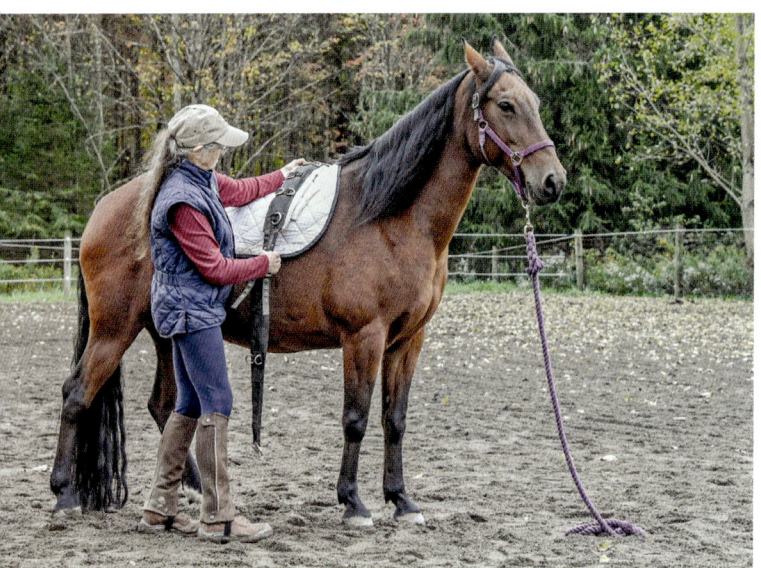

**8.1 A** Brandy's posture and expression show concern as I place a lungeing surcingle on her back.

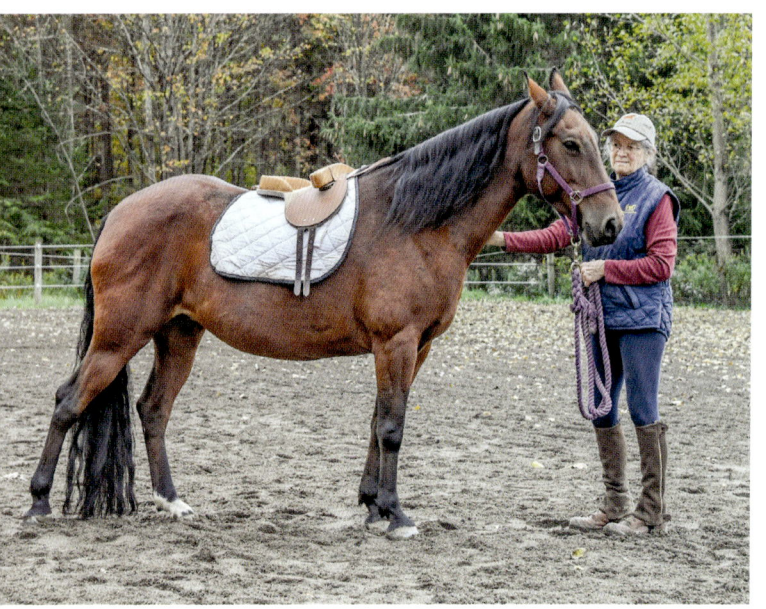

**8.1 B** She is actually a bit more relaxed with the felt toddler saddle. Before girthing anything, I picked up her lead so that if she became too anxious, she could not run off with equipment attached to her.

### Shiloh's Behavior Reinterpreted

In contrast to Bronzz, Shiloh's unwanted behaviors had a long and interconnected list of underlying causes. Lyme disease caused *pain and stiffness.* Poor conformation contributed to *insecure balance.* Lack of training led to *confusion* so she did not know how to relieve the *pressure* of ordinary cues. Multiple owners guaranteed *inconsistent expectations.* All of this created many *stressful situations,* and ongoing *anxiety.*

### Brandy: Dangerously Unpredictable

In chapter 2 (Earning Trust—p. 16), I described how Brandy progressed from being touched with a folded towel in her stall, to wearing a saddle pad while loose in our arena. In another two weeks of short sessions, we progressed through bareback pad, lungeing surcingle, a soft felt toddler saddle, and finally my synthetic dressage saddle (figs. 8.1 A & B). I gave her time to relax with each new piece of equipment before moving to the next.

Between saddle lessons I bridled her, trying different bits to see what she was most relaxed with (an ordinary D-ring snaffle). We practiced yielding to gentle touches on the reins. I was actually getting optimistic about riding her.

Then we had two dramatic bucking incidents in which she exploded without warning. One was in the barn aisle and the other occurred as I led her across the arena. Both times she was saddled. The second time, she dashed wildly back and forth past me, bucking so hard that manure landed on top of her saddle. Each time, she stopped as suddenly as she'd started. After the first incident she calmed quickly. After the second she came to stand beside me trembling and sweating, flinching violently when I reached for the girth.

Never again did Brandy relax with anything strapped around her. She stood for me to put a saddle on, but remained tense and alert.

This is the "Hidden Anxiety" that can really get you in trouble. Had I looked only at her cooperative behavior, I would have tried to ride her. That could not have ended well, yet whatever happened would not have been Brandy's fault. She was simply doing her best to comply with what I asked.

I tried hand-grazing Brandy with the saddle on, hoping she would relax, and maybe even develop a positive association with saddles. No luck. The tension never abated. I tried a new strategy. She had learned to dribble a ball with her nose, and seemed to consider that a fun game. I put her saddle on, took her to the round pen, and turned her loose to play ball. The moment she put her nose down toward the ball, she jumped and took off racing, bucking, kicking, and twirling. I scrambled out of the round pen, barely getting the gate shut as she tried to follow me.

The whole wild episode lasted just a minute or two, then she stopped. I went in, clipped her lead on, and she politely walked all around with me, but she would not lower or turn her head. I took the lead off and free-lunged her. She did all I asked except to canter. She would canter one stride with her hind feet, acknowledging that she understood, then resumed trotting. After I took the saddle off, she cantered on cue better than she ever had before, as if trying extra hard to please me.

Anyone seeing one of Brandy's bucking episodes out of context might conclude that she was dangerously aggressive. Yet my husband, who witnessed each incident, made the same observations I did. Each time, we saw terror in Brandy's eyes. The wet manure on her saddle confirmed intense fear. And at no time did Brandy injure me. Even in her panic, she remained aware enough of my presence to avoid kicking or crashing into me.

Wondering if a different type of saddle would change anything, I pulled out a small leather jumping saddle. By the time I set it on her, she was shaking so hard that if I had let it go, it would have vibrated right onto the floor. I was humbled by the fact that she still trusted me enough to let me put a saddle on her, and mightily impressed with her self-control.

I now had an ethical dilemma. I did not want to subject Brandy to any more saddles, and I feared that anyone trying to ride her would be seriously injured.

Yet the rescue organization still owned her, and the director continued to assure me that she herself had ridden Brandy with no problem. I told her she needed to come here with the saddle she used on Brandy, and show me.

I was holding Brandy in the barn aisle, and Donna had the cinch just tight enough to keep the saddle on when Brandy turned her head to the left, and went up on her hind legs so suddenly she yanked the lead out of my hand. Brandy pivoted away from me and shot down the aisle. She ricocheted off the gate at the back of the barn and into an empty stall where we slammed and latched the door. When she stopped spinning, we removed the saddle by leaning over the partition.

As soon as the saddle was off, Brandy stood still. Tentatively I sidled into the stall with her. She came to stand beside me, head down, body shaking.

We all agreed that nothing short of intense pain would provoke such a violent reaction. We scheduled an evaluation with a veterinarian who specializes in sports medicine, and who coordinated her appointment with an equine chiropractor.

Meanwhile, I described Brandy's behavior to four well-respected local trainers. Two saw it strictly as a training issue. Bucking was dangerous and disrespectful and must not be tolerated under any circumstances. It did not matter if the horse was in pain. The third trainer suspected severe emotional trauma.

Fritz, Bronzz's breeder, was the only trainer who homed in on pain. He pointed out that since Brandy was trusting and obedient in everything else I asked of her, she must have a very compelling reason to behave as she did with a saddle on.

The sports medicine vet and chiropractor found pain in Brandy's back, and evidence of soft tissue injury that could explain severe pain with something girthed around her. They observed that Brandy moved comfortably without a saddle and that exercise reduced her pain, so they cleared her for any activity that did not involve saddle, surcingle, or anything else girthed around her.

Pain can come and go, explaining why our regular vet had not gotten a reaction, and why Brandy sometimes winced when I curried her back, and sometimes did not. Another practitioner observed that Brandy's behavior was consistent with a pinched nerve that causes severe pain. Distressing as that is for people, it would be terrifying for a horse who has no way of understanding what is happening. Finally, soft tissue injuries can worsen over time, explaining the change in Brandy's tolerance for being ridden.

There is no lack of explanation for how Brandy could have sustained such an injury: a too heavy rider, a too large saddle, too much weight behind her last rib, a fall, a fight with another horse (one of her scars is hoof shaped), carrying a foal as a yearling. It's anyone's guess.

## Brandy's Behavior Reinterpreted

Brandy's unwanted behavior was solely a result of *pain* and *fear of pain*. We have not had a single incident of "aggressive" behavior in the six years since she last had a saddle on her back.

Her history shows how easily signs of pain can be mistaken for aggression. It also shows that pain cannot always be diagnosed definitively, even by qualified practitioners. That does not mean there is no pain. It means that we have to be all the more alert to the behavioral signs that tell us it is there. Finally, Brandy shows that even a horse who appears dangerous may be very different when the cause of the problem is removed.

We proceeded slowly and cautiously, with extra supervision, but Brandy proved herself to be gentle, patient, and careful around children. My little grandchildren's favorite chores when they visited came to include feeding and grooming Brandy, cleaning her hooves, and leading her to and from pasture (figs. 8.2 A & B).

Now I had a dilemma. I had never intended to keep Brandy, and I most certainly did not want to fill my last stall with a horse I couldn't ride. But adoption prospects are nearly non-existent for horses who cannot be ridden, and Brandy presented an additional complication. She was young enough to live another 25 years. Odds were that someday, someone would decide that

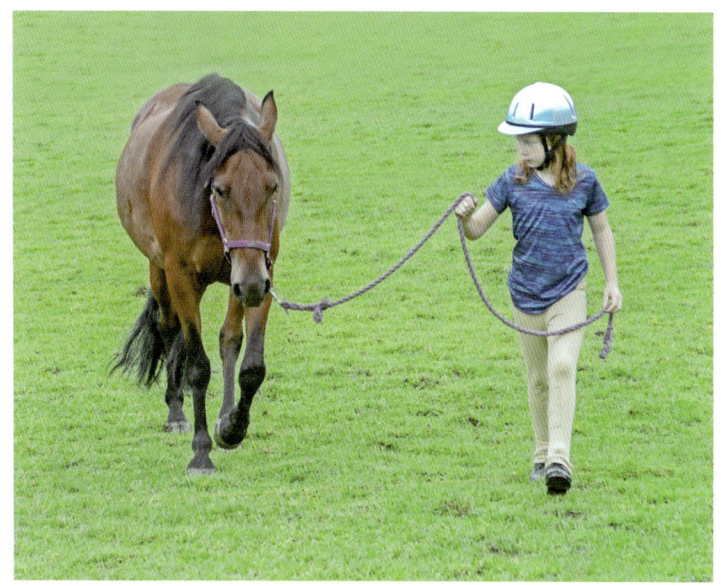

**8.2 A** Eight-year-old Camille can lead Brandy to the barn at dinnertime because Brandy knows it is her responsibility to watch out for her handler.

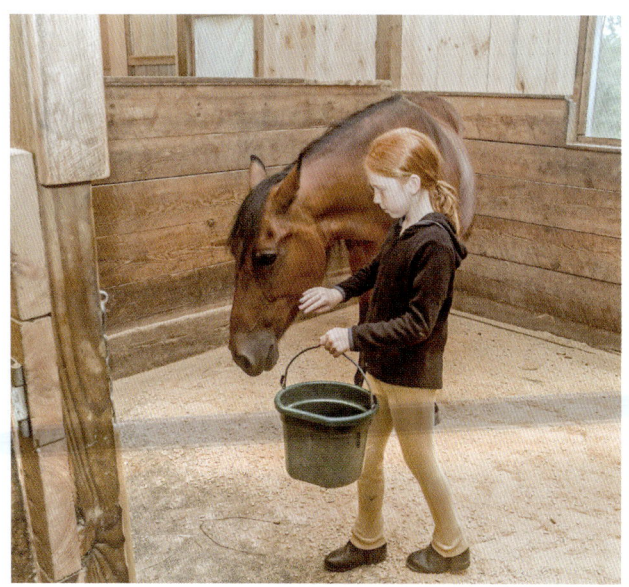

**8.2 B** Brandy politely steps away on cue as Camille serves her dinner.

such a nice pony could surely be ridden. The consequences could be disastrous. Added to that, Brandy *trusted* me. Sending her off to an uncertain fate felt like a betrayal. I couldn't decide what to do.

## In Retrospect

I would have done better with Shiloh when I was a teenager. I was strict with dangerous behaviors, but otherwise friendly. I assumed that horses misbehaved because they didn't know better, or because they were defensive from previous rough treatment. I assumed they needed reassurance that I would be fair, and that once they knew the rules, they would do their best to cooperate. Such attitudes are self-fulfilling prophesies.

More than one woman has told me that she has never, as an adult, had the special relationship with a horse that she did as a teenager. I wonder if that's because as kids we were better Protector Leaders, less worried about being in charge, and more inclined to treat horses as friends.

I will be forever grateful to Fritz for helping me establish a friendlier relationship with Bronzz, and to Thistle's young trainer for showing me the way to do even better with Brandy.

## Summary

Each of my horses has shown unwanted behaviors that are often addressed with training or "discipline." In each case, training failed to resolve the problem because it did not address the root cause. Having addressed the underlying causes of the problems, we have horses who are both happier and reliably well-behaved.

### THINGS TO TRY

- Consider a behavior your horse does that is a problem for you. List as many possible causes as you can. Take into account whatever you know of his personality, history, and current living circumstances.

- When you see someone else's horse "misbehave," put yourself in the horse's place (not the person's) and imagine what he might be trying to say.

# PART FOUR: Communicate Like a Horse

> "Since horses communicate primarily through body language and feel, they interpret our actions in their own terms. That's why we need to learn their language—not only to understand what horses are saying to us, but also to know what our position, posture, and movements are saying to them."
>
> —Cherry Hill *(How to Think Like a Horse)*

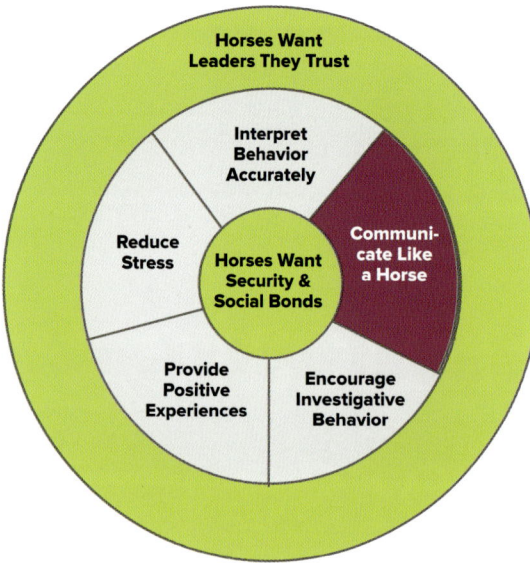

Horses want clear communication. It is part of a secure relationship. The previous three chapters were devoted to listening to horses and interpreting their behavior accurately. The next three chapters are about the other side of our two-way conversation: how we can communicate with horses using body language that makes intuitive sense to them and invites trust and cooperation. Only then can we discover how willing they are to work with us as partners.

Horses naturally tune in to those around them. The complex social system of a wild herd depended on fine-tuned communication to maintain group harmony and coordinate movement. Their ability to read the body language and intent of other species was a survival skill for them as prey animals.

Horses notice subtle nuances of our posture, gestures, and facial expressions. This makes our body language a powerful means of communication, *if* we are saying what we intend to say. The catch is that what we think we are saying is often at odds with horses' intuitive interpretation of our body language. The result is confusion and anxiety.

People most often use body language that applies pressure. That is a basic part of our communication with horses; it can provide clear, precise instructions, or provoke a fight or flight response. Chapter 9 (p. 102) describes what makes the difference so you can maximize the benefits and minimize the risks.

Chapter 10 (p. 113) demonstrates how to use body language that makes intuitive sense to horses, so you can communicate with less pressure and more clarity. Chapter 11 (p. 128) shows that rewards are not only useful training aids, but powerful motivators and relationship builders.

Skills from these chapters are applied in later chapters to help horses become more confident, responsive, and reliable.

**Part Four Key Points:**

- Pressure is both our main communication with horses, and a common source of stress that provokes unwanted behavior.

- People typically use body language based on pressure that tells horses to move away from us, not stay with us.

- Friendly Body Language provides clear communication that invites horses to stay with us. Based on horses' natural inclination to follow a trusted leader, it has been successful for centuries.

**You will learn how to:**

- Turn pressure into clear communication instead of stress.

- Use Friendly Body Language to encourage your horse to stay with you, watching for your guidance and direction, especially when he is nervous.

- Use rewards to communicate, motivate, encourage learning, and improve your relationship with your horse.

*chapter 9*
# The Power and Pitfalls of Pressure

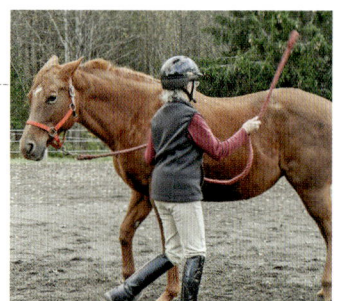

> "You can never rely on a horse that is educated by fear. There will always be something that he fears more than you. But, when he trusts you, he will ask you what to do when he is afraid."
>
> —Antoine de Pluvinel *(1552–1620)*

Pressure is a fundamental part of our interaction with horses. Used well, it can provide the easy communication of friends who practically read each other's minds, or dance partners whose bodies flow effortlessly together. Gone wrong, it can trigger fight or flight responses and thus all sorts of unwanted and even dangerous behavior.

*Section 1* of this chapter describes how horses use pressure with each other, and *Section 2* explains how they perceive the pressure that people typically use. The contrast shows where many problems arise. *Section 3* describes the dynamics of pressure gone wrong, and *Section 4* explains how you can turn pressure into communication that inspires cooperation.

## How Horses Use Pressure with Each Other

Horses use pressure to move other horses away from them. This can be a gesture so subtle we may not notice: a glance, a change in ear or head position, a flick of the nose. The horse on the receiving end might move so casually that it does not even appear to be in response to the gesture.

Bronzz and Shiloh demonstrate pressure as communication: no drama, no

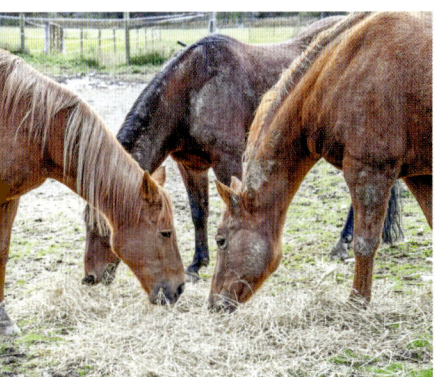 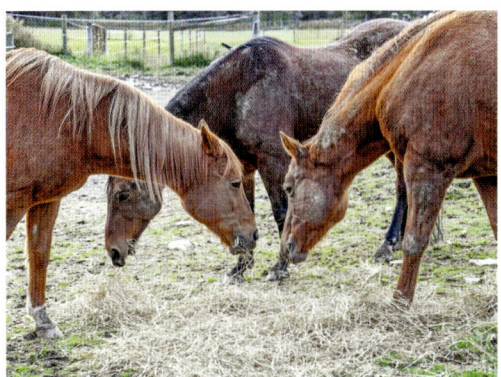 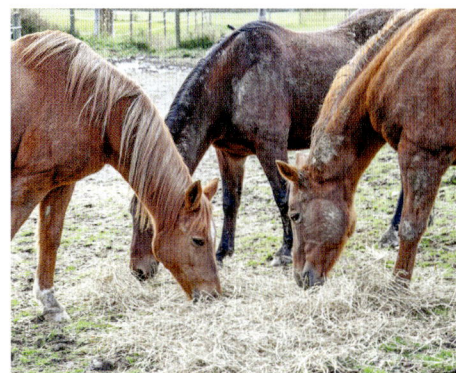

**9.1 A** Shiloh has eased a little too close to suit Bronzz.

**9.1 B** Bronzz flicks his nose toward her, asking her to move; she is already turning her head away.

**9.1 C** Both horses resume calmly eating, with Shiloh's face a few inches farther away from Bronzz's.

stress. Additional hay piles are off camera. We happened to catch a cozy family dining moment (figs. 9.1 A–C).

Pressure as communication meets these four criteria:

- **The pressure is gentle**. Bronzz used mild pressure. His feet did not move.

- **The meaning is clear**. Shiloh understood that meant move her face away from his. She also correctly gauged how far she needed to move.

- **The horse is comfortable doing what is asked**. Shiloh had plenty of room to move without leaving the hay. Her body language shows no distress.

- **The pressure is released promptly.** Bronzz immediately went back to eating.

When Brandy exerts stronger pressure, her whole body moving toward Bronzz (fig. 9.2), this elicits a bigger reaction.

A lunge with pinned ears and snaked neck is the equivalent of a person shouting, "Get *away* from me!" It can mean that multiple requests have been ignored or, as in this case, the "lunger" is seriously irritated. It can also mean that one or both horses never learned proper etiquette, or they are in a high stress situation.

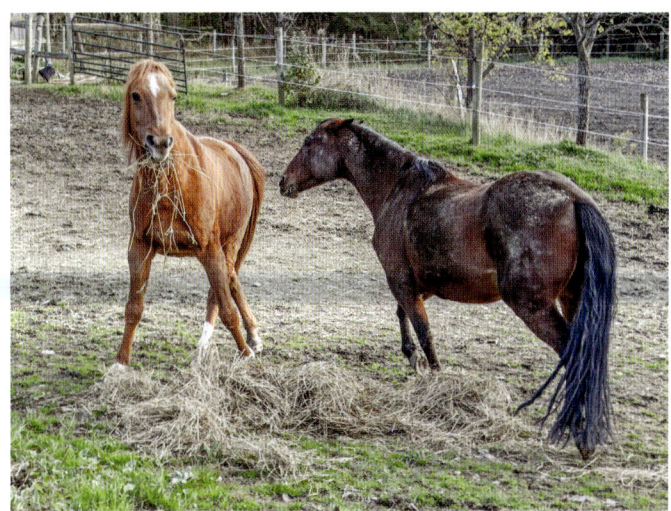

**9.2** Brandy has already moved multiple times at Bronzz's request. Apparently her patience has run out. This time, she says, he is the one who is moving!

PART FOUR: COMMUNICATE LIKE A HORSE — 103

## How People Inadvertently Turn Pressure into Stress

Whether we touch a horse or not, our pressure often fails to meet the four communication criteria listed above. The result is unnecessary stress and the unwanted behavior that it provokes.

### Pressure That Is Too Strong

If you judge your horse's response only by whether the feet go where you want them to, you miss important information. You must look at the whole body. In both photos (figs. 9.3 A & B) Shiloh has stepped under herself with her left hind leg, starting a turn-on-the-forehand. In the first photo, however, the tension in the rest of her body says I used too much pressure. Shiloh is reacting to me much like Bronzz reacted to Brandy in fig. 9.2. Only the lead rope, already going tight, stops her from leaving me.

I apologized to Shiloh, took her for a little walk, and used a different approach. Her response (fig. 9.3 B) was not only more relaxed, but more correct.

The same dynamics apply when we ride. Riders often use arm motions to stop or turn when a finger squeeze would do. They use taps or kicks for forward instead of a hug with their legs. You might claim that most horses do not respond to finger squeezes or leg hugs. And why is that? Because people have taught them to expect the stronger cue.

Horses are so sensitive they feel fly feet walking on their hair. A horse is never more sensitive than the first time he is ridden. He is tuned in to *everything* his rider does. Instead of taking advantage of this sensitivity and teaching horses the meaning of subtle cues, many trainers use bigger motions as if that will make their meaning clearer. In fact, it just teaches horses to tune out quieter cues.

Strong or abrupt movements are sometimes meant to encourage swift obedience. Instead, they startle the horse, cause tension and discomfort, and disrupt the horse's and rider's balance. The horse's focus naturally shifts from the job at hand to avoiding more unpleasantness. He might, for example, attempt to preempt kicks by charging forward every time he thinks his rider is even thinking about kicking him. Now he is harder to stop. Or he might try to disengage from the whole process by refusing to move at all.

When you ride, you need to notice how your horse's body *feels* as he responds to your cues. Relaxed and fluidly responsive? Or tense, hesitant, jerky?

On the ground, you need to watch your horse's whole body, just as he watches yours.

Horses notice our *posture and energy*. That is why we approach a hard-to-catch horse with a low-energy slouch. The more upright, speedy, and assertive our approach, the more likely our pressure will prompt the horse to move away.

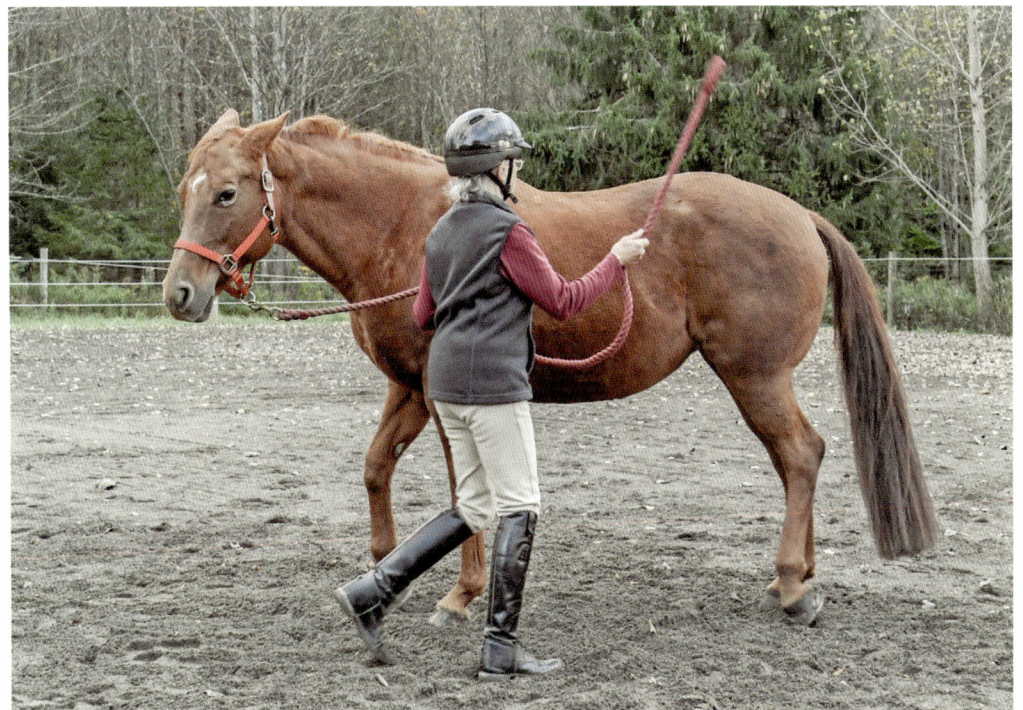

**9.3 A** My cue is too strong as I step toward Shiloh swinging the rope. Her head and ear positions show tension, and she is moving her front end away from me before she begins to step under with her left hind.

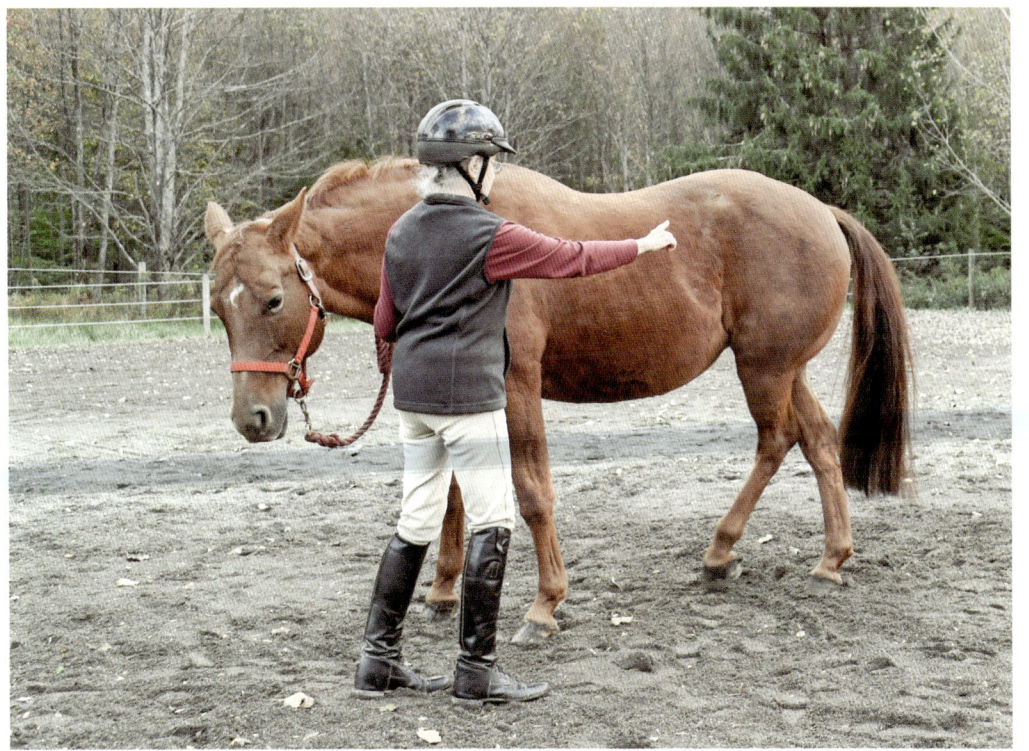

**9.3 B** My body is quiet as I point to Shiloh's hip, giving her a clear, gentle cue to move her haunches. Her body is relaxed, head down, left ear attuned to me. Her front feet are still as she steps her left **hind foot under** in the beginning of her turn-on-the-forehand.

They react to *where you look, which way your body points, and which way you move*. Directing any of these toward a horse's back end sends a message to move forward or away from you. Toward the front encourages him to slow down.

A horse's interpretation of *eye contact* depends on the context. He may seek it in a friendly situation, but hard eye contact is pressure, especially along with assertive posture.

*Facial expressions and tone of voice* are another part of the image you project. One study showed that horses were distressed just seeing *photographs* of angry faces,[72][73] and another showed that stern voices created distress.[74]

Horses can feel pressured when you enter their *personal space*, just as you do when another person gets uncomfortably close. Yet many people fail to take the extra few seconds to approach horses courteously.

Horses are acutely attuned to all of this body language. Use it with subtlety and you have communication. Use it too strongly, and you make them uncomfortable.

While you normally want to use much less pressure than most of us were taught, understanding how horses perceive your body language gives you the vocabulary to notify a horse when he has overstepped a limit or, better yet, warn him before he does. You can use any combination of hard stare, upright body posture, stern voice, and/or stern facial expression. You can also stamp a foot, something horses understand because they use it themselves to express annoyance or impatience. These send a clearer message to a horse than yelling, hitting, pulling on his lead line, or other forms of punishment, none of which make intuitive sense to him.

## Pressure That Does Not Have a Clear Meaning

Because horses' instinct is to resist pressure, they can easily feel trapped. For instance, if a gate catches a horse partway through, his instinct is to push forward against the pressure, possibly with enough force to hurt himself.

A horse must be *taught* to yield to the pressure of something touching him. He must also be taught that different types of pressure mean that you want him to perform specific actions. The first time a horse is ridden, he has no way of knowing that pressure from the rider's legs means go forward. Repeating a cue more forcefully is not teaching. It is more like shouting at someone who does not speak the same language. It not only fails to clarify your point, it makes the other individual less able to focus, and perhaps actually afraid of you.

Each cue should have a specific meaning. "Go faster," for instance, is not specific. This problem is often seen in lungeing. A horse is sent forward with a twirling rope, a waving whip, or arm movement, but he is not told what gait is wanted. Being left to guess creates anxiety, especially if he anticipates a "correction" for a wrong guess. Meanwhile, the unnecessary motion raises his energy level. A horse who appears to be obediently zipping along at the handler's direction may actually be moving only because his flight reflex has been triggered.

When you're riding, unintended shifts of weight, leg pressure, or bumps on the reins can change the meaning of the cue you think you are giving. (More on this in chapter 19, Being a Considerate Rider—p. 236.)

### The Horse Is Not Comfortable Doing What Is Asked

When you ask a horse to do things that make him uncomfortable, physically or emotionally, you put him in a no-win situation. He must choose between obedience and self-preservation. This invites behavior you do not want.

### Pressure That Is Not Released Promptly

Releasing a cue tells a horse he is doing what you asked. Without the release, communication is lost, and a horse can feel trapped.

For instance, when riders use constant leg pressure, horses either tune it out or continue accelerating. When pressure is tuned out, riders need more and more leg to get the same response. As horses become dull to that, whips and spurs come next.

If horses continue accelerating from constant leg pressure, riders need more and more rein pressure for control, while horses get increasingly frustrated with conflicting faster/slower cues. Stronger bits make horses feel more miserably trapped, and a vicious cycle is in motion. In *Know Better to Do Better*, Denny Emerson points out that riding a horse "…between the driving aids and the restraining aids," as many of us were taught to do, can make a horse feel practically claustrophobic.[75]

## The Pitfalls of Pressure

Pressure is inherently problematic for several reasons.

### Pressure Is a Tricky Training Method

The standard horse training method is pressure and release, a form of *negative reinforcement*. We apply an unpleasant or irritating stimulus (pressure) to get a response, then "reward" the horse for a correct response by removing the stimulus (releasing the pressure). In theory it is simple and effective. In practice there are many ways it can go awry.

One problem is that as a training method, pressure/release requires more precise timing and greater consistency than most of us can apply. Otherwise we get stress and confusion.

Another problem is that pressure can be distracting, and releasing it is not a reward that inspires enthusiasm. If you asked me to solve a tough math problem, for instance, I might work diligently for a piece of good chocolate. But if my only reward was that you would stop squeezing my arm, I would not only be less motivated, I would get stressed trying to think while you were squeezing my arm.

Finally, pressure alone does not show a horse what we want him to do. He might experiment and figure it out *if* he understands there is an answer to be figured out, *and* he feels safe experimenting, which he might not if he has been punished in the past for wrong answers. As he develops a vocabulary of cues he already understands, he has more information on which to base guesses, and a better idea what actions are not appropriate. The less experience and confidence a horse has, the more guidance he needs.

*When we make ourselves a source of stress, we forfeit trust.*

### Pressure Has a Negative Impact on Relationships

A review of multiple studies showed that horses who are trained exclusively with negative reinforcement develop a negative association with people.[76] This is an important factor to consider when choosing a trainer.

This was apparent in the study in which two groups of ponies were taught to back up on the verbal cue "back" (see p. 86). One group was trained with reward, the other with pressure (a shaking whip). When the ponies were turned loose in a paddock with their trainer, the reward-trained ponies chose to hang out with her. The pressure-trained ponies avoided her. Five months later, the pressure-trained ponies still avoided their trainer *and other humans as well*.[77]

The implications for leadership are huge. Such studies document experimentally what Delgado and Pignon say in *Gallop to Freedom*. When we make ourselves a source of stress, we forfeit trust. It also validates that lack of trust is transferred to other people. This explains many difficulties that people have with new horses.

Happily, this works both ways. The reward-trained ponies not only learned faster and performed more reliably, they chose to hang out with their trainer and with other people. I saw this dynamic in Bronzz who readily extended his trust from his breeder to me. All I had to do was not blow it.

### High-Pressure "Training" Methods Can *Appear* Dramatically Successful

You can intimidate most horses into doing what you want if you apply enough pressure. This makes for impressive "training" demonstrations that actually result in more anxiety than learning.

## Horses Can Be Overwhelmed By Pressure

Horses vary greatly in how much pressure they can tolerate, but any horse can be overwhelmed if he anticipates pressure that is too constant or too strong *for him*.

Some horses fight back, and make no mistake about it, even the nicest of horses might fight. Bronzz is described by all who know him as gentle, well-behaved, and reliable. Yet I have no doubt that if Bronzz were placed under constant high-pressure demands, he would fight back hard enough to be declared dangerous. That is not because he is mean, but because he is bold enough to resist treatment he would consider unfair.

At the other end of the spectrum are horses who shut down emotionally into a state of *learned helplessness*. Dr. Sue McDonnell describes them like this, though it can happen in any discipline:[78]

"Standing quietly with head lowered, unresponsive to normal social and environmental stimuli, and moving only on release command or directive of the handler. Considered basic training in certain Western show and working disciplines."[79]

This behavior is often mistaken for obedience, but it is closer to that of a traumatized person who is dissociated from his emotions. It is dangerous because the horse no longer gives the normal warning signs of stress. If he is sufficiently stressed to provoke a reaction, that reaction can be violent and appear to come out of nowhere.

Learned helplessness also dampens a horse's sense of self-preservation so he may not resist doing dangerous things. I have seen horses slip and fall rather than risk punishment for disobedience.

## The Power of Pressure as Positive Communication

It is not your goal to avoid pressure altogether. Yielding to pressure is one of the most important lessons horses need to learn. It makes them safer and pleasanter to handle, thus encouraging people to treat them more kindly. It can save them from injury. I have known two horses who became entangled in fence wires overnight and were found uninjured in the morning because they yielded to pressure as they had been taught, and waited for trusted caretakers to rescue them.

Your goal is to turn pressure into communication that meets your horse's need for clarity and security.

## Pressure Should Be Gentle Enough to Be Comfortable for the Individual Horse

There is great individual variation in how horses respond to pressure. For instance, the amount of leg pressure that would tell Shiloh to leg-yield one step would send Bronzz halfway across the arena. Good riders automatically recalibrate their cues on different horses so they use just enough pressure to clarify their meaning while leaving the horse *relaxed*.

Many of us were taught to escalate pressure if we do not immediately get a response, but this can create a bigger reaction that requires a bigger response from us, and so on. It is more effective to allow horses time to think through what we're asking and realize that we will keep asking until they comply. *Patience is more powerful than more pressure.*

### Pressure Should Be a Clear Cue That the Horse Understands

The clearer your communication, the less pressure you need. Ideally, on the ground, your whole body projects the same message. When you're riding, the horse should *feel* the same message from your legs, weight, seat, and reins.

However, no one is perfect, and mixed signals are inevitable. This is not a big problem as long as the horse is not punished. When a horse does the "wrong" thing, I assume it is my mistake or an honest misunderstanding. Then, I rethink how to ask more clearly.

When we ride a new horse, we cannot assume that he understands cues the same way we use them. My friend and mentor Betsy had a brilliant way of dealing with this. With a delicate touch, she'd try different cues and see what the horse did. She called it "playing" with the horse. Whatever the horse's response, she accepted that as his interpretation of the cue she'd used. Instead of "correcting" the horse, she adjusted her cues.

Horses adored her. I once saw a horse side-pass across an arena with an expression that said almost as clearly as words, "Wow! I didn't know I knew how to do that!" More than one horse she test rode when we were horse hunting was ready to climb in her truck and go home with her.

### Horses Should Not Be Pressured to Do Things That Make Them Uncomfortable

Yes, they often need to step out of their comfort zone, just as we do. But horses do not push each other into scary situations. A braver or more experienced horse leads by example (see Part Five—p. 139).

A horse who hesitates because he is uncomfortable is not being disobedient. If you push, you can expect resistance that will only increase in the future. As Sharon Wilsie points out in *Horse Speak*, "Keeping pressure on a horse, even inadvertently, is the fastest way to create resistance." Avoiding pressure means you don't provoke resistance (figs 9.4 A & B).

### Pressure Is Released Promptly

The timing of this is counterintuitive. We naturally want to hold a cue until the action is done, like we keep the wheel turned on a car until we complete the turn. With a horse we need to think of it more as if we're sending a message. Leg

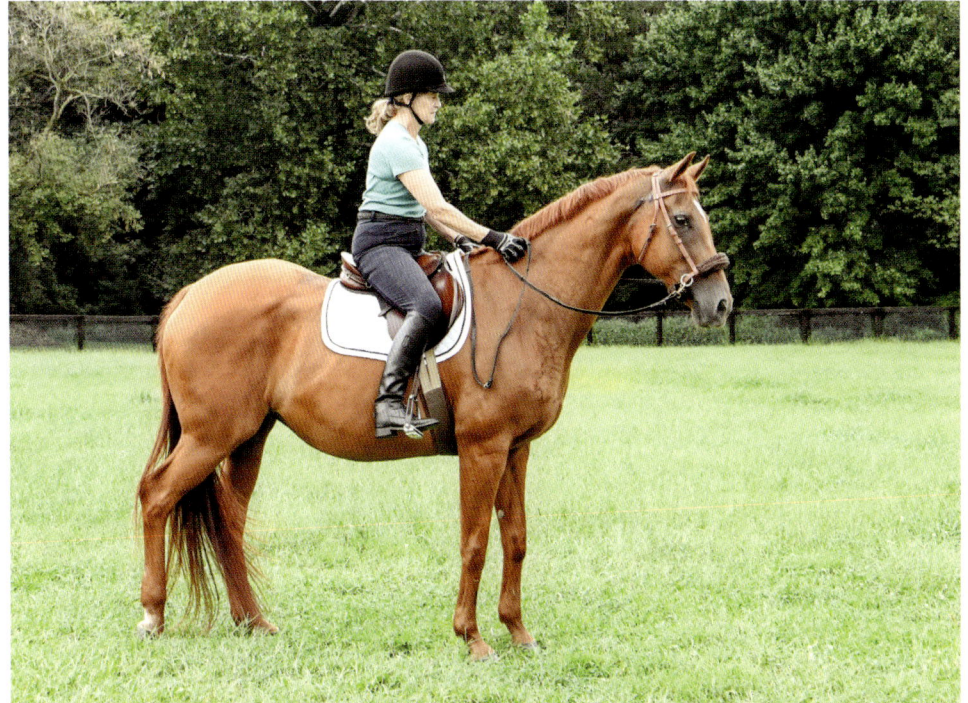

**9.4 A** Gracie stops, staring with concern at something strange in front of her. Dani places a reassuring hand on Gracie's neck and quietly waits for her to assess the situation.

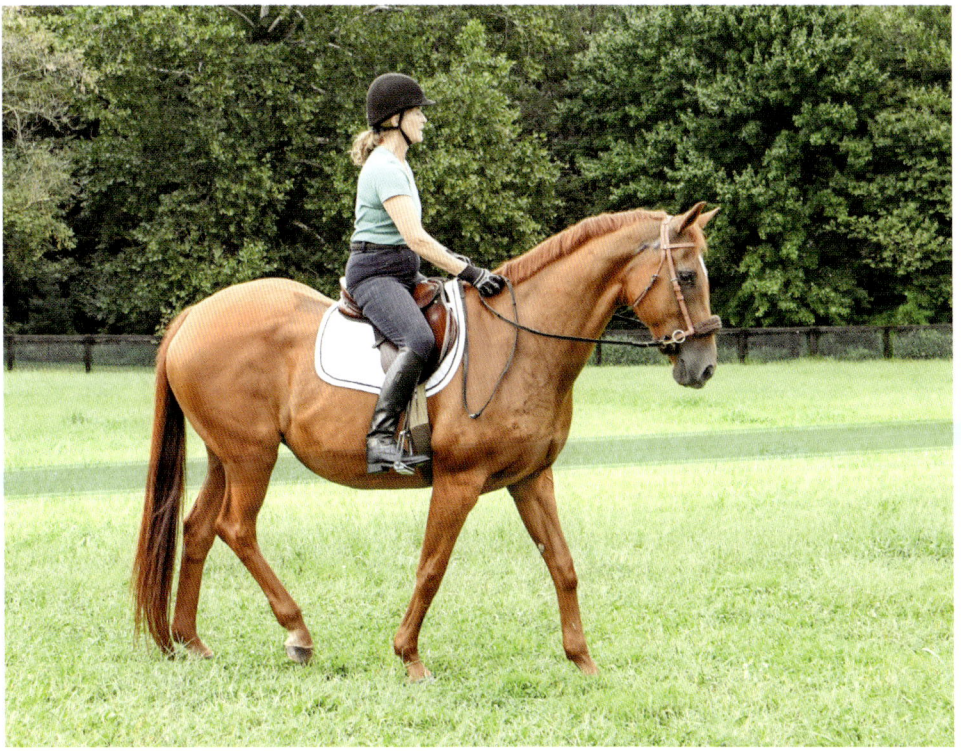

**9.4 B** In less than a minute, Gracie offers to move forward, now more curious than concerned. No pressure, no resistance.

PART FOUR: COMMUNICATE LIKE A HORSE — 111

squeeze to say, "Start walking." Horse *starts* to move, legs relax. We can always add another leg squeeze if he's not walking fast enough. Gentle rein pressure to say, "Slow down." Release pressure as soon as he *begins* slowing down. Repeat as needed.

Using gentler pressure and releasing it promptly can go a long way toward resolving problems. Rein pressure was Sapphire's pet peeve. She wanted a loose rein, and a gentle check-release for slowdown cues. If her rider forgot, she threw her head down and slung it side to side while humping her back. Jerry quickly learned to keep a light hand on Sapphire's reins to avoid being catapulted over her head. End of problem.

## ◆◇ Summary

*Pressure and release* is an essential part of your communication with horses, but it can easily make them feel trapped and anxious, thus provoking unwanted reactions.

In order to qualify as communication, pressure must meet these criteria:

- The horse recognizes the pressure as a cue
- He knows what that specific cue means
- The cue is given clearly and gently
- Pressure is released promptly

### THINGS TO TRY

▶ Notice your horse's responses to signals based on pressure, such as tension on the lead or reins, or leg cues as you're riding. Is his response relaxed and correct? Or does tension or bracing suggest he might be uncomfortable or confused?

▶ The next time a horse doesn't do as you meant to ask (riding or on the ground), pause and mentally review whether you could possibly have given a conflicting cue at the same time.

▶ As you are riding, experiment with how gently you can use a cue. If your horse does not respond to a gentle cue immediately, hold the cue and pause for five or 10 seconds. If he still has not responded, use your regular cue. Repeat this procedure as needed, and notice how quickly your horse starts responding to the new gentler cue. You are reawakening your horse's sensitivity, and horses catch on quickly when you are consistent.

## chapter 10
# Friendly Body Language

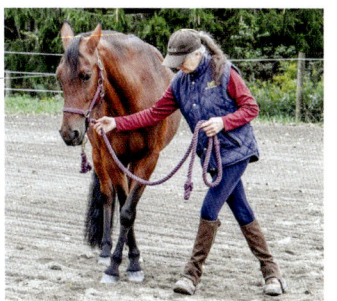

> "If your object is to become the lead horse you have to develop signals or body language that will be clearly understood."
>
> —Magali Delgado and Frédéric Pignon *(Gallop to Freedom)*

Clear communication gives horses the security of knowing what's expected of them and of understanding our guidance when they are anxious. Our body language is a powerful communication tool, *if* we use it to speak our horses' language in a positive way. Many people do not.

Two factors interfere. First, much of the body language people use is pressure-based and tells horses to move away from us. Second, we often send confusing messages because horses, watching what our whole body is doing, can be influenced by actions we are not even aware of. This is especially problematic when horses are corrected for misunderstandings.

The solution is body language that makes intuitive sense to horses, *and* encourages them to stay with us instead of moving away. That is why I refer to it as "Friendly Body Language." It is not training exercises. It is a way of interacting with horses that transforms our relationships.

The benefits go far beyond communication: better manners and performance, stronger bonds of trust and leadership, more efficient training and, perhaps most dramatically, horses look to us for guidance when they are frightened instead of trying to escape.

First I'll explain why it works so well. Then Brandy and I will demonstrate how it worked for us.

## Synchronizing: Body Language That Promotes Trust and Leadership

Among horses, when one of them chooses to go somewhere, friends are free to follow or not. We normally need to be more direct to accomplish our plans but, as Frédéric Pignon puts it, we want to be decision-maker, not enforcer.[80] We can do this by emulating the first leader a horse learned to follow, a leader whose rules and decisions he trusted implicitly: his mother. Foals quickly learn to watch and copy mama (fig. 10.1).

Communicating with horses through their ability to synchronize with us is not new. It has been around for many centuries and is still used by some world class trainers whose demonstrations with their horses at liberty are awe-inspiring. More importantly for most of us, it is the foundation of clear, positive communication.

## How Synchronizing Is Different from Learning Through Pressure

When horses copy us, they do not need to learn a variety of pressure-based cues that have no inherent meaning to them. We use one concept that makes sense to them from birth: *Watch me and do what I do*.

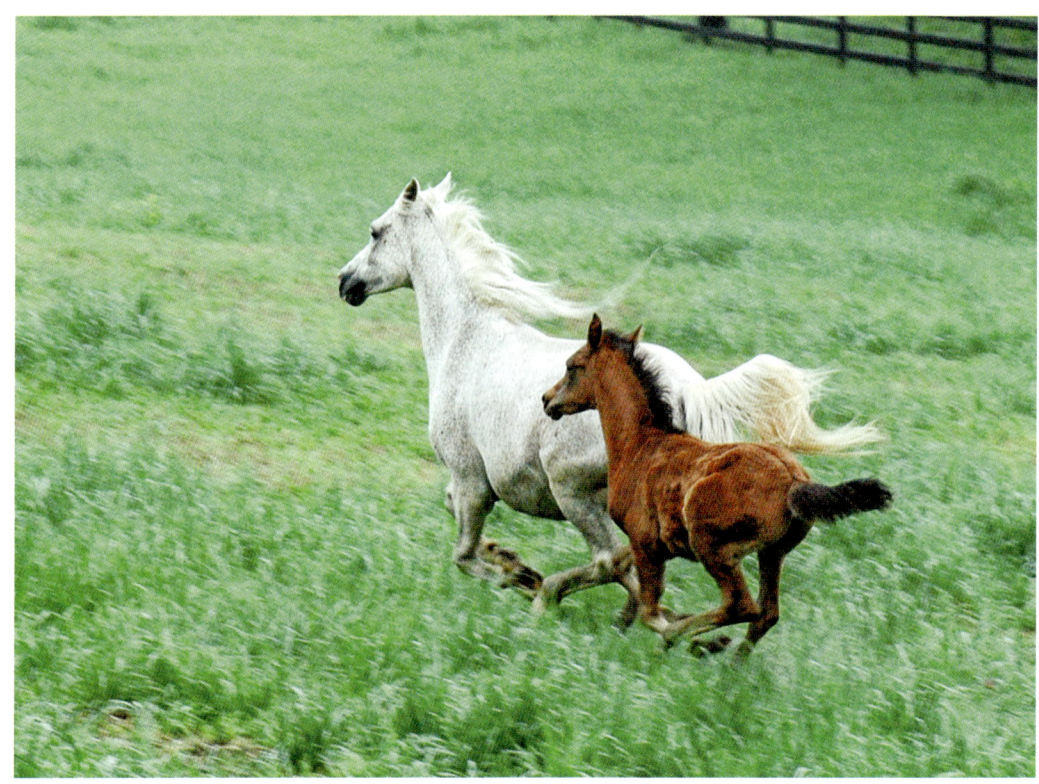

10.1 Saikana's six week old filly mirrors her mother's body position and footfalls at a gallop, right down to the way she flags her little tail, demonstrating horses' innate ability to match the actions of another individual.

At first they might need encouragement to watch us, especially if they've already been trained to wait for pressure cues. Once they get the idea, however, they need little coaching, provided our body language is clear to them.

In order to make our body language clear, we exaggerate our signals at first. This is the opposite of cues based on pressure, especially cues we use while riding. Those should always start whisper soft. To encourage horses to *watch* us for signals, we must be more dramatic until they develop the habit of tuning in.

If we use voice commands and hand signals along with body language, horses learn them by association, not by pressure. Now we have additional cues to use in other situations, such as lungeing, riding, liberty, and teaching skills that we cannot demonstrate.

## Brandy Demonstrates Synchronizing with Me

Brandy and I will demonstrate what worked for us. Other horses might respond best to slightly different signals than I used with Brandy because individual horses' interpretations of our actions can vary, just as two people might interpret the same words differently. For example, when I cue a turn, Brandy watches which way my hand points. Bronzz watches which way my shoulders turn. If a horse does not respond to a signal, a variation often clarifies our meaning.

For consistency Brandy is on my right in each photo, but all of these skills should be practiced with the handler on both sides. My lead line is loose, and my goal is to keep it that way at all times. A tight lead is a warning that we are relying on pressure, not our body language.

Brandy's ears are rotated back in many photos. This is an "I'm focused" expression, not to be confused with *laid* back ears that indicate distress.

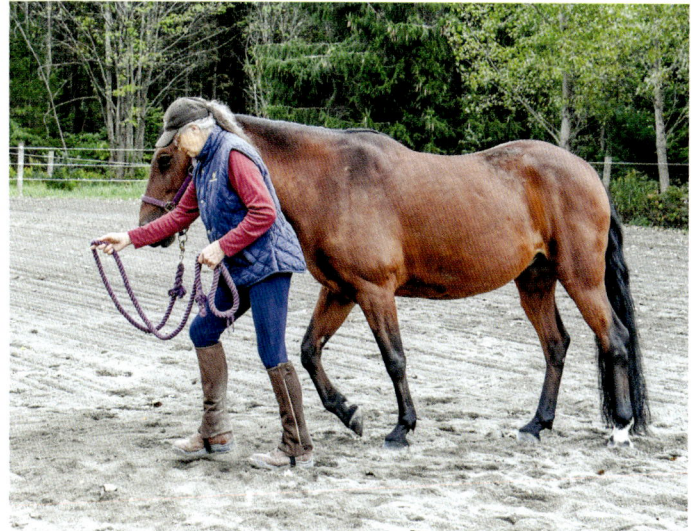

10.2 My hand and body say "forward," and I use the voice command "walk." Brandy is stepping right off with me.

### Walk

I lean forward, point ahead with my lead line hand, and say, "Walk." Confident posture and energy clarify my intent (fig. 10.2).

If Brandy wasn't with me, I made eye contact and clucked. If she still lagged, I *wiggled* the lead or used a light tug and release. The wiggle must remain a mild nagging wiggle, and not escalate to a fling. That would move the horse away, the opposite of what we want. A tug must be a check-release, not a steady pull, so the horse has nothing to lean on. It should also be gentle so it encourages forward motion instead of resistance.

## Leading Position

With Brandy's head at my shoulder, we can see each other clearly, and she can respond most easily to my signals (fig 10.3).

Many of us were taught to walk at a horse's shoulder. From a horse's perspective, he is leading because he's in front. He is also a step ahead, making right turns awkward, and leaving us little reaction time if anything happens. A horse behind us is in a driving or power position. This can be dangerous because, as Xenophon colorfully pointed out centuries ago, "…you have the least chance to look out for yourself, and the horse has the best chance to do whatever he pleases."[81] Later, as our communication becomes more refined, we can direct the horse from any position.

## Turns

I cue turns by turning my whole body, and moving my lead-line hand in the appropriate direction. Each turn toward Brandy reinforces that it is her responsibility to step out of my way. Each time I turn away, I reinforce that I assume she will follow (figs. 10.4 A & B).

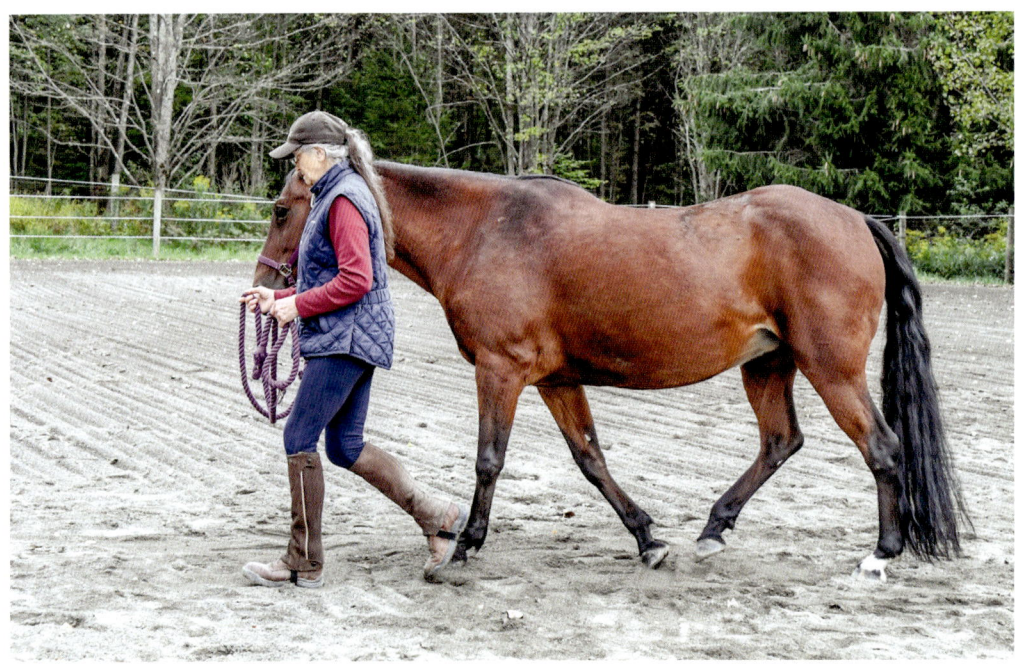

10.3 Brandy walks with her head at my shoulder, the leading position from which I can cue her most effectively. Her front feet are in step with me.

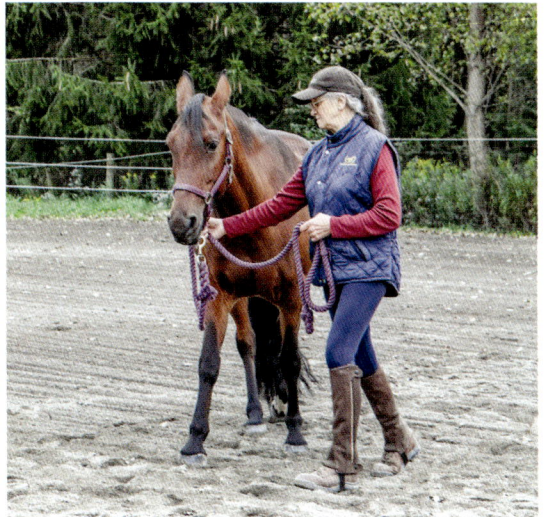

10.4 A  I turn my body in the direction I want to go, and "point" with my lead-line hand. Although my hand disappears under her head, Brandy can easily see my body turning.

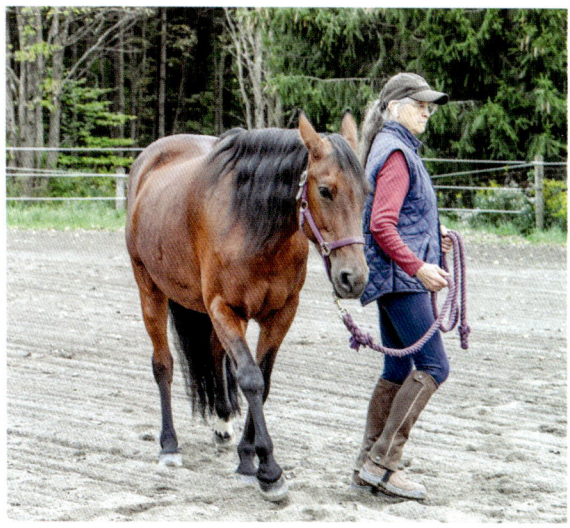

10.4 B  Accustomed to watching my body, Brandy makes a left turn here with just the slightest motion of my lead-line hand.

## Setting the Pace

She who sets the pace is leading. This is a crucial point. Many people unconsciously adjust their speed to that of the horse, telling him that he is calling the shots. Horses accustomed to walking with their shoulder next to the handler naturally speed up to maintain that position. We must set the pace and be sticklers about maintaining it. Encouraging the horse to walk in step with us helps control the pace. It does not matter if his hind feet or his front feet are in step with us.

If a horse doesn't match my pace, I deliberately do the opposite of what he is doing. When Brandy barged ahead, I slowed down or did a brisk about face and marched off in the opposite direction, letting her scramble to catch up. Or, I stopped, cued her to back up (without moving out of my leading position, as described below), and waited for her to reposition herself.

When Brandy had the hang of staying with me, I reinforced the idea of synchronizing by deliberately changing my pace. Faster, slower, bigger or smaller steps, random stops. I was careful not to make changes so abrupt or frequent that Brandy got confused or felt harassed. We must never set horses up to make mistakes; just make enough changes to keep their attention. Better yet, turn it into a game where the horse wins lots of praise.

## Halt

The halt must be decisive: shoulders back, hips forward (fig. 10.5). I stamp my feet once, left-right, and say "Whoa." Coasting to a stop does not send a clear signal. We must change our energy and

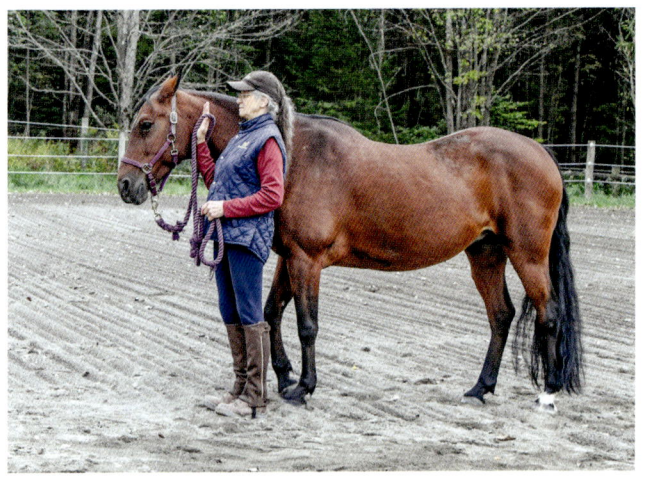

10.5 I halt with my weight back, feet planted, my body language clearly saying we stop *now*. The upward motion of my hand wiggles the lead, but there is no pressure on it.

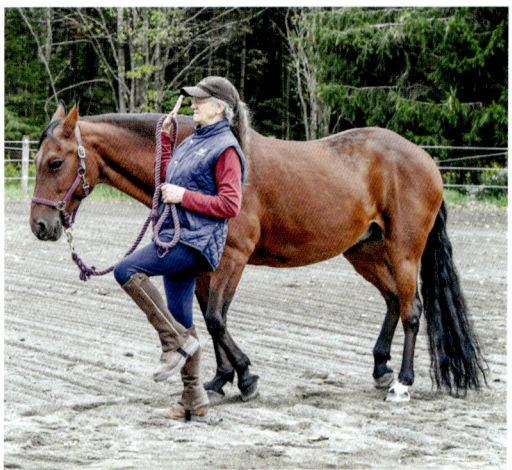

10.6 Brandy is lifting her left front/right hind feet to back up in step with me.

posture dramatically. My raised hand later becomes part of my signals for back up and "stay." However, if a horse is uncomfortable with motion around his face, I put my hand in front of his chest instead, or skip the hand signal altogether.

If Brandy hit the end of the lead, I just parked my feet and let her go around until she realized I wasn't going anywhere. At first, I accepted a stop one step ahead of me, but later I expected her to stop *with* me. If she did not, I asked her to back into position.

Once my horses developed the habit of stopping with the dramatic body, hand, feet, and voice command, they began responding to it remotely. I have used it to stop loose horses who had spooked and were revving up to race around, or who were staying one step ahead of me in the pasture when fresh grass overruled good manners.

### Back

I lean back, lift my knees high to call attention to what my feet are doing, pat the air with the back of my raised hand, and say "Back."

My lead-line hand in "Stop" position signals that we are not going forward (fig. 10.6). Patting the air with the back of my hand wiggles the loose lead to encourage backward motion. Backing from this position helped Brandy understand that her head-at-my-shoulder leading position is a constant, and it is her responsibility to maintain it, not mine. As soon as we turn around to back the horse up, we've changed that position.

Once horses learn the verbal command, "Back," it helps them learn other backup cues that are useful in different circumstances.

### Trot

I leaned forward, pointing forward with my lead-line hand, saying, "Terrrot," as I began to jog. Later, we practiced changing pace between slow jog and faster trot. To trot more slowly, I slowed my feet and added the voice command, "Eeeasy," in a soothing tone. Later when I lunged her, Brandy understood that "Eeeeasy" meant slower in the same gait, while a cluck meant faster without changing gaits.

### Canter

When I was lungeing Brandy and felt she was ready to canter, it was absurdly easy to cue her. I ducked forward and "cantered" a step. Off she went.

### Head Down

Brandy had been with us just two months when I saw her copying actions I had not even realized she noticed. I turned her loose in my arena one day as I went around to pick up the cones we used for steering practice. She walked with me as if attached with an invisible lead. Then, as I bent over to retrieve each cone, she lowered her head along with mine, her nose touching the ground (fig. 10.7).

After this, I noticed that she routinely

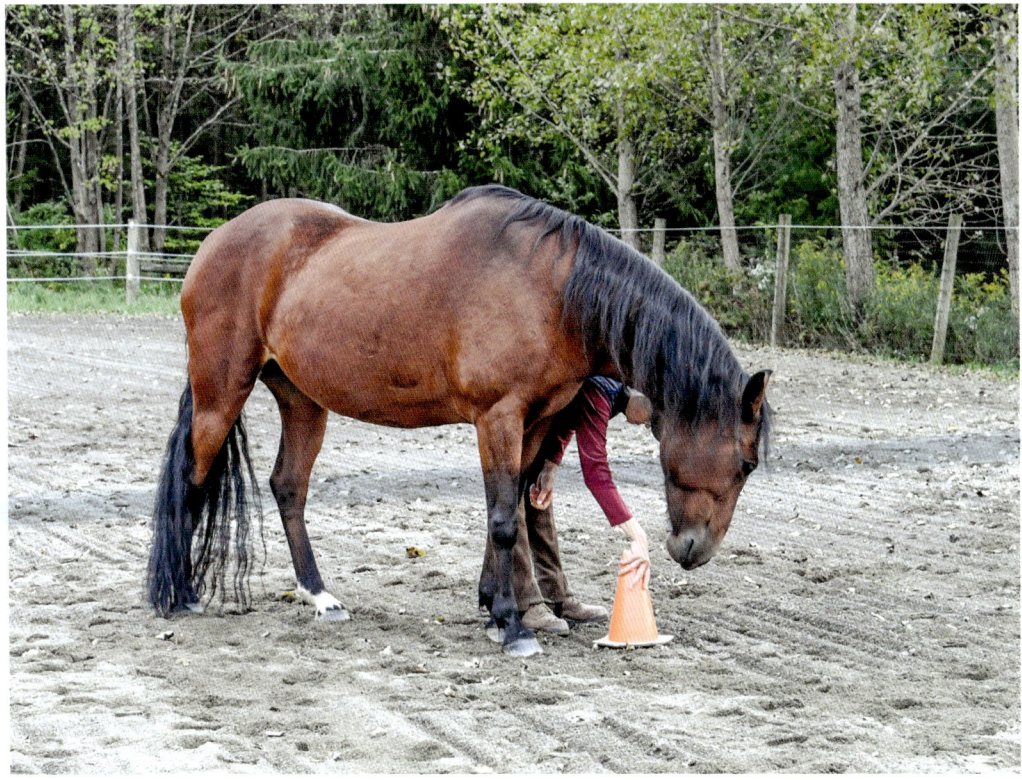

10.7 Off lead Brandy chose to follow me. When I bent over to pick up cones, she copied me by lowering her own head.

## Standing Still: Influencing Energy and Emotions

Our energy level influences our horses, and this can work for us or against us. Common reasons horses fail to stand still are:

- They do not know that's what you want.

- They are anxious.

- They have too much energy.

Typical responses are making them move, circling, yanking on reins or lead, or scolding. When his leader is busy moving around, why should a horse think that *he* is supposed to stand *still*? Instead, he gets more confused, anxious, and revved up.

It is more effective to model what you want. I assume the posture of a horse who is falling asleep. Yawning ostentatiously is a nice touch. The quieter you are, the faster the horse can calm himself (fig. 10.8).

When a horse crowds, I casually use chicken wings or windshield wipers to move him out of my space (see p. 24). If he tries to turn away, I gently turn his nose toward me. The lead should be just short enough that he cannot turn his butt to me or pull away. If he needs to move his feet, which horses naturally do when they are distressed, he can dance and fidget as long as he stays in the zone between my personal space and the end of the lead.

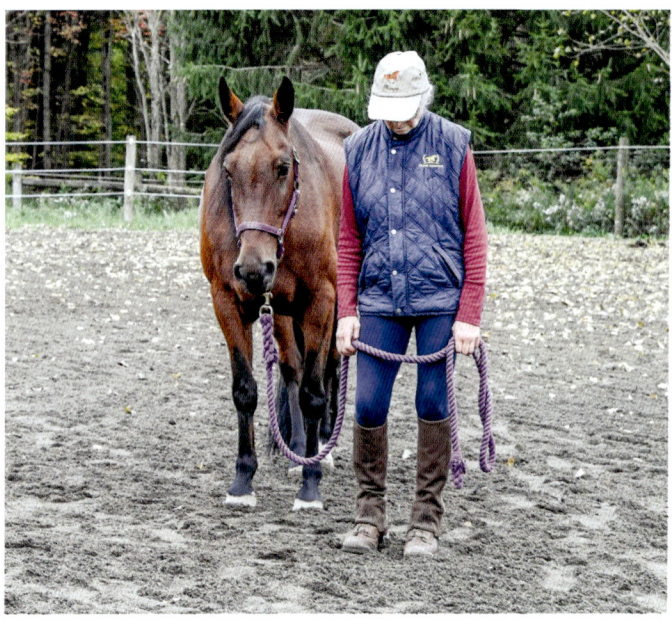

10.8 I show Brandy that I want her to stand still by pretending I'm falling asleep. Her body is relaxed, yet her ears show she is still attentive.

lowered her head when I bent over. Bending over is not always a convenient cue, since her head naturally popped up as soon as I stood up, so I held my hand above her poll as I bent over. With a little practice, Brandy was lowering her head with my hand just above her poll.

When Brandy and I started working at liberty, she sometimes became overly exuberant and playfully reared. I simply lowered my head. Instantly, Brandy's front feet touched down, and she dropped her nose to the ground. I use the same head-down cue if Brandy forgets to lower her head when small children want to halter her. I just need to catch her eye and bow my head. This shows how our communication generalizes to other situations even when a horse is excited or at a distance from us.

This is a radical change from the idea of *controlling* a horse's motion, but the fact is that we cannot *make* a horse stand still, and the more revved up he is, the less able he is to make himself stand still.

Practice in quiet circumstances helps horses understand and build the habit of responding to our calmness, so they are better able to do so when they are excited. The time this takes early on is a good investment in future calm behavior. We now have better control over our horses' actions because we have a calming influence on their emotions.

## Recall

Having a horse come when called is a convenience when he is at the other end of a pasture or arena. It can be invaluable if a horse is loose, frightened, and potentially in danger. I taught Brandy by building on the foundation I had started when I invited her to catch me (see p. 18).

My horses, like dogs, recall better when I use a distinctive sound, not just words. This is especially true when they are grazing and are in a meditative zone that is not on the same channel as human voices. Since I can't whistle, I make a high-pitched "whup" sound, followed by the name of the horse I want. When the horse looks at me, I do one of two things. I use my unthreatening "catch me" posture and back away (fig. 10.9). Or, I turn and walk or jog away. This is much like the way we teach a dog to recall. Recall became a game that Brandy likes to play. She knows that coming to me rates a treat and a nice scratching.

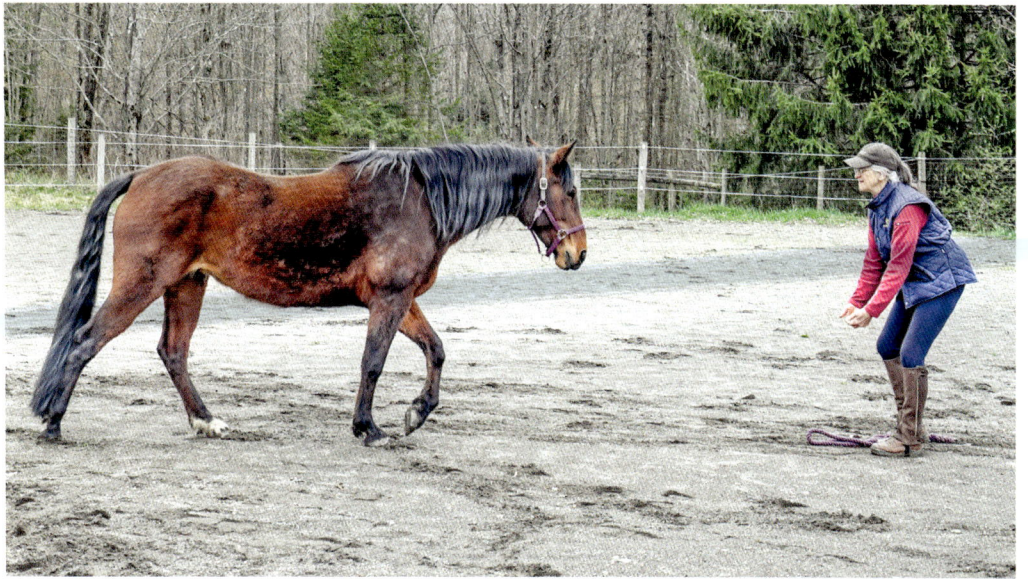

**10.9** My posture (Sharon Wilsie calls this "O" in *Horse Speak*) and backward motion invite Brandy to come to me. If I turned and jogged away, she would follow me at a trot.

This is quite different from the common round pen method of training horses to approach or follow a handler. That is based on pressure/release and conditioned response. Horses learn to relieve pressure by approaching or following the handler. It works in confined spaces where a horse cannot escape, but not where a horse has room to avoid the handler's pressure.[82][83]

In contrast, a Friendly Body Language recall is based on a trusting relationship and the horse's *understanding* of what we are asking. It does not require a confined space to be successful.

The ultimate test of recall is what happens when a horse is loose and scared. Happily, we've tested that only once. One summer evening at dusk my husband, heading to the manure pile with the wheelbarrow, left the back paddock gate partially open. In a flash, Brandy had ducked out to sample the grass, which was undoubtedly superior to any in a pasture. She came when I called her, but before I could slip a lead around her neck, excitement won out, and she dodged away, trotting up the pasture fence line toward the trail Bronzz and I take on our rides in the woods. Brandy reached the trail, turned right, and disappeared into the woods.

Not good. While Bronzz has loved woods since our first rides, Brandy seems to find them scary even in broad daylight. I could not imagine what she was thinking. By now it was dark. Find a dark bay pony in dense woods in the dark? More likely I would scare her by bumbling around, and hurt myself in the process.

I stayed at the gate and used my high-pitched recall sound. She turned but not sharply enough. We heard her crashing through the underbrush, heading for a small, but steep and rocky ravine where a seasonal creek runs. I called again. She altered course again and the crashing now came directly toward us but she had not turned soon enough. We cringed as we heard her scramble over rocks and through the ravine. A moment later, she popped out of the woods and trotted over to me, miraculously unscathed and apparently undaunted by her adventure.

Brandy does not always come when I call her. Sometimes she decides her own agenda is more important. "I'm busy eating grass, snoozing with my friends, whatever…." I don't make an issue of it; I just go to get her. So why did she come from the woods when I called her? Aren't horses normally *less* obedient when they're scared?

The answer has to do with security, not conditioned obedience. She did not come back because I had trained her to obey automatically every time. She came because when she didn't know what to do, she listened for my guidance, and she already understood what my recall signal meant.

> *The ultimate test of recall is what happens when a horse is loose and scared.*

## An Exciting New Perspective

Friendly Body Language dramatically changes our interactions with horses. We're looking for *understanding*, not a conditioned response. We do not drill; everything we do with our horses is practice. We get reliability by being reliable ourselves, using our Friendly Body Language every time we handle them. Practice sessions are optional, and should be short and focused, not long and boring.

Friendly Body Language is effective because it is the *horses'* language. We do not decide what our actions mean; *they* do. Therefore, it is our responsibility to be sure we make sense to them. If their responses are not what we want, we do not correct them. We figure out how to send a clearer message, and correct ourselves. This means less pressure and stress for the horses. It also means that we have to trust each horse's responses.

## Trusting Your Horse's Responses

Fortunately, I already had some experience with this concept, thanks to Bronzz's breeder who graciously mentored me through the first year of Bronzz's training. I could not guess how many times Fritz said, with a kindly twinkle in his eye, "Well, Lynn, Bronzz just did exactly what you told him to do. I'm not sure it's what you *meant* to tell him…." Thank goodness for his patient and astute feedback. Without it, I would have undermined my relationship with Bronzz over and over by "correcting" him for my mistakes.

Bronzz gave a dramatic example of doing what he thought I wanted the day I decided to teach him to turn on the forehand. I touched his hip. He didn't move. I touched harder. I tapped. I leaned. I all but shoved him. He continued to stand calm and relaxed.

A glimmer of understanding came to me. When I groomed his hind legs, I rested a hand on his hip. Had he learned that a touch on his hip meant *do not* move? Testing this, I turned and braced my shoulders against his hip, digging my heels in and pushing with all my 125-pound might. Bronzz leaned back against me, gently and precisely holding me up. He looked thoroughly pleased with himself, as if he'd figured out the rules of some strange human game.

When Fritz and I got done laughing, I touched Bronzz's hip with a fingertip and *clucked*. He stepped right over.

I kept this sort of miscommunication in mind as I worked with Brandy, trying to observe her responses with a non-judgmental attitude of, "Oh, so that's what that means to her." If it was not what I meant to say, I adjusted my signals.

How did I know she wasn't scamming me, ignoring me, or goofing off? At first, I didn't. I had to take her word for it. That was a big leap of faith for me. Then I began to see that Brandy was indeed following my directions as best she understood them. This was especially obvious when I got the same "wrong" response every time I used a given signal. For example, if I signaled, "Stop," with my hand, but my body leaned forward, she kept moving.

## The Benefits of Friendly Body Language

What we *see* as a result of Friendly Body Language is excellent ground manners. What has really happened is far more profound.

## Horses Feel More Secure

With more clarity and less pressure, we represent security. Brandy demonstrated this early on when I inadvertently let her lead get too loose. She put her head down to investigate something, and stepped on her lead. When she tried to raise her head and found herself trapped, she panicked and jumped back, freeing her head with a mighty fling. Then she scooted to my side and stood there. Though her body was quivering, her feet were still. Her fear had not prompted her to run away; she had run *to* me, and

10.10 After standing still for six-year-old Leora to braid her mane, Brandy remains carefully attentive as she walks with her on a loose lead.

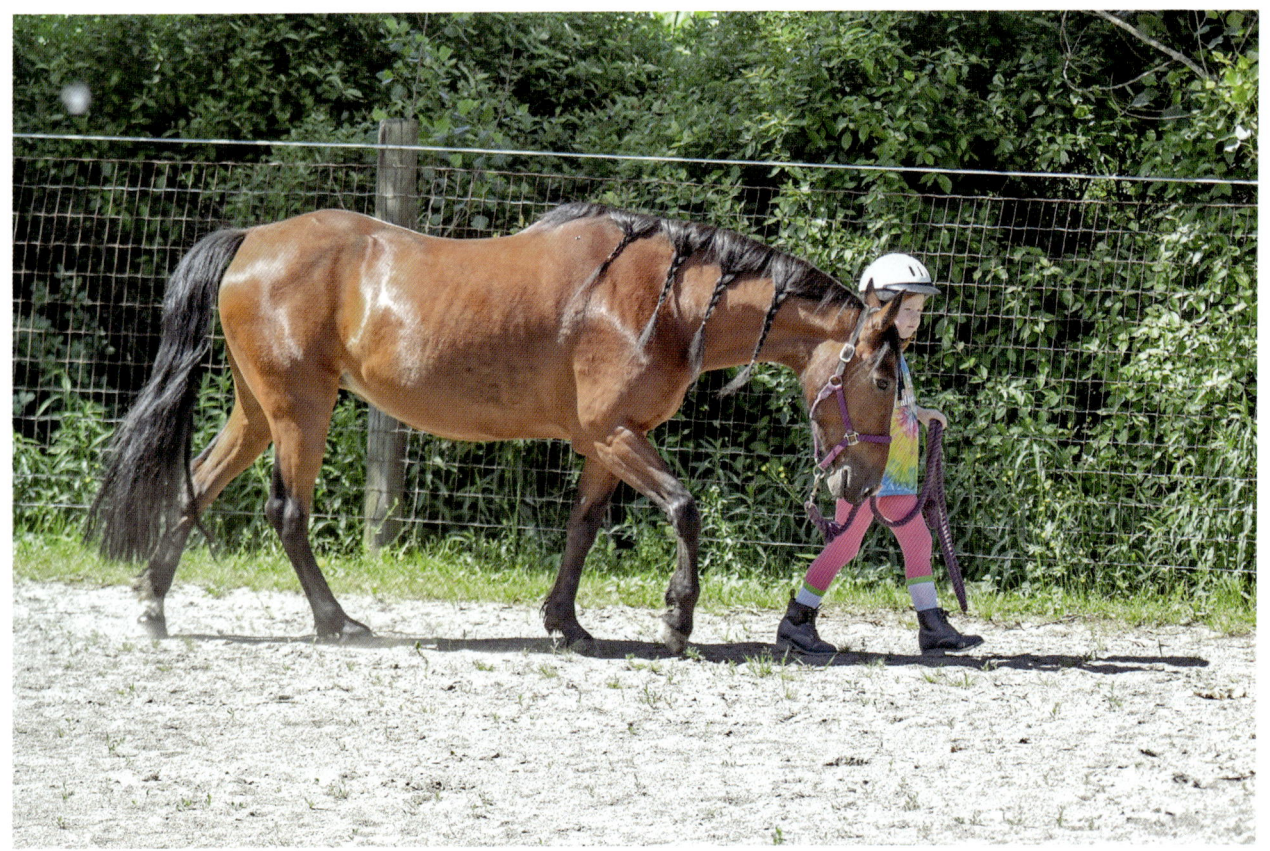

calmed quickly because I stood quietly offering a safe haven.

## Horses Reliably Focus on Leaders

Understanding that it was her responsibility to keep me on her radar at all times, Brandy learned to anticipate my actions and be ready to respond, such as when I turn around to close a gate and need her to step out of the way. This focus carries over to everything we do with horses, and to new and potentially scary situations. It also transfers to other handlers. Soon even novices and children could handle Brandy because *she* watched out for *them* (fig. 10.10). Close supervision is, of course, recommended with children, even after we have coached them on safe handling skills.

## Cues Learned by Association Expand Skills

When you teach new skills from the ground, horses have the advantage of seeing your body language and of not having to manage your weight while learning something new. Once they know the skill, the ridden cues for it make sense more easily. Brandy learned shoulder-in, and turns-on-the-forehand and haunches from watching my body language (fig. 10.11).

Brandy's original trot was speedy and unbalanced with high head and hollow back. When I began lungeing her, I slowed her down ("Eeeasy") and encouraged her to lower her head by

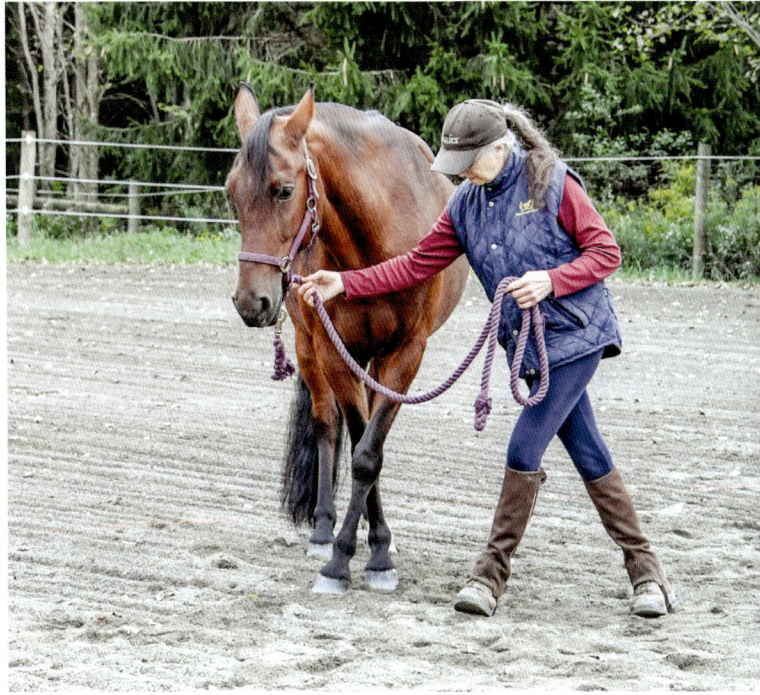

10.11 Brandy turns on her haunches by copying me as I cross left leg over right.

bowing mine. I reinforced an increasingly better balanced trot with Clicker Training (see chapter 11—p. 128). Her posture is improved and her trot better balanced, with no restrictive equipment ever used.

## Training Myself

The hardest part of using Friendly Body Language was training myself. At first, I had to consciously think about my posture, which way I turned or leaned, what each arm was doing, and where I was looking. This was a challenge for me since I am neither well-coordinated nor visually oriented. I would probably not have bothered with such a "radical idea" if I had not seen the transformation from terror to trust in Thistle, the pony described in chapter 2 (p. 20).

Instructions were hard to come by. The trainer who had given me the original demonstration had moved away. Books and videos on liberty work seemed to rely heavily on pressure. I was winging it on my own until I discovered *The Horse Agility Handbook* by Vanessa Bee.

The ultimate goal of Horse Agility is to work a horse over obstacles *at liberty*, in large open areas. This requires both the communication and the relationship I was trying to achieve. Though I was not interested in obstacles, I was thrilled to find clear, step-by-step instructions. *The Horse Agility Handbook* became my "body-language dictionary."

I also studied videos of people who used Friendly Body Language, noticing both their actions and their horses' responses. I experimented with Brandy and my other horses. I watched videos of myself and got feedback from my husband, who is visually observant.

Learning to use Friendly Body Language means experimenting as we observe how horses interpret what we do. This was a new concept for me. I was used to giving a cue and judging the response either "right" (praise) or "wrong" (correction). As I got better at reading my horse's responses and deciphering how to adjust to clarify what I wanted, I went from skeptical to amazed and delighted.

Each new horse I handle catches on faster as I get better at using Friendly Body Language, reading their responses, and adjusting accordingly. I had wondered at first if this worked so quickly with Brandy because her anxiety prompted her to stick with me, but I have found that calm, confident horses catch on just as well, and seem just as happy to realize that someone is finally speaking a language they understand.

A by-product of learning Friendly Body Language is that we are more aware of our body language when we ride, so our cues can be more subtle and precise.

## Expanding Your Fluency in Friendly Body Language

As you encourage your horse to cue from your body language, he may do so even when you are not asking him to, as Brandy did when she copied me and learned "head down." This can be handy, amusing, and occasionally disconcerting. I suspect that Brandy learned to duck under her stall guard and escape her stall by watching me do it.

Brandy's demonstrations in this chapter are only a glimpse of what is possible. *The Horse Agility Handbook* gives detailed instructions, from simple leading skills to complex communication at liberty, including problem-solving when things do not go as hoped. You will also find many insights on two-way communication with horses in *Conversations with Horses* by Hertha James and *Horse Speak* by Sharon Wilsie.

## Summary

Horses notice everything you do, including your posture, gestures, facial expressions, tone of voice, and where you are looking. You can take advantage of this by using body language that makes intuitive sense to them, while encouraging them to watch you and stay with you. Friendly Body Language:

- Clarifies communication.
- Reduces pressure and the resulting anxiety.
- Improves focus and learning.
- Reinforces leadership and supports a trusting relationship.
- Encourages consistently cooperative behavior.

### THINGS TO TRY

- With a human partner, take turns leading each other with one of you playing the role of a horse. Try walking, turning, and stopping casually. Then try precise body language signals. When you are the horse, notice how much easier it is to coordinate with your human partner when her body language is clear.

- When you handle and lead your horse, count how often the lead goes tight, indicating he is relying on pressure for guidance instead of watching your body language.

- If your lead goes tight, try using more precise, exaggerated body language to encourage him to tune in to you. If your lead stays loose, indicating your horse is already tuned in, see if he copies other actions such as bowing, turning around, or lifting your legs higher.

- Watch videos of people using Friendly Body Language to give horses precise cues. Good examples are online horse agility (OLHA) competition courses posted for the International Horse Agility Club, especially the liberty courses.

*chapter 11*
# Rewards are Positive Feedback

> "Horses do not learn by repetition. They learn by reward."
> —Alois Podhajsky *(My Horses, My Teachers)*

Reward completely changes the focus of your interaction with horses. Instead of watching for mistakes to correct, you watch for the horse to do the *right* thing—or to do the right thing better than usual.

Instead of trying to figure out how to avoid correction, the horse is motivated to understand what you *do* want, and to perform it reliably. This engages his ability to problem-solve and to generalize information. It reduces anxiety because he is not worried about negative repercussions if he makes a mistake. The horse now has a keen interest in his own success, and in your success together as partners.

Rewards have a long history in horsemanship. Xenophon (430–354 BC) recommended treats as part of building a friendly relationship with the horse to whom you entrust your life when you ride into battle.

Colonel Alois Podhajsky (director of the Spanish Riding School from 1939 to 1965) is famous for his role in saving Lipizzans during World War II. As a cavalry officer during World War I, he was wounded in battle and credited his horse with saving his life; that is the ultimate in reliability. In his writings, Colonel Podhajsky often mentions rewarding horses with kind words, gentle touches, and treats.

Research supports Colonel Podhajsky and Xenophon.[84] Rewards promote:

- More positive associations with people.
- Faster learning.

- Better reliability.
- Less stress.

## Is Your Approval a Reward?

Why not? It is taken for granted that dogs, also a domesticated social species, will work for human approval. Research with dogs indicates that in some instances an owner's praise is a *better* motivator than food.[85]

As a teenager, I assumed that the horses I rode tried to please me. In adulthood, I was more skeptical until Snickers came along. As his skills and confidence grew, he began to ignore the treats his good behavior earned. Yet his ears told me that he was always attuned to my words of praise. Snickers left me with no doubt that he was working for my approval as his main reward.

Snickers' lack of interest in treats was unusual, but I believe his interest in pleasing me was not unusual at all. Watching other horses with their people, I often see them making an effort to please the people they trust even when tangible rewards are not forthcoming.

This does not mean that tangible rewards are not useful. It might even mean they have more value in the context of a trusting relationship where they signify the leader's approval.

## Basic Facts about Rewards

Before discussing specific rewards, let's clarify a few points.

- **Rewards are not bribes.** A reward is earned, like a paycheck. Shaking a grain bucket to catch a horse is bribery. A treat produced from your pocket after a horse has allowed himself to be caught is a reward.

- **Horses *do* use rewards in their own social interactions.** It is sometimes claimed that rewards do not work with horses because they do not use them with each other. The aggressive behaviors sometimes seen among domestic horses might lead you to this erroneous conclusion. However, in well-socialized herds, aggressive behaviors are outnumbered by friendly interactions that are inherently rewarding. Behaviors such as sniffing, rubbing, or sharing a hay pile (see fig. 5.3, p. 59) are often discounted because they lack drama. Mutual grooming (see fig. 5.2, p. 55) actually produces endorphins!

- **Rewards must be something the horse appreciates.** You must tune in to what matters to each horse,

---

**Typical Rewards**

1. Praise
2. Stroking or scratching
3. Rest break
4. Fun break
5. Food

and provide rewards he considers worth working for.

- **The timing must show a horse what he has done to earn it.** If it does not happen while the horse is performing the action you want, or immediately after it, you're rewarding the wrong thing.

When you're training, a reward might mean a full stop in your activity while a horse enjoys his reward and has a break to process what he did to earn it. At other times, rewards might be woven seamlessly into your program so that a horse

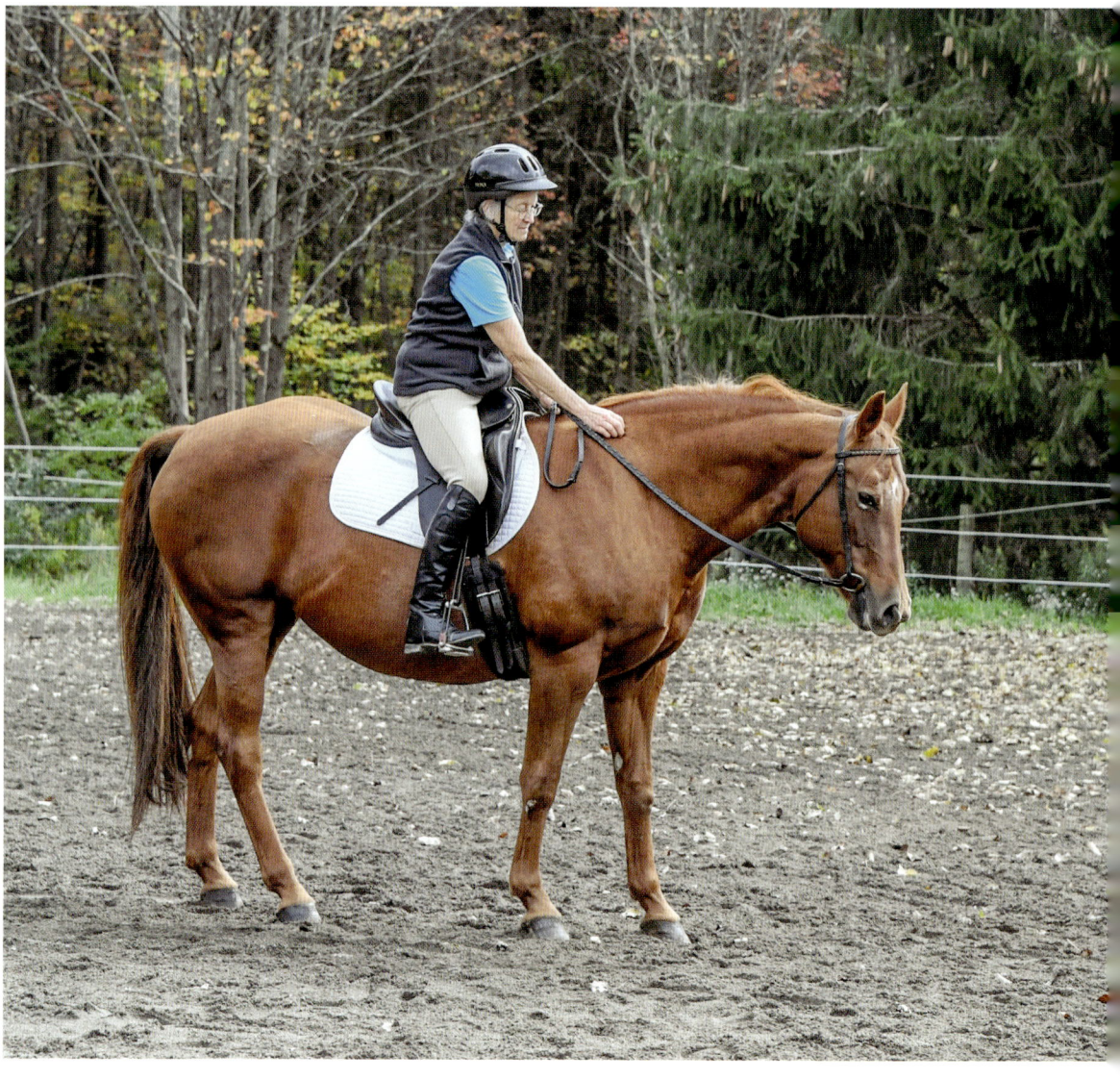

11.1  A rest and scratch break is Shiloh's second most favorite reward (after treats). Her enjoyment shows in her relaxed posture and soft expression.

receives the positive message, such as a quick stroke or word of praise, without missing a beat.

## Typical Rewards

### Praise

Praise is meaningful only when delivered in a positive tone of voice. Think of the soft nickers you hear when a horse is happy. By using the same word(s) and inflection, you help the horse to recognize praise easily.

I routinely thank or compliment my horses even for mundane actions I expect of them, like having a hoof in the air waiting for me as I pick out hooves. It lets them know I am tuned in to them, while reinforcing good behavior.

### Stroking and Scratching

Nothing in horses' innate body language tells them that enthusiastic pats and slaps are rewards, as you can see from the common raised-head startle reaction. Even gentle pats meant to show approval or affection may escalate to slapping when a person is excited.

In contrast, stroking, rubbing, and scratching mimic mutual grooming (fig. 11.1). This lowers heart rates and produces endorphins. This kind of touch may be a valuable reward that is generally underused.[86] [87]

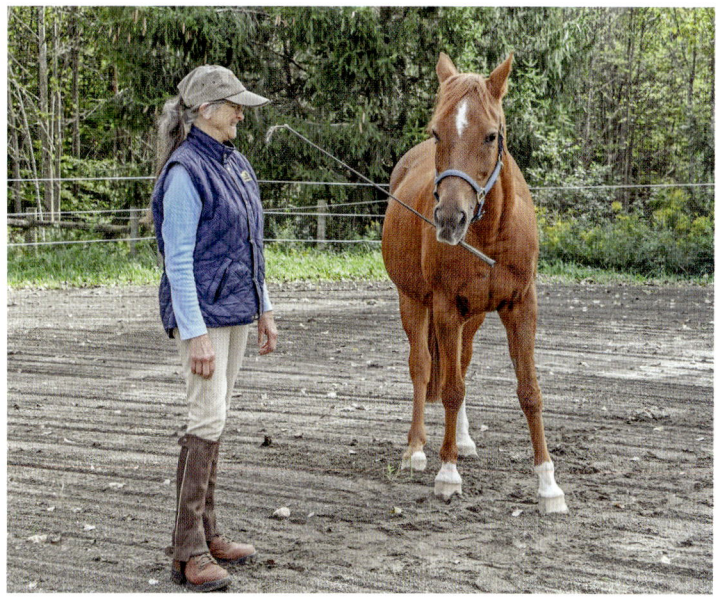

11.2 For a fun break, Bronzz likes to take my dressage whip and watch me laugh.

### Rest Break

A rest break can be appreciated not only after hard physical work, but after focusing intensely on something new or challenging. A break allows time to process new information, so it can be retained better.

Walking on a loose rein is sometimes considered a reward, but that depends on whether the *horse* thinks it is. After all, it is supposed to be his reward, not yours.

### Fun Break

You can reward a horse by asking him to perform an activity that he enjoys. Snickers' favorite was a turn-on-the-forehand. My sister's Appaloosa-Oldenburg considered jumping a reward. Brandy likes to go through some agility obstacle at a fast trot. Bronzz likes to pick things up (fig. 11.2).

## Food

Correctly used, food is a powerful motivator that engages most horses' enthusiastic cooperation. Poorly used, it means bribery, permissiveness, and pushy horses. No wonder food rewards are controversial in the horse world. It has been suggested that food rewards do not promote reliable behavior but the real issue is with *how* food is used. Food rewards are now common in dog training, including Personal Assistance, Search and Rescue, and Law Enforcement dogs whose reliability can mean life or death for people.

The successful use of food takes into account several potentially sticky issues:

- **A reward is *earned***. Horses who get random, unearned treats may feel entitled to constant treats. Horses who score treats with nuzzles and nudges are in training to become cookie monsters.

- **The timing of delivery is crucial**. To reward a horse for standing still, for example, you should give the treat *before* he moves. If he steps toward you and reaches out for it, you have just rewarded him for stepping toward you and reaching for the treat. This timing issue limits your ability to use food rewards when the horse is in motion or beyond arm's reach. I will describe an effective way to overcome this limitation with clicker training (see p. 133).

- **Horses must be taught to accept food politely**. They should stay out of your space while you extend the treat, and they should take it gently. No reaching, grabbing, or mugging.

- **Food can be a distraction**. While other rewards can be incorporated into whatever you are doing, food often means a full stop, however brief, in your other activities. Food also tends to generate more excitement than other rewards. This is part of its value, but the downside is that it can divert a horse's attention from the job at hand to second-guessing what will score him the next goodie.

Since food can be a marvelous motivator or a recipe for trouble, it is worth looking at how to address these issues so you can enjoy the benefits. One way is with structured routines. Another is the use of Clicker Training.

### Structured Routines

Predictable routines and expectations offer reward opportunities without encouraging food-related problems. You might offer one treat when you first put a horse's halter on. Or right after hooves are picked. Or at a specific point after a ride, say between removing the bridle, and giving the much-appreciated face rub. One treat, at the same time in the sequence of a routine.

Treats can reinforce safe behavior. One served after a horse has stood still for mounting, and before he is asked to walk off, can do wonders for mounting manners. At turnout time, a treat offered as the horse is turned loose gives him an incentive *not* to dash off.

Treats are nice consolation prizes for unpleasantness. Sapphire was prone to static electricity under her winter blanket. As I slid it off her rump one day, I saw sparks. I could not have blamed her if she'd reflexively kicked out, but instead she shot forward, slipping on the hard ground and landing on her knees. I felt awful. Next day, I folded her blanket forward onto her shoulders, a safer plan, anyway, and showed her one of her favorite peppermint candies. Happily anticipating the candy, she was less concerned about the static when the blanket slid off her shoulders. (Lifting it off would have been better if I were tall enough to do that.)

Insulin resistant Bronzz is a trooper to have blood drawn for glucose tests. We reinforce his good manners with a mouthful of hay to munch while he's stabbed, and a treat to look forward to afterward. Chewing the hay, by the way, relaxes his neck muscles so the jugular vein is easier to find.

When grass season means muzzles, our horses stuff their faces right into their muzzles because they know there is a primo treat in the bottom.

In each instance the treat is clearly part of a routine, so the horse knows when to expect it. He also knows that he can expect just one, so there is no point lobbying for more.

When we want to use a treat to reward good behavior or performance aside from routines, we can connect the treat to the behavior by using the same distinctive word or phrase just before the treat, like "Yes!" or "Good boy!"

This kind of structure usually sets up clear expectations and heads off trouble. But not always.

Shiloh arrived with the impression that humans were mobile vending machines activated by nuzzles, nudges, and nips, in that order. Nothing I tried altered this conviction. My veterinarian recommended Clicker Training. I was skeptical, but it proved to be remarkably successful.

### Clicker Training

Clicker Training is one of the few truly modern innovations in training, introduced to the horse world only a few decades ago. While a horse is doing something you want to reward, you produce a unique sound, typically a click but anything distinctive will work. The sound tells the horse that whatever he is doing at the moment he hears it has earned him a reward. This allows some lag time between the behavior and the reward because the horse now knows that a treat is forthcoming, *and* what he has done to earn it. Thus, it works

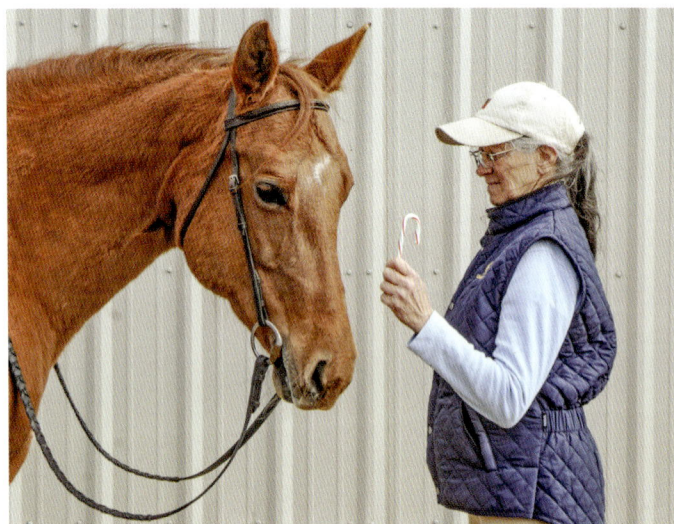

11.3 A  Shiloh is *not* reaching for the candy cane that I am holding right in front of her face. She knows the way to earn a treat is to wait politely until I click and serve it to her.

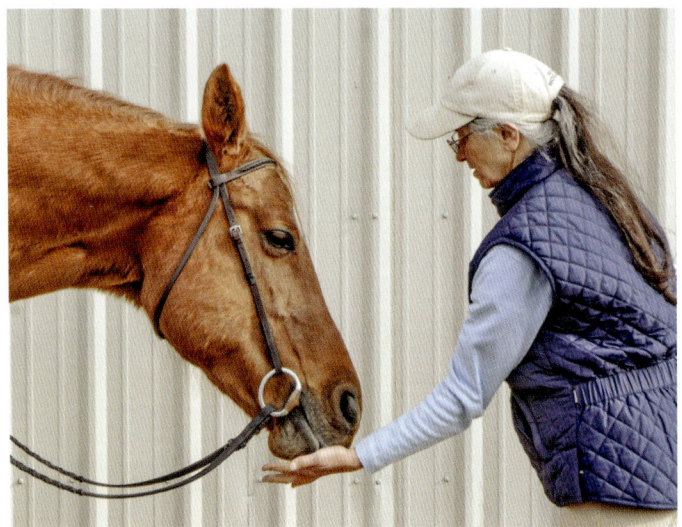

11.3 B  I click, and then Shiloh takes a piece of candy cane gently from my out-stretched hand.

even when a horse is in motion or at a distance from us.

Clicker Training has gotten a bad rap, sometimes associated with frivolous tricks and rude horses grabbing for treats. "Tricks" can be useful (see p. 215), and Clicker Training can actually solve food-related problems when used correctly. I have found Clicker Training to be a powerful way to engage my horses enthusiastically in their own learning, and to have a lot of fun with them. I will share how I use it, with the caveat that I do not consider myself a skilled clicker trainer. I hope that if you are unfamiliar with it, my experience will convince you that it is worth learning more about.

First I showed Shiloh that when I clicked the little gadget, she was about to get a treat. Then I taught her to earn the treat by touching a target, a simple first task. Soon she was reaching every which way to put her nose on the old stuffed toy I used as a target. Shiloh was thrilled with the game. I was disgusted; her treat grabbing was worse than ever.

When I consulted a skilled Clicker Trainer, it was immediately obvious where I'd gone wrong. There is a critical difference between Clicker Training a dog and Clicker Training a horse. We cannot lob treats for horses to snatch mid-air as dogs do. We need to add another step that teaches horses right from the start to stay out of our space and accept the treat politely. It must be crystal clear to the horse that this means every treat, every time, no exceptions.

So, I now taught Shiloh to stand at attention, face front and center. I showed her the position by holding my hand where I wanted her mouth to be, my fist closed around the treat, and the back of my hand up. If she grabbed my fist, I bopped her mouth lightly with it. I turned my fist over and opened my hand only when she was standing quietly in position and not touching me. Some people emphasize the "out of my space" rule by having the horse turn his head away from them to receive the treat. With pushy horses, it is safer to start with a barrier such as a stall door or fence between horse and handler.

Shiloh soon stopped mugging people, and started standing at attention to ask for treats, adding a little nicker ("Please?") if we were slow to notice how politely she was asking (figs. 11.3 A & B).

Beware—it is easy to hold treats too close to the horse's chest. This overflexes neck muscles and ligaments, causing enormous strain and potential damage, like that shown in Sapphire's neck in fig. 7.4 B (see p. 83). Instead, the horse's face should be vertical or somewhere in front of vertical, as Shiloh's is in both photos.

The successful resolution of the mugging problem inspired me to experiment with other uses for Clicker Training. It was as simple as keeping a few treats in my pocket because once my horses had the hang of it, I could just click my tongue on the roof of my mouth. In my experience, we need to start with a clicker or some other very distinct sound so horses do not confuse it with the "cluck" that means move, but once they understand they can easily hear the difference.

Clicker Training can be used by itself or in conjunction with any other type of training to teach new skills, and to refine or reinforce skills the horse already has. A few examples of how I have done this are mentioned in chapter 16. Clicker Training also provides a way to encourage spontaneous behaviors that are difficult to train, such as Bronzz's Downward Dog yoga stretch (fig. 11.4).

What I like most about Clicker Training is that horses are motivated to figure out what earns the click and reward. This makes them enthusiastic participants in their own learning.

## Making the Most of Rewards

Special rewards are a particularly good investment when:

• You have a stressful situation like a vet visit. Rewards reinforce good behavior, offer diversion from the unpleasantness, and add a positive association to the situation.

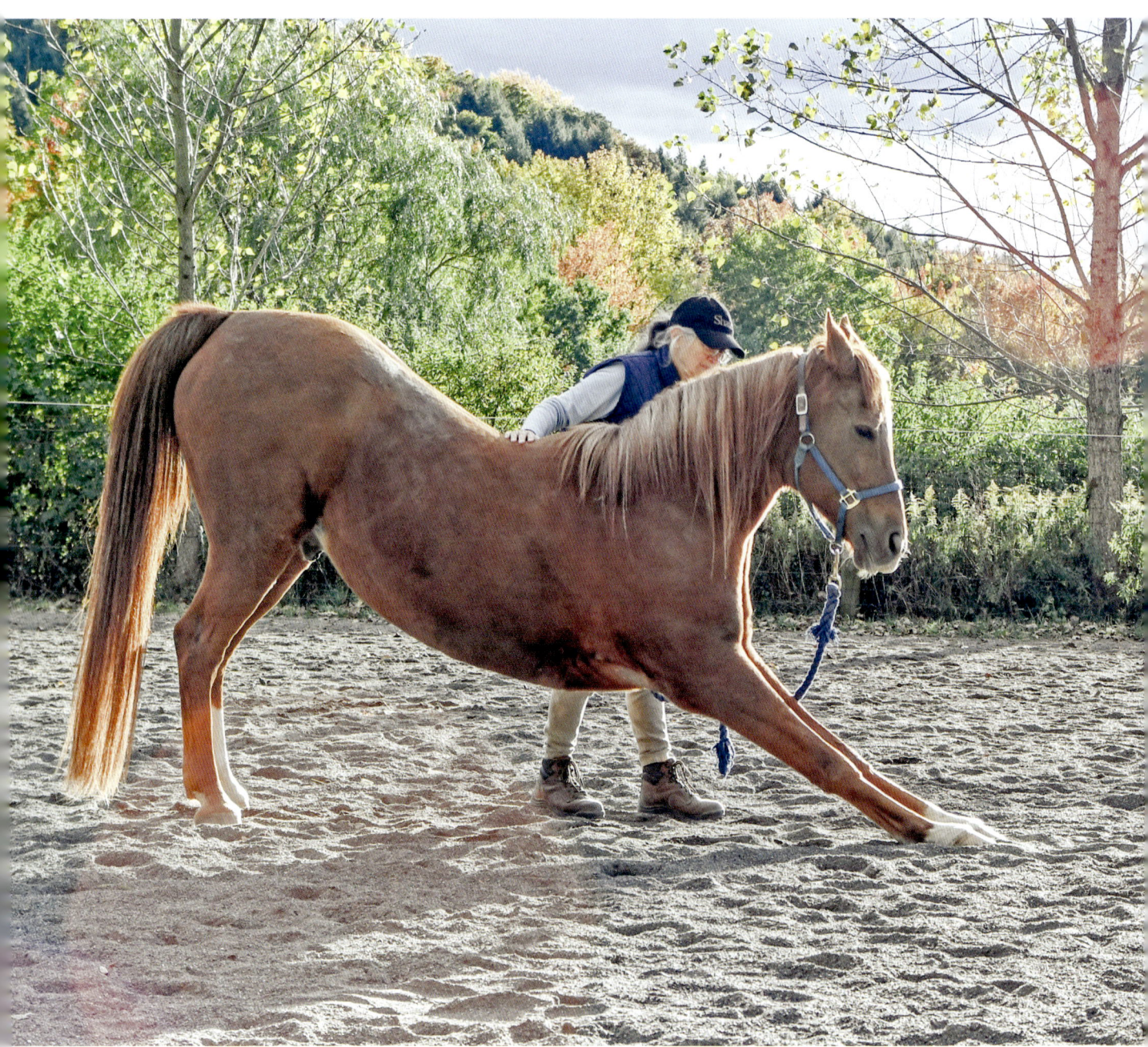

11.4 Bronzz started doing this stretch spontaneously. His chiropractor says it is good for his back, so I encourage him to do it with a Click and Treat.

- A horse is learning something new or difficult. Rewards encourage effort and clarify correct responses. When a horse performs a skill reliably and with confidence, special rewards are phased out.

- A horse has done something exceptionally well. Colonel Alois Podhajsky suggests that when this happens in a training session, you might jump right off, reward generously, and end the session.

On the other hand, when a horse finds an activity inherently enjoyable, fewer tangible rewards are needed to encourage reliable performance. Low-key rewards such as scratching, stroking, praise, rest breaks, and fun breaks can be woven seamlessly into whatever you are doing. Gentle touches and kind words can easily become part of your everyday Friendly Body Language. Thus, your Friendly Body Language itself becomes an ongoing reward, and often that is all the reward a horse needs to keep him engaged in whatever is on your agenda.

## Limitations of Rewards

- Rewards do not replace the need for good leadership, sound basic training, clear expectations, or consistent limits. Horses must know how to behave properly and do their job even when no rewards are forthcoming.

- Rewards do not replace pressure and release as an efficient means of communication; they do make the learning of pressure-and-release cues more efficient and less stressful.

- Rewards do not replace Investigative Behavior or Confidence Building exercises (see Parts Five and Six—pp. 139 and 175). These are educational activities that engage horses' innate learning abilities. Too much focus on treats can distract from learning.

- Rewards do not teach concepts such as Intelligent Disobedience. A horse focused solely on earning rewards is not fully processing other information.

- Rewards do not replace the need for security. A horse who is fearful might be frightened by a touch instead of being rewarded. In this instance, earning the horse's trust needs to come first.

## ➤ Summary

Rewards are a powerful means of positive communication, and have been used with horses for many centuries. They give horses information ("Yes, you just did what I wanted") and incentive to repeat the action. They encourage horses to proactively figure out what you want, thus engaging more of their cognitive learning abilities. Rewards also encourage a positive attitude about you and whatever you ask your horse to do.

An effective reward is something the horse wants; the timing shows him what he did to earn it. Common rewards include:

- Praise
- Stroking and scratching
- Rest breaks
- Fun breaks
- Food

If food is used, horses must be taught to receive it politely. Rewards do not replace good leadership, appropriate training, clear expectations, or consistent limits. They must always be earned by good performance or honest effort.

### THINGS TO TRY

▶ Count how many times you reward your horse compared to how often you correct him. Do this for a set period of time or for a specific activity, such as a ride, drive, grooming, or groundwork session.

▶ Count how many different rewards (from the list above) you use with horses.

# PART FIVE:
# Investigative Behavior Expands Horses' Comfort Zone

> "The paradoxical thing about novelty is that it can be extremely attractive to an animal when he can voluntarily approach it."
>
> —Dr. Temple Grandin *("Thinking the Way Animals Do")*

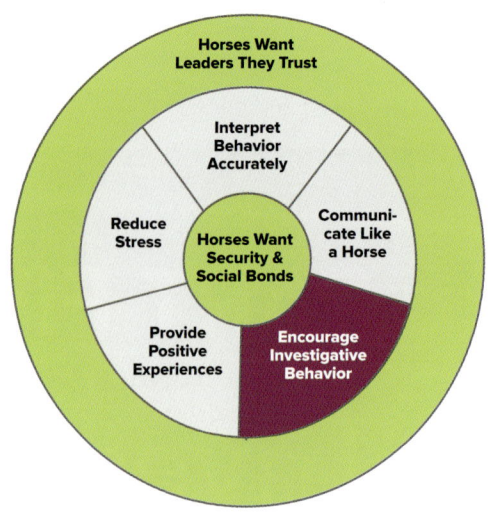

Horses are naturally curious. Their wild ancestors could not afford to be afraid of everything; they needed a healthy balance of caution and curiosity. Dr. Temple Grandin, author of *Animals Make Us Human*, describes curiosity as essential for horses' mental health.[88]

Investigative Behavior expands horses' comfort zones, making them less fearful and more reliable. They evaluate what they discover in the context of previous experiences, and retain information to apply in the future.[89] [90] The more they learn, the more quickly and confidently they evaluate new situations. People are often unfamiliar with this process because most training systems discourage giving horses the freedom to investigate.

Chapter 12 (p. 141) shows how horses use Investigative Behavior on their own without interference from people. Chapter 13 (p. 154) shows how you, as a Protector Leader, can encourage Investigative Behavior. The trust and communication you have developed through Friendly Body Language helps you maintain safer control of a horse while he is investigating a potentially scary situation. Spontaneous events related in chapter 14 (p. 166) show the variety of situations in which Investigative Behavior can reduce or overcome anxiety, encourage learning, and enhance your status as a Protector Leader. Photographs in these chapters show how Investigative Behavior follows consistent patterns among different horses and in different situations.

**Part Five Key Points:**
- Horses are naturally curious. This curiosity can prompt them to investigate scary objects or situations using Investigative Behavior.
- Investigative Behavior reduces fear and anxiety because it is a natural learning process, not a training technique.
- The pressure of common training techniques can shut down curiosity and provoke anxiety, causing horses to focus on escape instead of learning.

**You will learn how to:**
- Reawaken your horse's curiosity and ability to learn in new and potentially scary situations.
- Use Friendly Body Language to encourage and support Investigative Behavior so you can turn spooks and "resistance" into learning opportunities instead.

*chapter 12*
# How Horses Explore the World

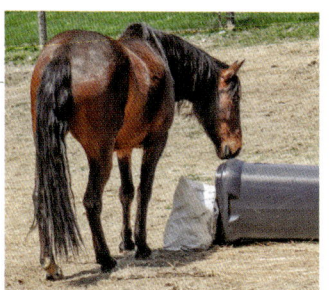

> "Most training systems don't allow the horse to move far enough away or give him the time he needs to make decisions about whether something is dangerous or harmless."
>
> —Hertha James *(Conversations with Horses)*

**I**nvestigative Behavior is not a training technique; it is a *learning process*. Before I learned the term "Investigative Behavior," I called it "horses training themselves."

Free-roaming ponies investigate visitors to their home territory at Assateague Island National Seashore (figs. 12.1 A–C). The confidence with which they explore is not a result of training; it is built on life experiences they gained by investigating new things.

When these ponies were young, parents and older herd members provided guidance and reassurance. As they learned, their confidence grew along with their store of knowledge, so that fewer and fewer things were frightening. Domestic horses, having little scope to explore, often grow up more fearful of new situations.

The good news is that the experience of exploring seems to be more important than what horses get to investigate. There is much evidence that when we provide adult horses with opportunities for "remedial" learning, Investigative Behavior becomes a powerful way to turn their fear to curiosity and ultimately to confidence.

## Why Confidence Matters

Training is not the same thing as confidence. Training teaches horses the skills to do what we ask of them. Confidence is their trust in their own ability to perform those

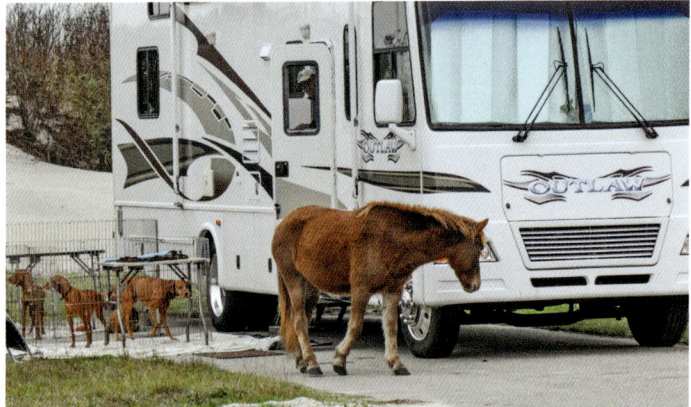

12.1 A  This pony wandered into a campsite, past the dogs, and strolled around to inspect the side and front of the RV.

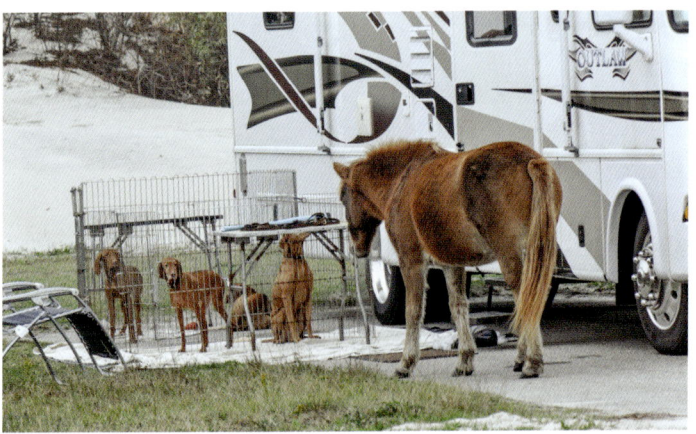

12.1 B  Then she turned around and went back to the dogs' pen, and stood quietly observing them for several minutes. The dogs, who barked at first, stopped barking and observed her in return.

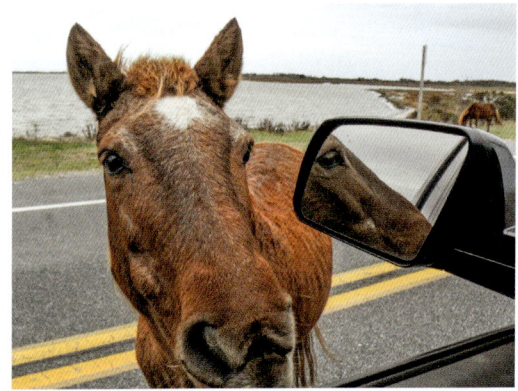

12.1 C  This pony's curiosity about the photographer's long telephoto lens overcame her initial caution about approaching the truck.

skills, and cope with new or stressful situations. When horses lack confidence, their training tends to fall apart when they're frightened even if we're there to guide them. In any case, I do not want a horse blindly dependent on my guidance. I'm not always with him and I'm not always right. We get maximum reliability when a horse is well-trained, trusts our leadership, *and* has confidence in himself. That is a thinking partner.

For instance, let's take two horses for a ride in the woods. One has confidence in himself; the other does not. We come around a bend and see a fallen tree across the trail. Both horses have the same skills; both are equally capable of stepping over a log and weaving through underbrush. But their reactions are not the same. The not-confident horse's body language says, "Scary thing ahead, time to go home!" The confident horse's body language says, "That's different. Let's check it out. What's the plan? Step over the log on the right, duck under the low branch, turn left, and squeeze between the saplings? Sure, I can do that."

The scenario could just as well involve taking a horse to a show or other event, or simply having some new object appear on his home turf. The point is that "stuff" happens, no matter how well trained horses are. Training alone does not prepare them to cope, but *we* can by encouraging Investigative Behavior. Every successful "adventure" our horses have with Investigative Behavior contributes to their knowledge and confidence. Every time we support their investigation we build their trust in us as Protector Leader.

## The Investigative Behavior Sequence

Horses start their investigation by assessing a situation from a distance. They observe, listen, and smell. If nothing appears too alarming, they ease in for a closer inspection. They might be satisfied with observation, or they might touch, taste, paw at, and even dismantle a new object.

Horses' emotional reactions vary in intensity. The casual demeanor of the Assateague ponies suggests that nothing they saw on that day worried them unduly. Brandy is going to demonstrate a more dramatic reaction, starting with the discovery of something alarming in her territory and culminating in an intense inspection involving all of her senses (figs. 12.2 A–O). You'll see that she does not home right in on the strange situation.

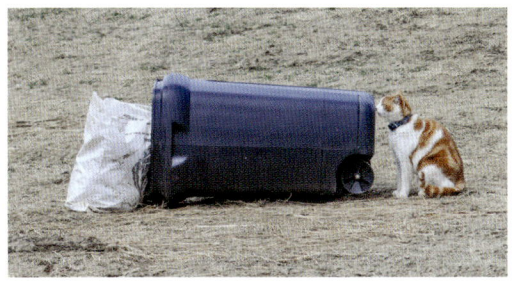

12.2 A  In the horses' paddock we placed an overturned trash can with bedding sacks spilling out. Columbus, the cat, is incidental.

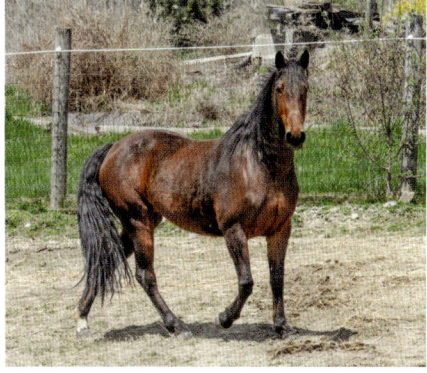

12.2 B  Brandy spots it as she returns from pasture, her alarm showing in her abrupt halt and head-high posture.

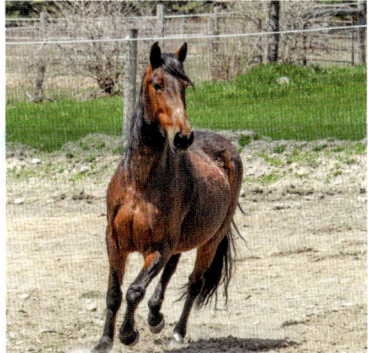

12.2 C  She starts around one side, keeping a careful eye on the suspicious situation.

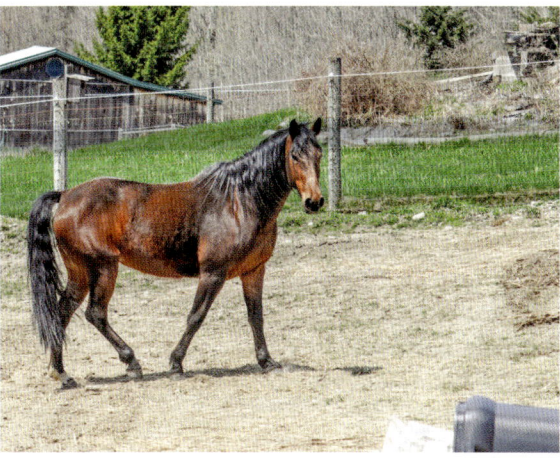

12.2 D  Then she goes around in the other direction, still keeping a cautious distance.

PART FIVE: INVESTIGATIVE BEHAVIOR EXPANDS HORSES' COMFORT ZONE — 143

She goes back and forth and around both ways, taking time to look it over from different directions. This is the opposite of the "walk straight up to it without stopping" approach that humans often expect of horses.

Brandy also demonstrates that ordinary things are worrisome when there is something "wrong" about them. She knows what a trash can is. She also knows that trash cans are supposed to be right side up and *not* in paddocks. Recognizing when something was different or out of place was a survival skill for her wild ancestors.

Although Sapphire makes only a

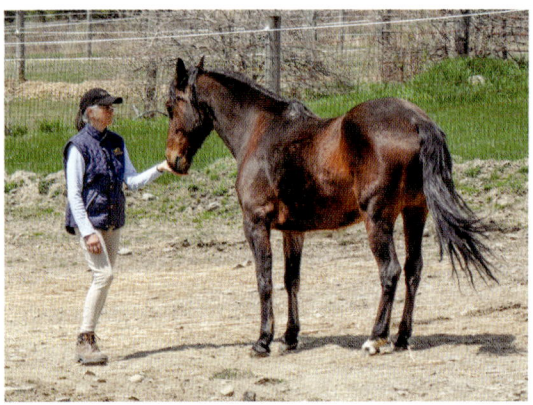

12.2 E  Brandy comes to me, her Protector Leader, for guidance. But this time I do not offer to investigate with her as I normally would.

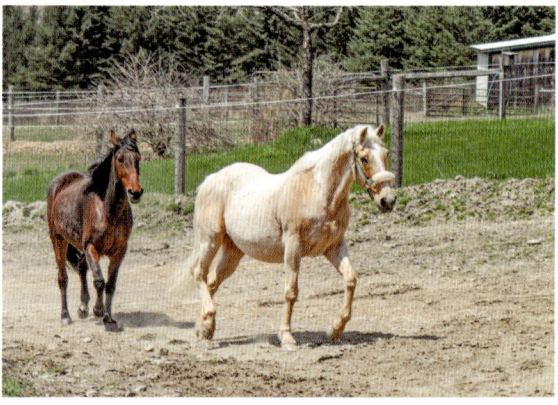

12.2 F  Reinforcements arrive. Brandy hangs behind Sapphire, trusting her older friend's judgment. Time elapsed so far is 6 minutes, 45 seconds.

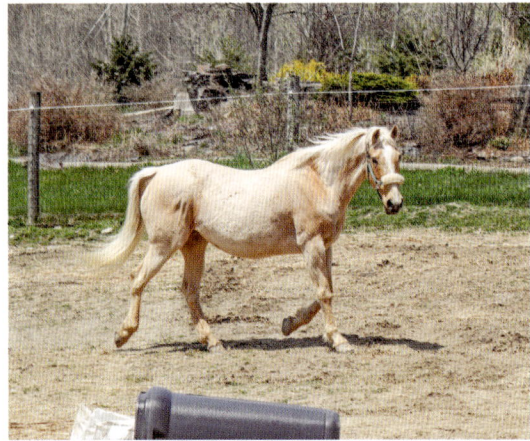

12.2 G  Sapphire looks the situation over but, not particularly concerned, circles on by to visit with the photographer. Notice what Brandy does in the next three minutes.

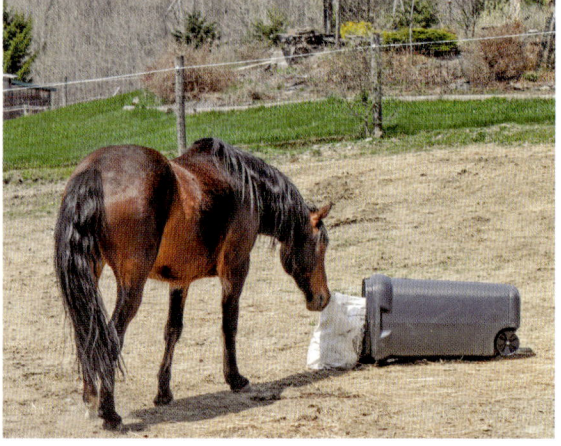

12.2 H  Reassured by Sapphire's lack of alarm, Brandy moves in for a closer inspection. First, she touches a bag.

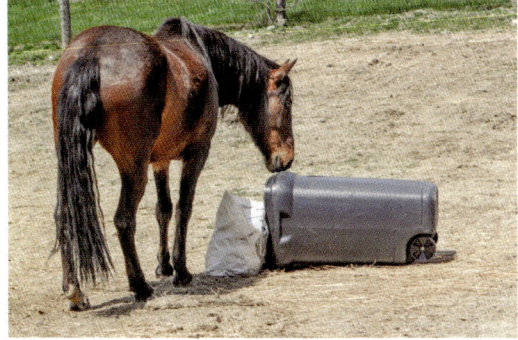

12.2 I  Next she touches the trash can.

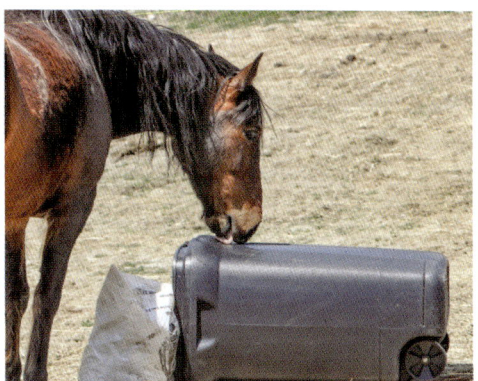

12.2 J  Brandy has her eye on the photographer as she licks the can, showing she is still aware of other things happening around her.

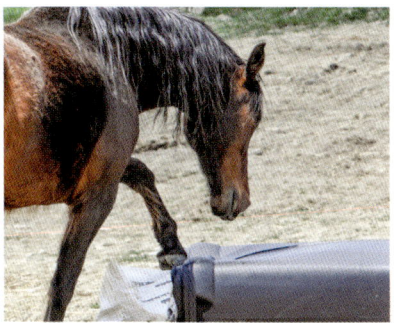

12.2 K  She paws at the can.

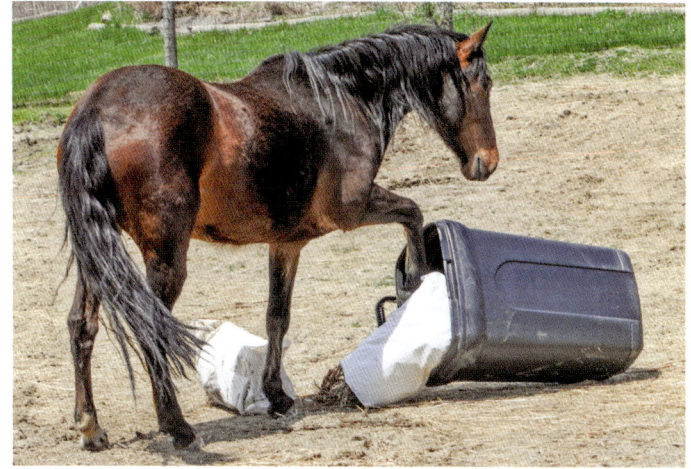

12.2 L  She digs the trash out of the can.

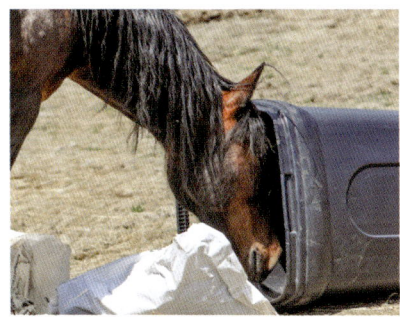

12.2 M  She peers into the can. By now, her manner is showing only curiosity, not anxiety.

12.2 N  She rolls the can around. The once scary object is now treated as a toy.

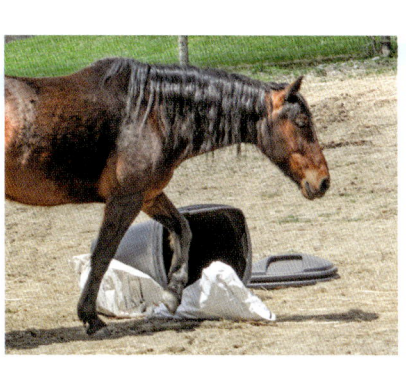

12.2 O  Brandy's demeanor is relaxed as she strolls away. The entire inspection took 9 minutes, 50 seconds from the moment she first saw the trash can.

PART FIVE: INVESTIGATIVE BEHAVIOR EXPANDS HORSES' COMFORT ZONE — 145

cameo appearance, her role is pivotal. She shows the influence of a trusted friend, the role we assume as Protector Leader. Once this trusted friend arrives, Brandy investigates more boldly and more quickly.

## A Successful Investigation

Brandy's investigation was successful, *not* because she touched and played with the trash can, but because she was relaxed and confident when she finished with it. In the course of her investigation she:

- Determined that something that looked scary at first turned out to be harmless.

- Learned new information to apply the next time she sees a trash can, plastic bags, or anything like it in a new place.

Every successful investigation helps shift a horse's default reaction in new situations further from, "That's scary; I'm leaving," and closer to, "That's interesting; let's check it out."

## Obedience vs. Learning

For many people, using Investigative Behavior requires a leap of faith. We have to trust our horses in a way that we are often told *not* to do.

It is a common assumption that when horses resist doing something, they are being disobedient and, if we allow it, the disobedience will escalate. Thus horses are pressured into situations that, from their perspective, are potentially unsafe. As pressure increases so does anxiety, until fear overwhelms curiosity, and the horse's priority shifts from investigation to escape. He is not trying to be disobedient; he just wants to be safe. If escape is not possible, the horse's fight reflex may be triggered, making his reactions dangerous. Many behavior problems are created by pressuring horses whose anxiety is mistaken for disobedience.

Even when a horse *goes* where we want, that does not mean he has learned anything or overcome his fear. Horses often obey in spite of anxiety. Horses also obey if they are more intimidated by the person than by the new situation. This can look impressive until the horse encounters something scarier than the person. That's the person most in danger of being bucked off or mowed down when the horse panics.

When a horse is investigating, your goal is learning, not obedience. When he has learned what he needs to know, *then* he is ready to return his attention to your agenda.

## Horses See Things Humans Do Not

As prey animals, horses are always monitoring their surroundings for possible danger. Anything unusual can be cause for concern. When they are accused of reacting to "nothing," it is likely they have spotted something that escaped human notice. This is not just because they have better peripheral vision than we do. Their vision also functions differently than ours.

Horses are often described as nearsighted, giving the impression that they see less than we do. This is misleading. Their visual acuity actually ranges from about 20/30 to 20/60, better than humans are required to have for a driver's license.[91] The significant differences in vision come from the fact that horses are partially colorblind, the equivalent of a person with red-green colorblindness. For them as prey animals, this is an asset, not a liability.

Remember those rods and cones we heard about in science class? Cones allow us to see color. Rods relate to depth perception and shape recognition. Fewer cones for color means more rods. The result is that horses spot shapes better than we do because they are less fooled by color camouflage (fig. 12.3). They are also better at detecting variations in texture that might signify unreliable footing.[92 93]

My optician, who also happens to be red-green colorblind, described how this works for him. When he hunts, he is the first person to spot a deer. The shape, he says, "jumps out at him." Think about that! He is also a better tracker because his eyes pick up small disturbances on the ground that other people do not see.

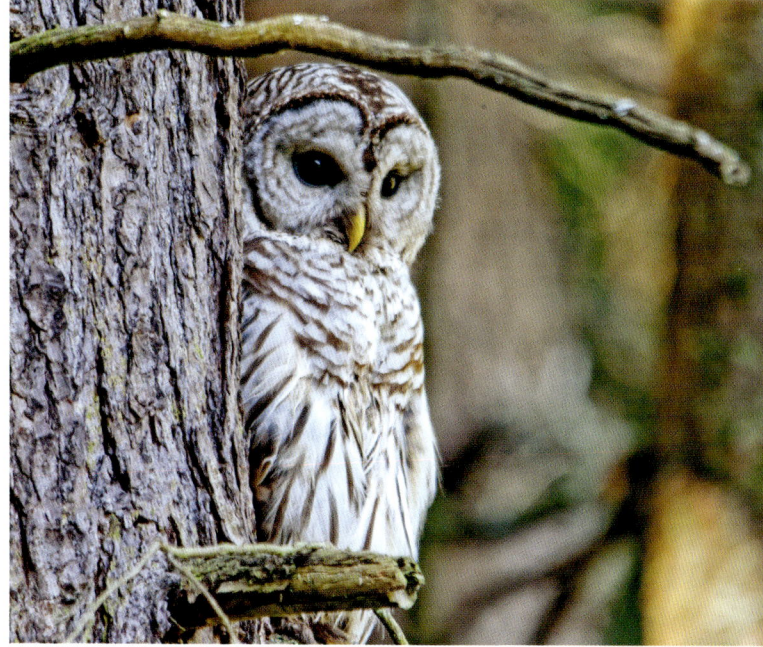

Horses' depth perception and ability to judge distance are also excellent. You see it when they squeak through tight spaces (fig. 12.4), sometimes at high speed, and every time a horse sails over a jump. Even when a rider sets a horse up with a good takeoff spot, the horse must calculate how high and how wide to jump.

## Horses See Things in a Different Context Than We Do

While we tend to focus on a specific object, horses seem to notice the bigger context. This is one reason they might spook at the same object when they see it from a different direction: the context

12.3 Most of us would ride right past this barred owl dozing in a tree, and never see her. Our horses, not fooled by her color camouflage, would spot her *shape* easily.

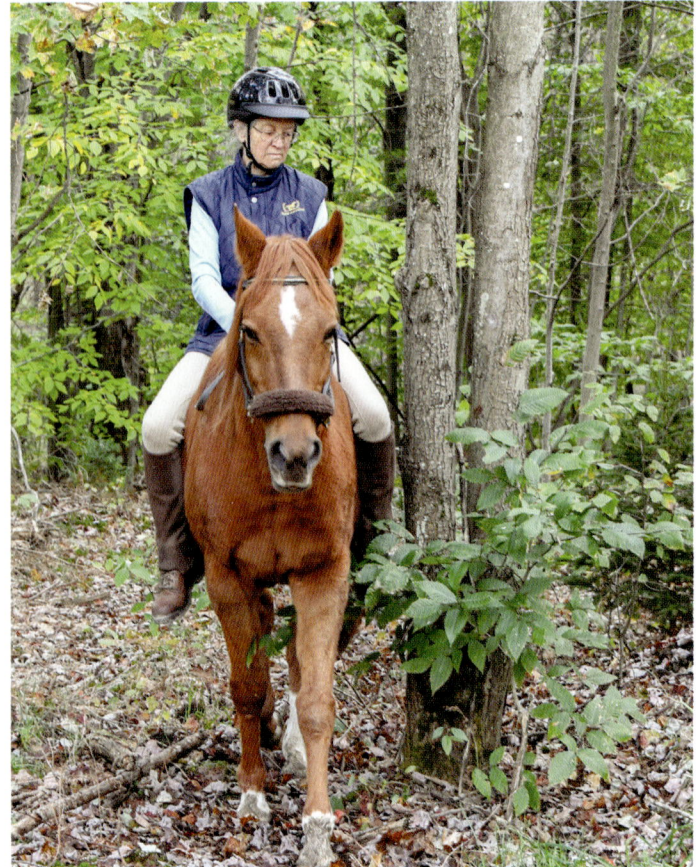

12.4 Bronzz squeezes between debris on the ground and a tree trunk with about an inch to spare for my leg. He has scraped my knee only once in 21 years, and that was when I insisted he squeeze between two trees where we really did not fit.

surrounding the object is different. They might also spook at the same object from another direction because the object itself looks different from another angle. Both of these scenarios reflect the fact that horses are visually observant, and have good memories for what they have seen. (It was once believed that when horses see something with only one eye, they cannot recognize it with the other eye. Research studies have demonstrated that this is not so. [94])

Then there is the "something is out of place" scenario that Brandy demonstrated earlier in this chapter (see p. 143) when she startled at the tipped-over trash can in her paddock. For their wild ancestors, survival required being suspicious of anything new, out of place, rearranged, or reoriented. Nature gave horses incredible visual memories so they recognize these changes. When a horse shies at a trash can, we might hear, "Stupid horse, it's just a trash can." A more accurate reaction would be, "Smart horse, you noticed we moved it."

Bronzz demonstrated this trait one day when our ride took us along a trail where my husband was cutting firewood. Bronzz didn't bat an eyelash at the noisy chain saw, but he went sideways past the newly cut and stacked wood, watching it with great suspicion. He remembered that the last time we took that trail, there were no logs piled beside it, just a fallen tree. This same visual memory ensures that he can unerringly find any obscure trail we have ever taken, no matter how long ago, or how overgrown it might be now.

The bottom line is that horses see things we do not. Add to that their superior senses of hearing and smell, and it is very difficult indeed to ever prove a horse has spooked at "nothing" (fig. 12.5). Protector Leaders trust their horses' perception instead, and allow them to observe or investigate as needed.

The benefit of our horses' powers of perception is that they are not necessarily taken by surprise even when we are. As Bronzz and I strolled through the woods one day, a pair of ruffed grouse exploded out of the underbrush right in front of his face. These are large birds who make a lot of noise when threatened. I spooked. Bronzz did not. Their color camouflage would not have fooled him.

## Investigative Behavior Study: Retraining Jumpers

Although Investigative Behavior has many practical applications, there seems to be remarkably little study of it. The first study I found, however, was very practical, and was conducted by a researcher who is also a skilled rider.

Angelo Telatin has international show jumping credentials and has competed his horse in hunter classes *without a bridle*. He observed that riders often increase their aids as a horse approaches a jump, especially if the horse shows even a hint of hesitation. This is what most of us were taught to do if we took jumping lessons. I can still hear my first jumping instructor yelling, "Leg, leg. Use your crop, and mean it!"

Telatin suggested that the pressure of increasing the aids could trigger the horse's fight or flight response and contribute to refusals. He hypothesized that horses would jump more reliably if allowed to investigate jumps first. Since jumps represent a fairly consistent set of shapes, colors, smells, materials, and textures, horses could generalize the information they learned at home to jumps in competition. To test this hypothesis he supervised the reschooling of 50 horses with a history of refusals.

During the retraining process, the rider did *not* increase the aids when a horse slowed or even stopped in front of a jump. Instead, the horse was allowed to investigate without pressure for as long as he wished (figs. 12.6 A & B). If a horse was too afraid to approach the jump at all (more likely with older horses), the rider dismounted and led the horse to it. A more experienced horse accompanied

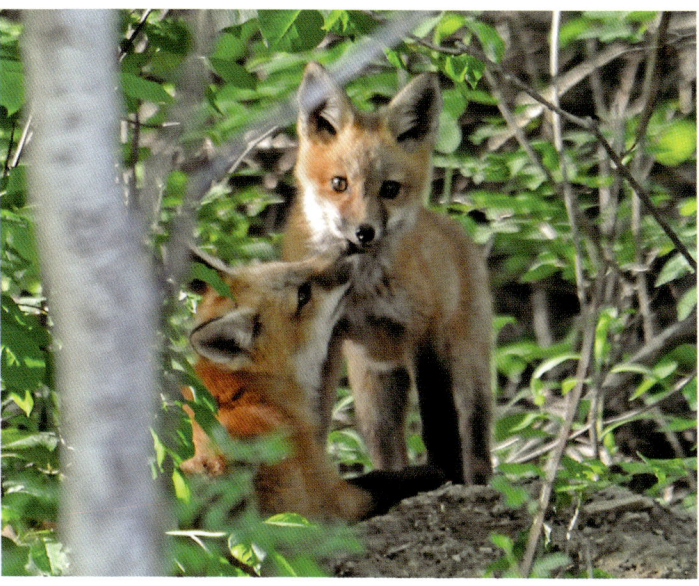

12.5 A horse would not only see these red fox kits playing in the underbrush long before most people would, he would also hear and smell them.

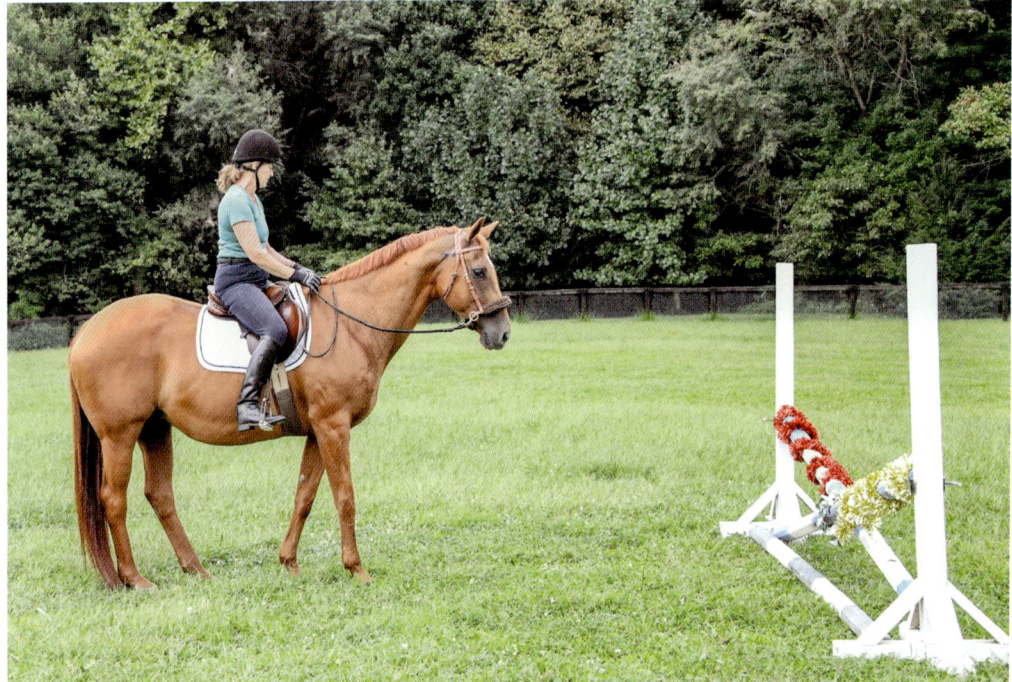

**12.6 A** Gracie hesitates at the strange sight of a cross-rail decorated with colored tinsel garlands. Dani waits quietly until Gracie offers to step forward.

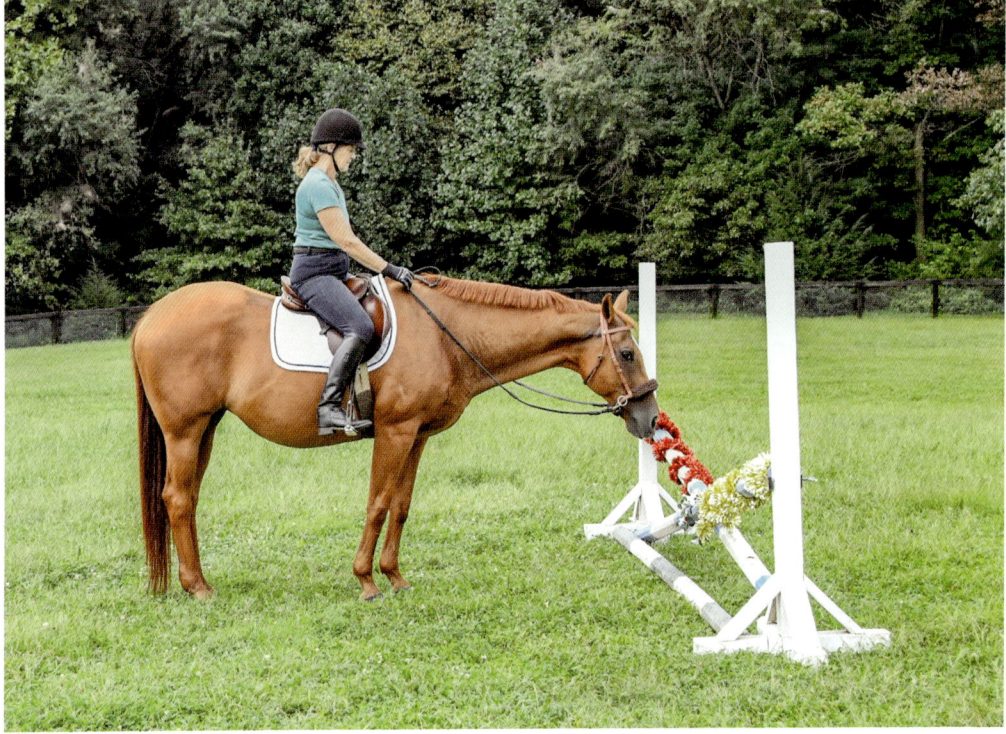

**12.6 B** Dani's posture is relaxed and her reins are soft as Gracie inspects the jump. The horse, not the rider, decides when the inspection is complete.

them, if necessary. When the horse's investigation was complete, the rider tried the jump again.

## Practical Application

After six months, the progress of the reschooled horses was evaluated by having them jump a course in a competition situation. Nearly all of the younger horses (eight and under) completed their course with *no* refusals. Older horses, who had more time to build up negative experiences, had a lower success rate.

This emphasizes that taking time to make sure horses' early experiences are positive is a good investment in future reliability. It also validates that when you acquire an older horse, extra time and patience may be needed to overcome prior negative experiences. Telatin observed that each horse's jumping success was influenced by his rider's ability to allow Investigative Behavior, suggesting this is an important leadership skill.[95]

## Other Reasons for Jump Refusals

Horses may also refuse jumps because of pain or anticipation of pain (a poorly fitted saddle or rider catching him in the mouth); horse or **rider off balance**; a **jump beyond the horse's training, ability, or confidence level**; or poor footing. Investigative Behavior is not a substitute for addressing other issues.

## Long-Term Benefits of Investigative Behavior

Long-term studies on the impact of Investigative Behavior do not seem to exist yet, but I have personal experience with its effectiveness.

I discovered the principles of Investigative Behavior the first year I had Bronzz. It was self-defense, pure and simple. Bronzz grew up on a quiet farm on a dead end road. When he was four years old, I moved him to a boarding stable on a busy road amidst a lot of noisy activity—not the safest place to ride an athletic young Arabian prone to flamboyant spooks.

Bronzz's lead-line manners, however, were rock solid. He had learned before weaning, at his mama's side while she was led. Since his breeder was a Protector Leader, his mares were calm and trusting with him, modeling for their off-spring that being led was a safe, normal part of life. Fritz's lead-line training instilled the rules that the horse must never pull on the lead or bump the handler, so it was second nature for Bronzz to watch out for me and yield to pressure.

Since I could safely lead Bronzz anywhere, we went for walks when there was no one else to ride with. The whole point of our walks was to let Bronzz see the sights, so I was relaxed and *laissez-faire*. Bronzz was constantly amazed and amusing. It soon became clear that he got over most of his anxieties with no help from me. Some of our adventures are described in chapter 14 (see p. 166).

The more Bronzz saw, the fewer things worried him. Since this approach worked equally well under saddle, it became my standard procedure. As Bronzz's confidence grew, observation replaced spook-and-bolt as his default response to surprises. This has made it possible for me to *enjoy* taking Bronzz many places that I would otherwise have found nerve-wracking at best.

The latest proof of Bronzz's confidence came when we wanted photos illustrating the rider's role when a horse is engaged in Investigative Behavior (chapter 13—p. 154). We were unable to find *anything* that alarmed him. I had to borrow a friend's horse.

My sister Dani's experience with Investigative Behavior goes back even further than mine. Her horses' early jump training always included courses of jumps of 18 inches (a half-meter) or less, incorporating as many unusual objects as she could safely assemble. After being allowed to look them over, they jumped hay bales, brush piles, and jumps decorated with things like balloons, streamers, pumpkins, cornstalks, cones, flowers, and barrels. Thus, they learned to jump strange things on their home territory, while developing the skills needed for negotiating courses, with jumps so low that they were neither physically nor mentally stressful. By the time they competed in eventing (which involves cross-country and stadium jumping), they confidently jumped whatever was asked of them.

This illustrates Angelo Telatin's points that horses trained without pressure learn to jump more reliably, and those who jump with confidence at home generalize those skills to jumping in other settings.

## ⇥ Summary

Investigative Behavior is a learning process in which horses' natural curiosity prompts them to explore novel situations and objects. As they do so, they apply knowledge they already have, and gather new information to apply in the future. An investigation might be calm and cursory, or it might start with a dramatic startle reaction and culminate in an intense investigation involving all of a horse's senses. An investigation is complete when the horse is relaxed and confident with the new situation.

People often interrupt horses' investigations with pressure, thus stifling their curiosity and triggering their flight/fight response. As a result many people are unaware that horses even have a natural curiosity, or that allowing them to exercise it can reduce anxiety and build confidence.

## THINGS TO TRY

- Place a strange object in a safely fenced area such as paddock, pasture, or arena. It must be something indestructible or expendable that the horse cannot hurt himself on, and he must have plenty of room to get a comfortable distance away from it. (A stall is too small.) We have found old stuffed toy animals to be a source of fascination.

- Position yourself outside the fence and simply observe what he does. Do not interfere. Does he investigate, ignore, or pretend to ignore it while eyeing it cautiously?

- If he investigates, how does he approach it? Directly or circling? What senses does he use? How long does it take until he is bored with it?

- If he does not investigate, is it because he's too anxious? Try a less scary object. If he is bored, try something different. Or try putting hay or treats near the object.

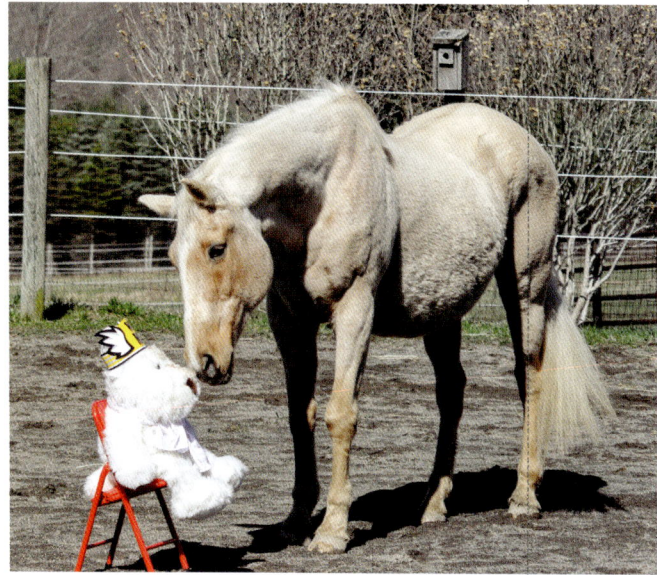

12.7 Sapphire, still curious at age 34, is intrigued by a toy bear wearing a cardboard hat. (I did determine that the folding chair was not a safe object of investigation since a horse could get a leg caught in it.)

- Try interspersing hay and/or treats among various strange objects to encourage horses to interact with the objects as they seek out the food.

*chapter 13*
# Encouraging Investigative Behavior

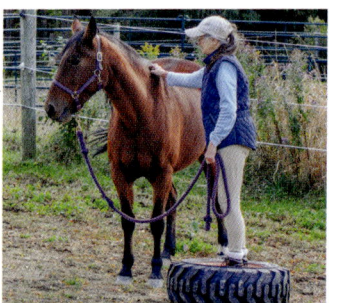

> "When we use ropes and small pens, we have removed the horse's primary way of feeling safe again – the ability to move away and reassess a situation."
>
> —Hertha James *(Conversations with Horses)*

In the last chapter, Brandy demonstrated how horses use Investigative Behavior on their own. This chapter shows how you can provide guidance that encourages Investigative Behavior while reinforcing your role as Protector Leader.

Many people already use Investigative Behavior. It is what we're doing when we let a horse observe a strange object or inspect a new jump or trail obstacle; or when we take a horse to his first show with no expectations to compete, just letting him watch the action instead.

## Your Role as Protector Leader

Most of us have been taught to be very much in charge when riding or handling a horse. Sapphire, as you saw in the last chapter, did *not* take charge or direct Brandy's actions in any way. She went off to visit with the photographer. The simple fact that Sapphire was not concerned provided the reassurance Brandy needed.

We are not quite so *laissez-faire* when we are handling or riding a horse, because we do not want him to decide he'd rather just leave and forget the whole thing. Our challenge is to direct the horse's *attention* rather than his *actions*.

Once he starts his investigation, let him focus on it.

Patience is the essential ingredient. You must accept that your agenda is on hold until the horse completes his investigation on his own schedule, not yours. It may seem that a horse is taking a long time while you are doing nothing. When I check my watch, however, I find that the time elapsed is shorter than it seems. People often spend far longer circling a horse past a scary object over and over. The result is just a tired horse who learned little or nothing useful.

In this chapter, I will demonstrate using Investigative Behavior in two situations, one in which the horse is led, and one ridden. Although we planned these scenarios in order to get photographs, the procedure is the same whether we set up a situation or it catches us by surprise.

## Investigative Behavior: General Guidelines

- **Lead by example**, conveying relaxed confidence.

- **Position the horse on the edge of his comfort zone**. That is, near enough to be concerned and focus his attention on the object or situation, but not frightened enough to try to escape.

- **Allow investigation with no pressure or distractions**, including verbal coaxing, tight lead, whip, twirling rope, or treats. A horse must *never* be tied or otherwise feel trapped.

- **Allow approach and retreat**. He may back away or walk around near the object, but not leave the vicinity.

- **Stay tuned in to the horse's emotional state** at all times. If the horse's fear level increases, back off immediately. Relieving the pressure on a frightened horse is not "letting him get away" with anything. It demonstrates that he can trust your leadership, and it helps keep you safe. If necessary, rethink how to make the situation less threatening and start over another time.

- **Plan for safety**. After all, your goal is to convince the horse that there really is no danger. A "too-easy" challenge builds confidence; but when a horse is overwhelmed, he has just learned that the situation is scary after all.

## Investigative Behavior on the Lead

### Skills Needed
- **The horse must have reliable lead-line manners** including respect for the handler's personal space. When a horse normally requires a whip, chain, or other special control devices, leading and handling practice with Friendly Body Language (see chapter 10—p. 113) is

essential before risking a situation that further challenges the horse's self-control or your ability to manage him.

- **You must have good horse-handling skills**, including the ability to give clear cues and to read a horse's body language and emotional state. This is necessary to judge his anxiety level, anticipate his actions, and respond safely to unexpected moves.

## Equipment

An ordinary nylon, leather, or rope halter is suitable. A long lead (10 to 15 feet) is needed for maneuvering room. A lunge line is too long and poses a risk of entangling someone. I do not necessarily wear a helmet when handling a trained horse I know, but a helmet is always a good idea. It is essential if a horse is particularly reactive, or any other factor

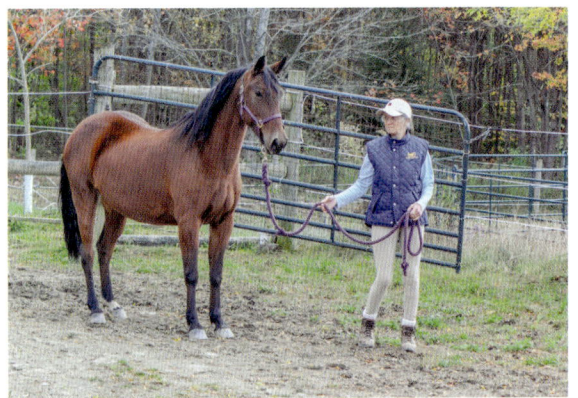

13.1 A  Brandy alerts on the strange object. I stop with her.

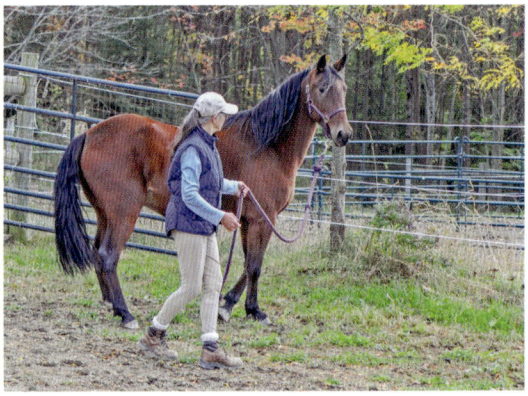

13.1 B  She circles behind me to observe it, a sign that she trusts my protection.

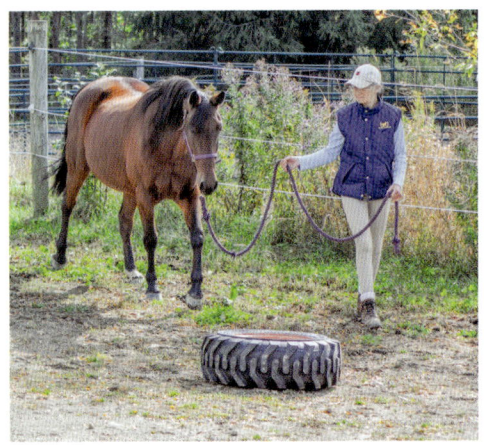

13.1 C  As she moves closer, I go with her.

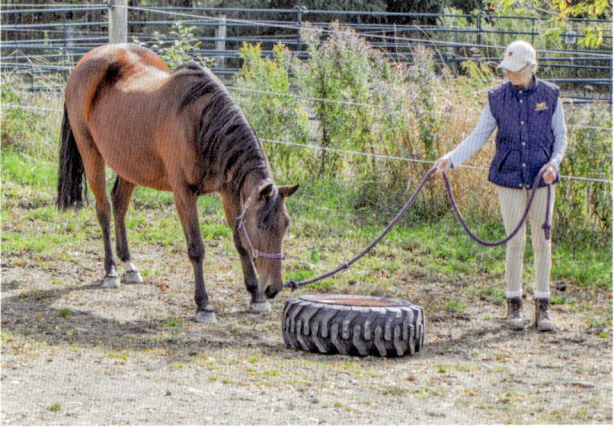

13.1 D  Her weight is back, ready for a quick getaway as her whiskers make contact.

creates a riskier situation. Sturdy boots are a given.

## Brandy and the Tractor Tire

It gets harder to find something that alarms Brandy, but again we have the "it does not belong here" scenario. If the tire were on the tractor, she would not have looked twice.

I move with Brandy as she investigates, staying closer to the object than she is. This demonstrates my leadership, and keeps me out of her flight path if she were to spook. I make no attempt to control her actions, reassure, coax, or reward her. All of those would distract her from investigating. Instead, I let her show me when she is ready to approach and when she needs to retreat (figs. 13.1 A–I).

*My lead line never goes tight.* Only

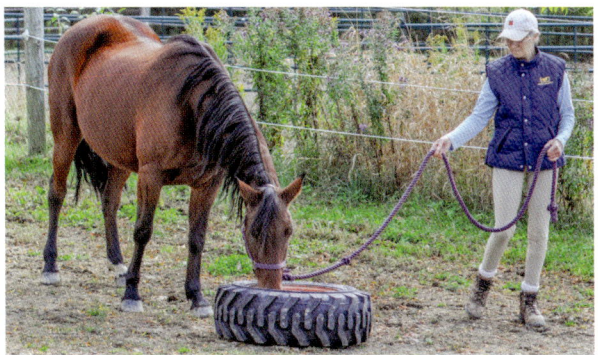

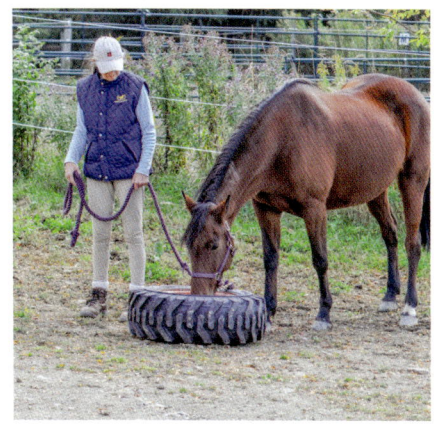

13.1 F She circles around, coming at the tire from a different angle, and moves in for a taste.

13.1 E Now she is comfortable enough to touch it. This has taken exactly three minutes since she first saw it.

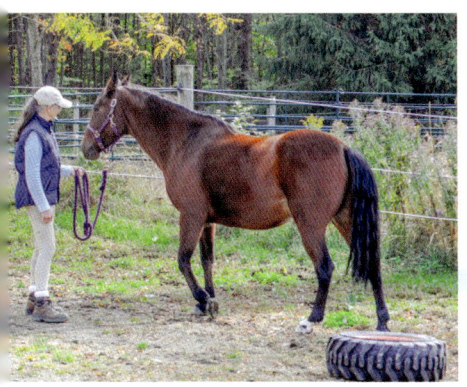

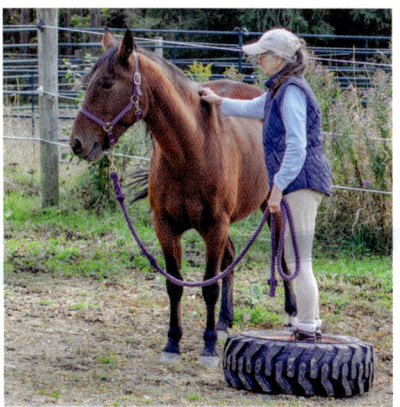

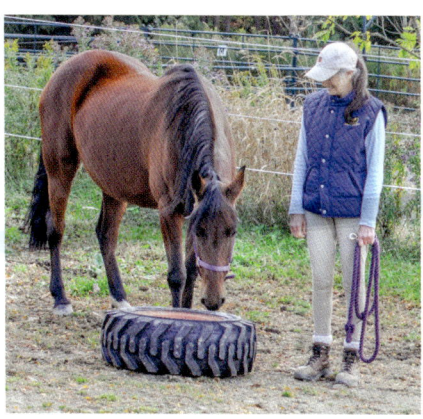

13.1 G Retreat and return is a normal part of the process and may happen several times. Some people lead horses to the object and away, but I prefer to let the horse show me what he needs to do.

13.1 H Now that Brandy has finished investigating, I reward her relaxation with a scratch on the withers. Four and a half minutes have elapsed so far.

13.1 I Another retreat and return, this time off the lead. In six minutes and 40 seconds, Brandy is ready to play with the once-scary object.

PART FIVE: INVESTIGATIVE BEHAVIOR EXPANDS HORSES' COMFORT ZONE — 157

if the horse attempts to leave the area should you put pressure on the lead.

## When *Not* to Get Ahead of the Horse

There is an exception to the rule of staying closer to the object of investigation, and that is when you want a horse to cross something, like a tarp, ditch, or creek. In that case, you should stay beside the horse's shoulder to be safely out of the way if the horse rushes across or takes a flying leap (figs. 13.2 A & B). Never cross something like a ditch or small creek ahead of a horse. If he is anxious, he might assume that the safest landing place is right where you are standing. I learned this the hard way.

## Investigative Behavior Under Saddle

### How It Goes Wrong

We would not normally plan to have a horse investigate something strange while we're on his back, but such circumstances often arise while we're riding. Although we can usually turn them into learning experiences that enhance our partnership, they are often turned into fights that undermine our credibility and create unnecessary resistance.

### Big Horse vs. Small Ditch

A few years ago, a friend asked me to accompany her when she rode her young Warmblood on his first expedition outside an arena. All went well for the first tenth of a mile. Then we encountered a ditch. It was a small ditch, barely more than a grassy swale. The tall gray Percheron-cross could have stepped over it easily, but he stopped dead, as if it were a deep, dark chasm.

Barbara firmly legged him on. He sucked back. She used her crop. He backed up farther. At Barbara's direction, I rode my mount, a sensible older mare, across the ditch and started up the hill on the far side. Faced with the prospect of being left "alone" in a scary situation, the gray got even more agitated, dancing in front of the ditch.

I rode the mare back, and we waited. For 15 frustrating minutes, Barbara did as she'd been taught, urging the horse forward with legs, crop, and voice. She tried crossing the ditch at different places. No go. The big gray danced to and fro, sashayed side to side, acting as if the ditch were surrounded by an invisible force field he could not penetrate. By the time he started humping his back, revving up to buck, I was worried enough about Barbara's safety to risk insulting her with a suggestion I knew would sound radical. She was anxious enough to agree, and she implemented the new plan perfectly.

She let her mount back away from the ditch until he was standing still, now focused on the ditch instead of escape. This placed him at the edge of his comfort

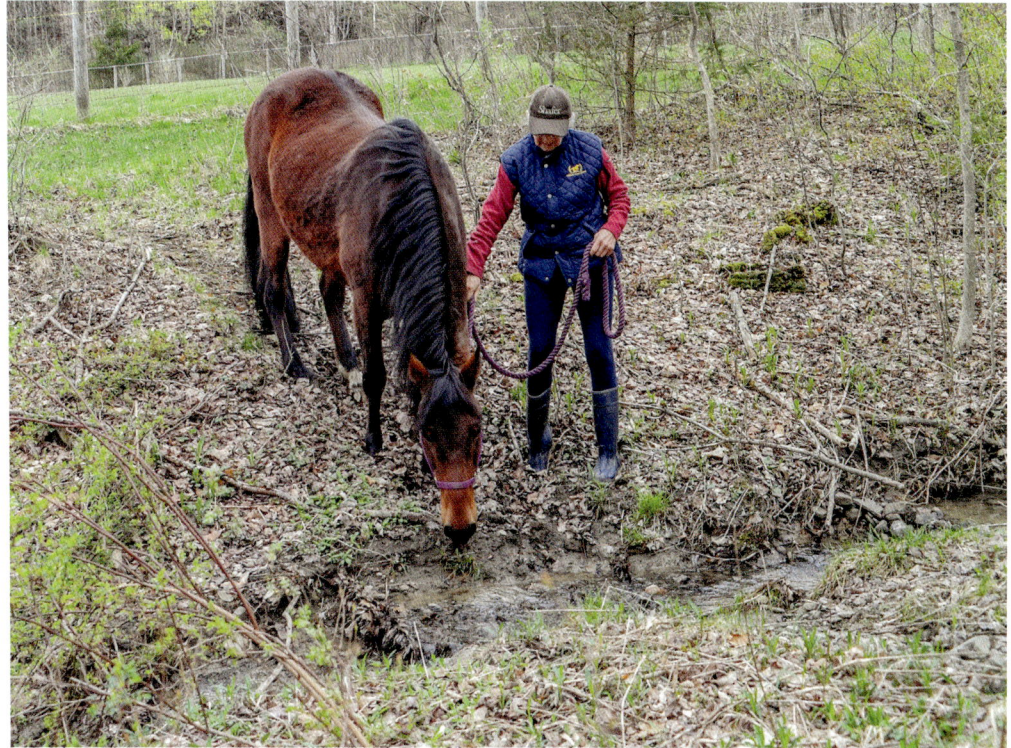

**13.2 A** I wait at Brandy's side as she investigates the creek.

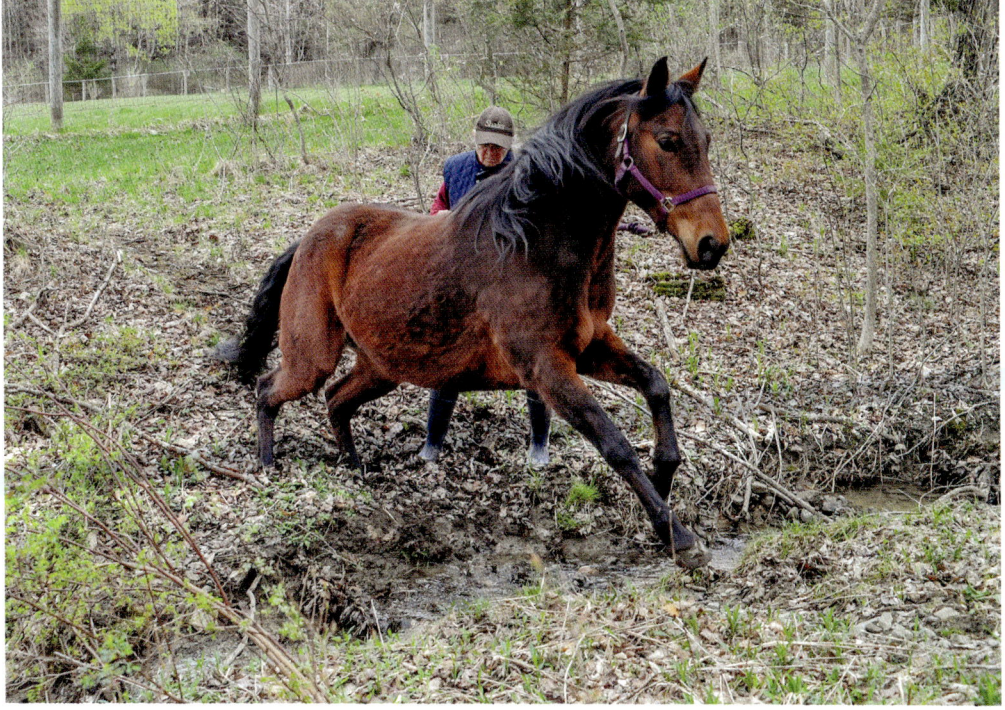

**13.2 B** I am safely out of her way as she leaps across.

zone, instead of pushing him into his anxiety zone. Sitting quietly, one hand holding mane in case he took a flying leap, Barbara did nothing except reposition him to face the ditch when he tried to turn away. She waited. He stared at the ditch. In less than five minutes, with no further drama, he strolled calmly across. Barbara laughingly observed that the hardest part of that program was doing nothing.

## When a Human Is Not Acting Like a Leader

Variations on this scenario are played out over and over. A horse is worried and needs a few minutes to investigate. The person interprets this "balking" as disobedience, and is determined to make the horse do as he was told *now* because she fears that if she lets him "get away with" hesitating, he will become increasingly disobedient and out of control. In the end, the fight was not over whether the horse would cross the ditch or not. It was over whether the horse would cross the ditch now or five minutes from now.

From the horse's perspective, the human is not acting like a leader. When a horse indicates that something is alarming, other horses take him seriously. No one, not even a higher-ranking horse, forces him into a scary situation. A horse's assessment of this dynamic might be summed up as, rider is a bully who is too clueless to listen when he tries to warn her of possible danger. At the next ditch or other scary situation, he is already braced for a fight.

As Protector Leaders we can have it both ways. We acknowledge his concern by allowing him to investigate. We still decide where we're going and what we're doing as soon as the horse gets done "training himself." Our payoff is that each new ditch is crossed with more confidence, less hesitation. When Barbara and I returned from the ride described above, her horse did not hesitate at the ditch. Instead, he marched right up to it and leaped across.

## Skills Needed

The same guidelines apply as for Investigative Behavior on the lead. The corollary skills needed are:

- **The horse must respond reliably to basic riding cues.**

- **The rider should be skilled and confident enough to stay physically relaxed while mentally alert**, able to redirect the horse as needed, and avoid giving unintentional cues. This requires a secure seat, steady hands, and good self-awareness. Holding mane or leather to avoid bumping a horse's mouth is prudent and considerate, but a nervous rider clinging for dear life puts herself in jeopardy while making her horse more anxious. Note: When in doubt, dismount! Most horses seem to feel safer with their person on the ground, and people are naturally calmer when they are not worried their mount will dodge out from under them. The exceptions are horses who are better controlled mounted than on the ground, and situations where we might actually be in more danger if we dismount.

## Bella and the Big Bad Ball

Our demo horse for Investigative Behavior under saddle is Bella (figs. 13.3 A–J). When Karen rescued her five years prior, Bella was emotionally shut down and unpredictably fearful. She has come a long way but remains hyper-alert to possible danger. It was easy to find things that she needed to investigate before approaching. If it sounds unkind to deliberately present her with such situations, remember that we are not out to scare her. Our goal is to engage her curiosity and offer her opportunities to discover that the world is not so scary after all. Her body language shows she is alert and cautious, but not overwhelmed with anxiety.

Bella looks over to Karen multiple times, as if assessing her trusted owner's reaction to the situation, much like Brandy checked out Sapphire's reaction to the overturned trash can.

I do not allow Bella to circle away from the object as Brandy did when she was inspecting the tire. This might work differently for someone else, but in my experience, when I allow horses to circle under saddle, they get busier moving than investigating. I do let them back up so they do not feel trapped, and I also let them pause and turn their head away, which Bella does multiple times. This seems to serve the same function as circling. Possibly they are "testing" what the strange object (or creature) will do if they do not appear to be watching it. This would be logical since some predators freeze when looked at, then creep forward when the prey appears not to be watching. Or they might be thinking things over, or "taking a break" from a situation that is emotionally stressful. The important factor is that the horse must never feel trapped.

We should always stop at a point when the horse is confident and relaxed, so that is her take-away message. For Bella, touching the ball was a big accomplishment. A good time to stop and let her process what she learned.

Bella completed her investigation of the ball with no sudden moves. If the wind had rolled the ball, however, she might have backed up speedily or tried to spin and bolt. That is why it is not normally advisable to set up mounted Investigative Behavior situations on purpose.

## Investigative Behavior Compared to Desensitizing, Bomb-Proofing, Spook-Busting, and Flooding

Investigative Behavior is unique in that it engages horses' curiosity and actively involves them in observing, exploring, and learning.

The term "desensitizing," when used by a skilled behaviorist like Dr. Sue McDonnell, means getting a horse accustomed to something ("habituated" is the official term) by "repeated exposure below the threshold for escape or panic."[96]

It happens all the time without human intervention as horses are exposed to different life circumstances. My horses, for instance, are used to loud noises because we have neighbors who enjoy target practice with loud guns. The horses got over their initial alarm on their own, as do all guest horses. At the boarding stable where Bronzz and Sapphire lived, all the horses became accustomed to the

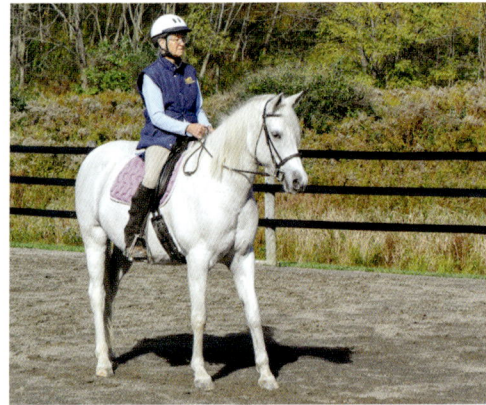

13.3 A Bella watches Karen roll a ball into the arena. She is leaning back, poised to move. I sit quietly with relaxed legs and soft reins, but ready to "catch" her with leg and rein if she turns.

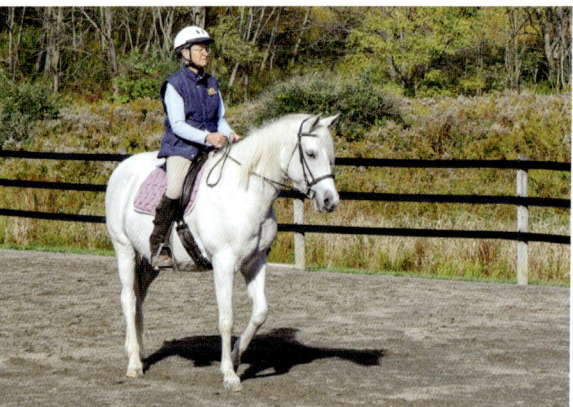

13.3 B I allow Bella to back up so she won't feel trapped. Next she tried to turn left. I straightened her with gentle right rein and left leg, then immediately relaxed again. Quiet cues are essential. Large, abrupt motions over-correct and make a horse more anxious.

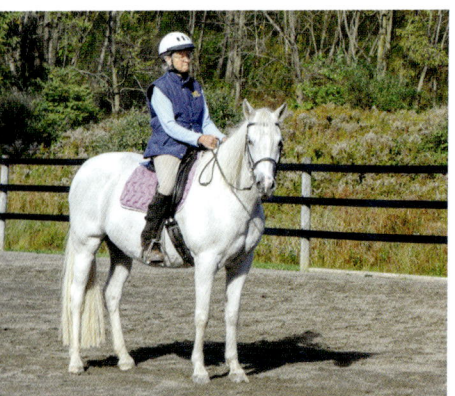

13.3 C Bella looks toward Karen, who is now standing next to the photographer.

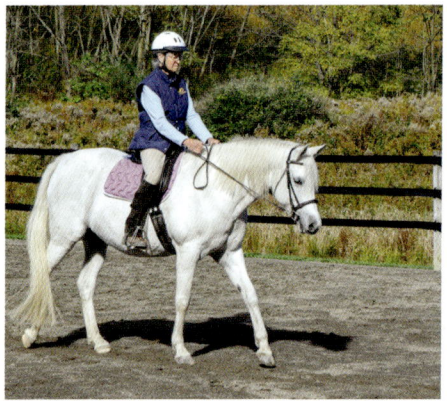

13.3 D Bella starts toward the ball, watching it carefully.

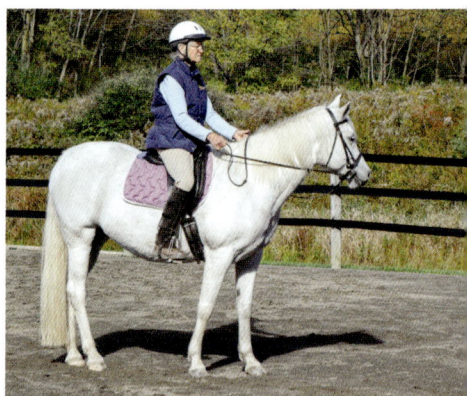

13.3 E She halts and looks away.

resident cows and guinea hen, railroad trains that ran adjacent to the farm, big trucks from the gravel pit up the road, sirens from emergency vehicles, and the noisy four-wheeler used to deliver meals to pasture-kept horses.

The danger of programs designed for bomb-proofing, spook-busting, de-spooking, and so on is that, if not applied with great care, they can push a horse so far out of his comfort zone that he thinks only of escape, and learning shuts down.

The most treacherous technique is one in which a horse is "flooded" with a scary stimulus, such as a plastic bag in the

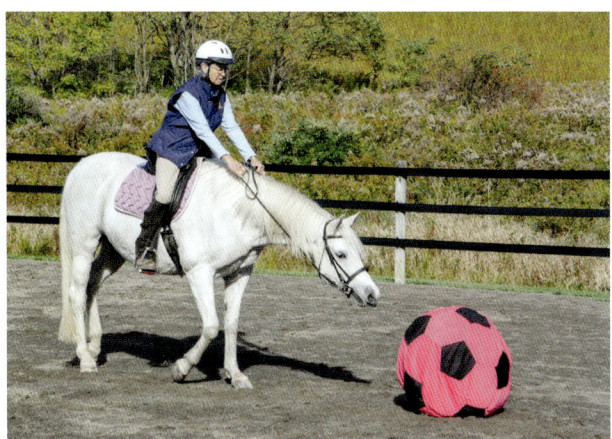

13.3 F  Bella steps forward, halts, and looks away twice more. Then she stretches her nose toward the ball.

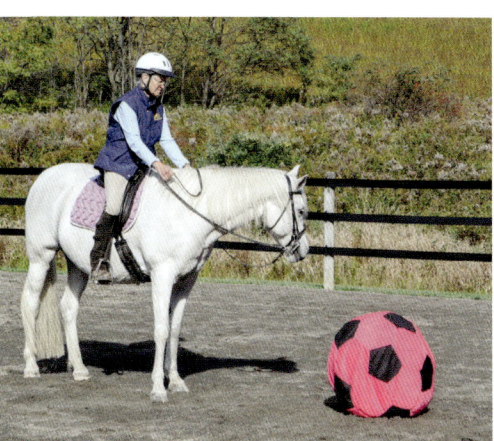

13.3 G  She looks away again.

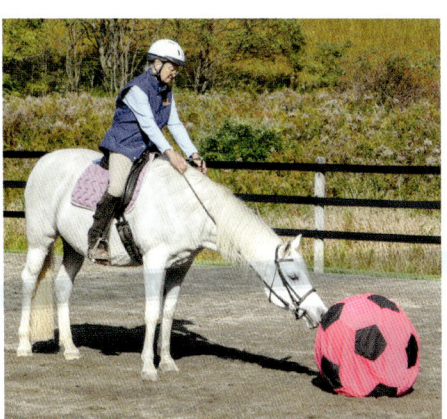

13.3 H  After more observation of the ball, and another look to Karen, Bella stretches her nose forward, tests with her whiskers, and touches the ball.

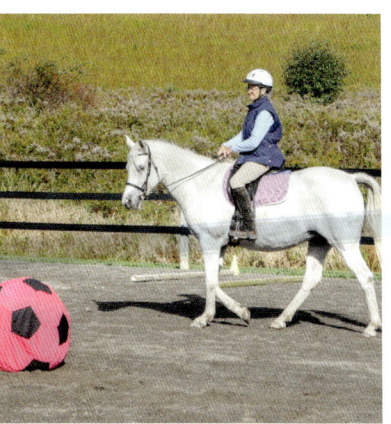

13.3 I  I walk Bella around the ball once in each direction for further observation.

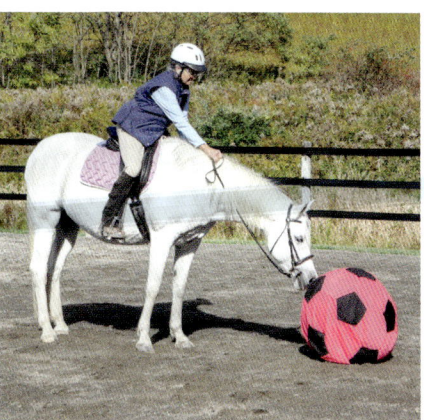

13.3 J  This time she is more relaxed with the ball, and touches it firmly enough to move it.

face, until he stops reacting. Though the horse may appear to have "gotten over" his fear, it can mean that he has been overwhelmed and shut down emotionally. This is the beginning of "Learned Helplessness," a dangerous condition described in chapter 9 (p. 109).

## Why Investigative Behavior Is Underused

Investigative Behavior is not typically described as part of good horsemanship. One reason is that horsemanship instruction tends to focus on controlling horses' actions.

Investigative Behavior, in contrast, *engages* horses' minds. We must be willing to give horses the freedom to *use* their minds. The principles that support Investigative Behavior are contrary to many common ideas of horsemanship, but research shows they are solidly based on how horses think, feel, learn, and behave:

- **Horses are curious.** This is often not apparent because horses who anticipate pressure go into escape mode as soon as they see something that worries them.

- **Horses learn in ways other than repetition or conditioned response.** They also learn by observing, investigating, experimenting, and generalizing information.

- **Anxiety is a common cause of problems.** I've heard that it does not matter what a horse is feeling, he has to do his job like anyone else. Humane issues aside, the flaw in this logic is that horses' actions, like ours, are influenced by their feelings. Ignoring feelings sets us up for ugly surprises.

- **Horses do not fake fear.** They are more likely to hide it. If they act scared, they *are* scared.

- **It is okay to let horses retreat, back away, look away, and/or circle around at their own discretion.** This is at odds with the typical human expectation that a horse should walk straight up to the object or situation of concern.

- **You need to *wait* until the horse tells you he feels safe.** It is not enough for you to be satisfied he is safe; *he* needs to feel safe.

- **You must not interfere with the horse's investigation.** Doing "nothing" is nearly impossible for many people!

- **You are not undermining your leadership when you let a horse focus on whatever is worrying him.** Quite the contrary, you are acting like a Protector Leader.

## Summary

The advantages of Investigative Behavior show why it is a valuable part of Protector Leadership:

- It is safer and less stressful because horses do not feel pressured or trapped.
- It takes less time because horses use innate ways of learning and processing information.
- It builds horses' confidence so they are more reliable in the future.
- It builds trust between horse and human because you become your horse's "moral support" instead of a source of pressure and anxiety.
- It is versatile because it does not require any special equipment or change in how you normally ride, handle, or train horses. It is simply a "time out" from whatever you were doing until they establish in their own mind that the new situation is safe. Then you return to your agenda.
- It's fun! You get to relax and enjoy watching horses train themselves.

### THINGS TO TRY

- The next time your horse spooks or balks at something, allow him to use Investigative Behavior, making sure you keep yourself and your horse safe in the process.

- If he is not immediately interested in investigating, he may be anticipating pressure. Your challenge will be to do "nothing" while you show him with your Friendly Body Language that you are not going to pressure him.

- Note what time it is when he starts investigating. Watch for his body language to show when he goes from curiosity to relaxed confidence. Check the time again.

## chapter 14
# Adventures with Investigative Behavior

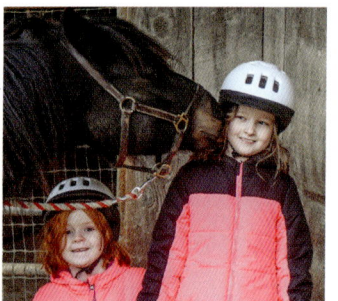

> "If Judith was frightened by anything... I allowed her ample time to take a good look at the object of her fear and even to sniff it...this sometimes took quite a while but nevertheless it was not a waste of time for gradually Judith gained confidence in me and lost her spookiness."
>
> —Alois Podhajsky *(My Horses, My Teachers)*

I learned about Investigative Behavior while taking Bronzz for walks to see the sights around his new boarding stable, as I described in chapter 12 (p. 141). In this chapter, I relate some of these and later adventures to show the variety of circumstances in which Investigative Behavior can be used and some different approaches that made it successful.

When a horse is reluctant to approach or investigate, we need to get creative, not forceful. I have stage-managed situations, play-acted, given demonstrations, offered incentives, and enlisted the assistance of other horses and people, including complete strangers.

### Enlisting Assistance: Alien on Wheels

As Bronzz and I strolled down the road one day, a boy whizzed by on his bike. Bronzz, having never seen a bike, went straight up in the air like a cartoon horse. Equally shocked, the boy screeched to a halt and apologized. I thanked him profusely for stopping, and asked if he would do me a huge favor: walk his bike back past us (safely on the far side of the road, of course), then ride by again. Bronzz watched, still bug-eyed but now recognizing that the cyclist was actually an ordinary human, not some bizarre wheeled creature.

## More Assistance: The Fly Fisherman

When Bronzz saw something alarming, we usually just stood and watched until he was bored. That did not work when we encountered fly fishermen. Things zinging through the air made him increasingly anxious and eager to leave.

As an excuse to engage a fisherman in conversation, I called hello, explained that my horse had never seen anyone fly fish, and asked if we could hang out and watch. One kind man set down his rod and came over to chat and admire Bronzz, who was learning to bask in such attention. By the time the fisherman resumed casting, Bronzz was satisfied that whatever this friendly human was doing, it must be harmless.

## Special Incentives: The Lean Mean Green Machine

We returned from a lead-line walk one day to find a lawn tractor parked outside the barn door. Never mind that where Bronzz grew up, a full-sized tractor was driven down the barn aisle daily for stall cleaning and that Bronzz had no trouble squeezing between said tractor and the wall to mosey out the barn door and hike down the driveway when no one was looking. This little machine did not look like any tractor he had ever seen, and its appearance, apparently by magic when he wasn't looking, was highly suspicious.

I let Bronzz hang out in his comfort zone at the end of his lead while I sat casually on the tractor seat. When it became obvious that he had no intention of coming closer to inspect the thing, I pulled a carrot from my pocket and ostentatiously inspected it. Bronzz soon decided that it was worth venturing forth for a bit of carrot, each bite held a little closer to the tractor. Then we circled and inspected it until it was deemed boring. I have since used our lawn tractor for a mounting block.

## Jackpot: The Sky is Falling

Bronzz's and my favorite lead-line adventure started with roofers tossing packs of shingles off a second floor roof. Things falling from the sky prompted Bronzz's slickest Arab teleport trick ever, as he suddenly materialized on the opposite side of me, placing me squarely between himself and the danger. Right where the leader belongs.

I called hello to the workers, using my standard excuse of asking if we could stay and watch. In response they swarmed down off the roof, provoking snorts of alarm from my shocked companion. As the men crossed the yard toward us, they explained that they rarely got to see horses and asked if they could pet him.

Could they, indeed? Make my day! By now Bronzz had identified friendly humans and gone into schmooze mode. The icing on the cake came when one of them produced an apple and asked permission to give it to Bronzz. For months after that Bronzz scanned rooftops hopefully, looking for friendly apple servers.

Events like this gave Bronzz a consistent message: behind that seemingly scary activity lurks a friendly human just waiting to pet and admire you. If you're really lucky you might hit the jackpot and score an apple!

## Three-Day Wonder: The Big Wide Scary Creek

Any trail ride from the boarding stable required crossing a wide creek. Bronzz had never seen any sort of creek, but he thought running water in ditches was plenty scary, so I planned a long, patient introduction as an investment in many years of reliable creek crossings.

**Day 1**: I put on my waterproof boots and hand-grazed Bronzz in a creek-side pasture. My husband led Sapphire, veteran creek-crosser, to the creek edge to graze. Bronzz naturally gravitated toward Sapphire, observing the creek as he went, and soon decided that the tastiest grass grew right in the water. In less than an hour he was standing fetlock deep in the running water, munching happily.

**Day 2**: When Jerry and Sapphire set out for a trail ride, I led Bronzz behind them as far as the creek. He would have followed them right across had I been prepared to get that wet.

**Day 3**: I saddled up and rode Bronzz to the creek behind Jerry and Sapphire. When she crossed the creek, he slogged along behind her. I let him go at his own pace, and play in the water.

Total time invested: less than 90 minutes. Result: Bronzz thinks creeks are *fun* (fig. 14.1). When we encounter a strange creek, he pauses on the bank to scope it out before wading in. That is only sensible; we humans do the same thing on foot. The amusing aspect of this is that on hot days, Bronzz looks for the deepest path across the creek.

Spreading Investigative Behavior over multiple sessions is powerful because it allows the task to be broken into smaller, less intimidating pieces, and gives the horse time to process the new information between sessions. A successful session ends at any point where the horse is relaxed and confident.

Arranging for a horse to follow another horse, as Bronzz followed Sapphire, is a very effective way to increase his comfort level and speed learning.

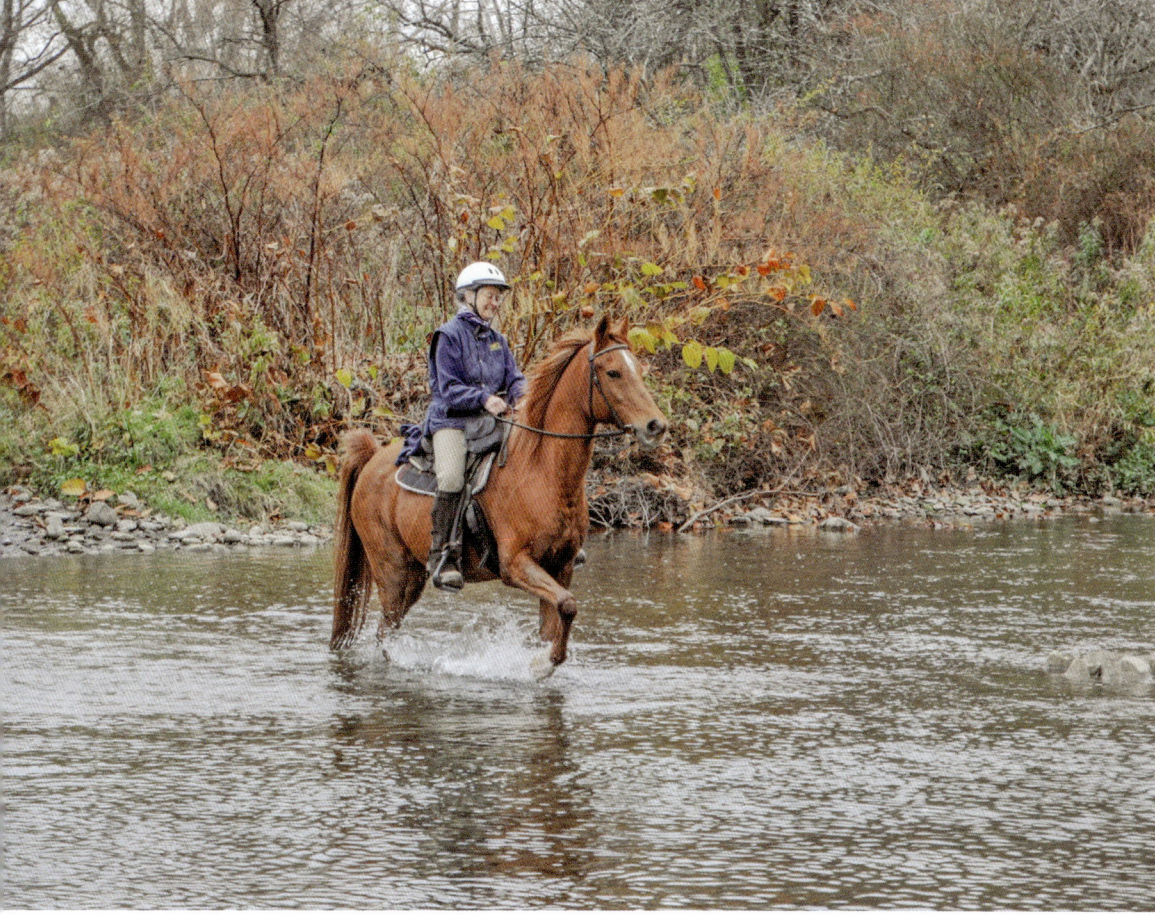

14.1 Bronzz returns for a visit and, with no hesitation, splashes into the creek he learned to cross 16 years before.

Horses learn best from horses who are older, more experienced, and higher ranking than they are, which made Sapphire a perfect demonstrator for Bronzz.[97]

## Positive Associations: Introducing Bugs on Wheels

When Bronzz was five, we moved him and Sapphire to the farm where we now live, adjacent to a state forest. We share the trails with mountain bikes, which are swift and quiet, like a stealthy predator. Hunched-over riders in cycling gear and helmets look more like giant insects than people. The gears sound suspiciously like the clicking of an electric fence, and sunlight flashes off the metal. From a horse's point of view, nothing about them looks safe or friendly.

Bronzz got his first sight of one as it whizzed along on a trail in the woods. Though Bronzz stopped as I asked him to, he danced anxiously, and looked to Sapphire for a second opinion. Her blasé reaction helped calm him. When the biker courteously stopped and removed his helmet to chat, Bronzz began to relax.

If I had it to do over, I would not wait for Bronzz to be surprised by a bike in the woods. I would ask a friend to bring a mountain bike to our place so he could see it up close and watch someone he knew put on a helmet and ride the bike. Preparing horses *in advance* to cope with such strange things is the topic of the next chapter.

## Observing from Afar: The Not-Quite-a Horse

As my husband and I rode along a quiet forest trail overlooking a farm, we heard a loud bray. Bronzz snorted and sat back on his hocks, ready to spin and bolt. Behind us, Sapphire was backing up in alarm. Both horses were staring at the pasture below us where a large donkey stared back.

Jerry and I did not allow our horses to turn around, but neither did we ask them to continue past the donkey, which was obviously a bizarre creature by their standards. Instead we waited, all watching the donkey while he watched us, the horses flinching every time he vocalized or moved his giant ears.

After about five minutes, Bronzz let out a huge sigh, and continued walking along the trail. Sapphire followed. They remained tense and suspicious, ready for action in case the strange creature made any threatening moves. When we passed the donkey again a few weeks later, the horses kept watchful eyes on him, but walked on by. The third time around, the donkey did not even rate a second look.

## Protecting the Leader: The Big Bad Recycle Mess

Brandy's first summer here, I took her for lead-line walks as I had Bronzz when he was young. One morning as Brandy and I started up the driveway, she went on full alert, head high, snorting and tap dancing. Her attention was focused at the top of the driveway where the recycle bin was overturned, its contents strewn far and wide. It looked like the raccoons had partied the night before.

Her fear was perfectly rational. This mess was not normal. The amazing thing was that she was not trying to bolt back to the security of the barn and the other horses. She was hanging tight to me instead! I saw an opportunity to reinforce my leadership and show Brandy that she could trust my judgment.

I tried letting her observe with no pressure to approach, but Brandy was too far away to see anything useful, and too frightened to go closer. When I casually moseyed toward the mess, she became more agitated, and actually moved ahead of me, blocking me from approaching it. I might once have interpreted this as pushiness or blatant disobedience, but from a Protector Leader perspective, I suspected she was trying to protect me by warning me not to approach something potentially dangerous.

Conveniently, my husband was within shouting distance, so I enlisted his help. Calling a cheerful greeting to Brandy, he strolled up the driveway and began slowly collecting the recyclables strewn along the road. Now Brandy's curiosity kicked in. Clearly Jerry was not afraid, and nothing bad was happening to him, therefore….

Brandy inched forward, observing intently. Minutes later she was standing next to the recycle bin, happily inspecting each item as Jerry placed it in. Gee, not only was the mess harmless, she got heaps of praise and petting just for looking at it. Meanwhile, my credibility as a protector went way up.

### Protector Leader vs. The Monster in the Woods

Our arena is bordered on two sides by woods, with barn and paddocks on the other sides. One day when Brandy was turned out in the arena, we heard a mighty crash in the woods. She shot across the arena toward the barn where I was doing chores, and whinnied loudly. I set down my pitchfork, and climbed through the fence into the arena where she was waiting anxiously for me.

"That was a big, scary crash, wasn't it, Brandy?" I said cheerfully. "Let's check it out." And I strode purposefully across the arena in the direction of the crash without looking back at her.

It might sound heartless to act cheerful in the face of a horse's fear, but unlike with people, it is the kindest thing to do. Petting, soothing, and making "there, there" sounds can come across to a horse as if you are worried, too. The most reassuring thing you can do is acknowledge the horse's concern by "noticing" the situation yourself; then demonstrate that you have a plan to deal with it.

You might not have a great plan if you're taken by surprise. You might be scared if there is real potential for danger. You might need to revise your plan as the situation develops. None of that seems to matter. What matters is that you are clear and decisive. That shows you are taking responsibility.

In this case, I had the advantage of knowing that my husband was cutting down trees for firewood. Another chance to show Brandy my competence as her protector. Brandy had the advantage of being in a safely confined space, so she was free to advance or retreat as she chose. As I crossed the arena, she hung back, stopping about half way to watch me. I leaned over the fence waving until I got my husband's attention and he shut off the chainsaw.

"Say 'Hello' to Brandy," I instructed him. "She's worried about what's happening out there."

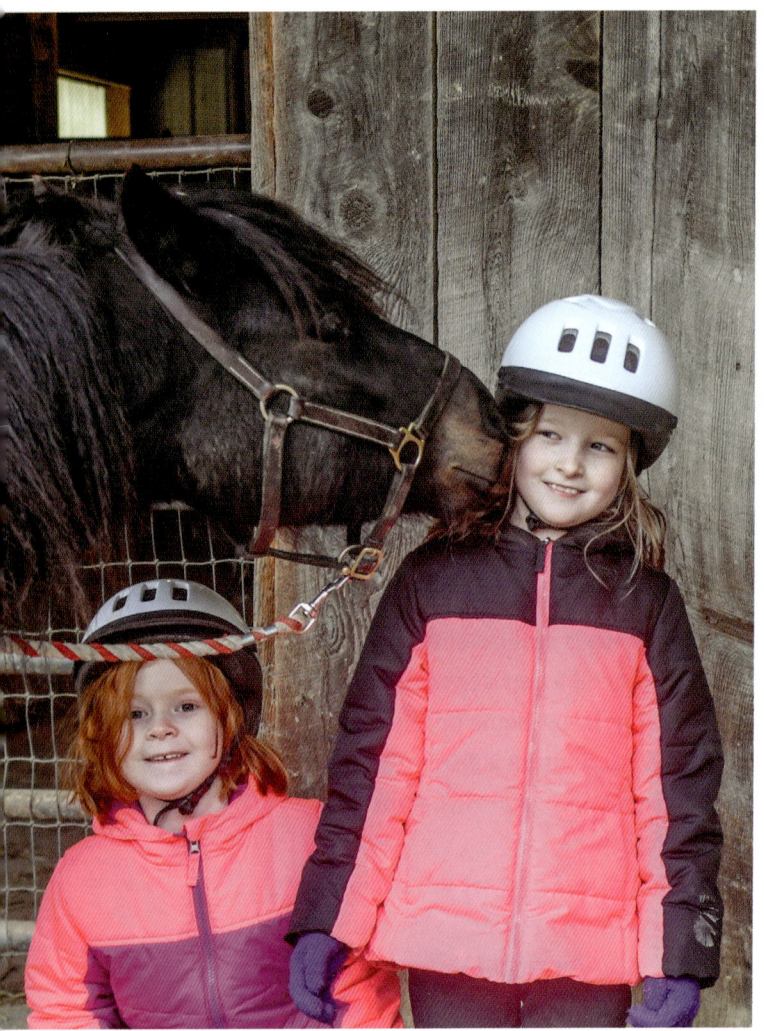

14.2 Visiting Dartmoor pony, Love, inspects Leora and Delia the same way Brandy once did.

self-appointed task of mowing edible weeds around the perimeter of the arena.

### New Species: Pint-Sized Humans

Brandy had been here about six weeks when grandchildren started arriving for summer visits. Brandy's wide-eyed astonishment at the sight of preschoolers suggested that they looked like a new species to her. We let her hang back and observe as the other horses stretched over their stall doors for little hay bouquets that the kids held up. When Brandy was ready, she inched forward and reached out for her share. Step One was accomplished: kids meant nice things happen.

Since bugs kept the horses in the barn on summer days, Brandy had plenty of opportunity to observe the children as they brushed the other horses, helped me clean stalls and replenish water buckets, served hay, played with cats, chalked pictures on the aisle mats, and did other kid things.

We made introductions cautiously. Before touching Brandy, the children stood still for her to inspect them, giggling as she sniffed their bodies and nuzzled their hair (fig. 14.2). I stood ready to body-block if necessary, or snag any child who even thought of going behind Brandy. Before visits were over, Brandy was relaxed almost to the point of dozing while small children brushed her and braided her mane.

"Hi, Brandy," he called. By now Brandy was beside me, watching Jerry. Brandy hung out with us while we chatted for a few minutes. When Jerry restarted the chainsaw, she barely flinched.

I went back to barn chores. Brandy hung over the fence watching Jerry until she was bored. Then she resumed her

## Taming the Trailer Terror

I do not know how Brandy was loaded to bring her to us, but she stumbled off the trailer shaking in terror and dripping with sweat. It was not a hot day. I could not tell if she was fearful of trailers or just the trainer who delivered her. I had my answer the first time I led her past our trailer. She scooted as far away as her lead allowed, head high, body tense, and produced a green cow pie.

A local trainer who is a genius at trailer loading says, "If you plan to take 10 minutes, it will take all day. Plan for all day, and it will take 10 minutes." Since I have not mastered his zen-like calm, I just tried to stay out of Brandy's way while she checked out the trailer and taught herself to load.

I would have liked to park the trailer in a paddock, and feed Brandy progressively closer to it until she was having all her meals inside it. I have seen this done with great success. Having no safe way to do that, I used a variation.

I put a hay pile as close to the trailer as Brandy was willing to eat. With her on a loose lead, I stood slightly closer to the trailer, ignoring her. Sometimes, at Brandy's suggestion, we took breaks to walk around the trailer, inspecting it from all angles. Gradually the hay pile went closer to the trailer, then farther and farther inside it. I went in the trailer ahead of her. Eventually, she was walking into the trailer, and quietly waiting for me to cue her to walk off.

It took about three hours, working in 10-minutes sessions over a couple of weeks. Someone else might have accomplished it faster, even without scaring her. On the other hand, I've seen people spend far longer and end up with a horse who's still scared and not in the trailer.

When it was time to return Brandy to the rescue farm for the winter, she walked right on the trailer with me, rode quietly for the hour-long trip, and arrived calm. When we returned to fetch her in the spring, she had not seen me or a trailer in five months. She walked right on the trailer with me.

The homeward trip involved a delay. As we were parked beside a sidewalk on a busy street, people came over to the trailer to admire the pretty pony. The pretty pony, who was terrified of people and trailers a year ago, calmly reached her nose over to the slats in the stock trailer and gently nuzzled the strangers' offered fingers.

## Is There a Downside to Investigative Behavior?

When horses are allowed to investigate the world, their curiosity blossoms, and their confidence along with it. They are now more likely to take the initiative to inspect new things. You might ask, if I let my horse stop to investigate things, won't he feel entitled to even when it's not safe or appropriate? While crossing a road, for instance, or in a show ring?

My experience has been just the opposite. The more I let horses investigate, the more they trust my judgment. That means that when I do need to say, "Not now," they are *more* likely to trust me and do as I ask even if they are anxious.

We just need to be extra careful with expensive or delicate items that might not fare well under close inspection, or items the horse could injure himself on. My husband left his camera on a fence post, imagining that it would be of no interest to a horse. Brandy thought otherwise. In the course of her investigation, she inadvertently knocked it off the fence post, with sad consequences for an expensive lens.

## Summary

Curiosity is the antithesis of fear. When horses encounter potentially frightening situations, people typically ask, "How can I stop my horse from reacting?" This focuses on trying to control an already anxious horse, often making him more anxious in the process.

It is more constructive to ask instead, "How can I transform this frightening event into an educational experience?" Staying mindful of everyone's safety, we focus on engaging our horses' curiosity and supporting Investigative Behavior. Some creativity may be required since each situation is unique, but patience is the main ingredient. A successful investigation leaves a horse more relaxed, and more confident in the face of similar situations in the future.

### THINGS TO TRY

- Think of a time your horse spooked, balked, or otherwise showed concern about a situation.
- If the outcome of the situation was a calm, confident horse, review in your mind what you did that led to success, and whether you can apply the same approach in other circumstances.
- If the outcome was not so successful, write down three things you could safely do in a future situation to promote success.

# PART SIX:
# Positive Experiences Build Confidence and Reliability

> "I've learned that people will forget what you said, people will forget what you did, but people will never forget how you made them feel."
>
> —Maya Angelou

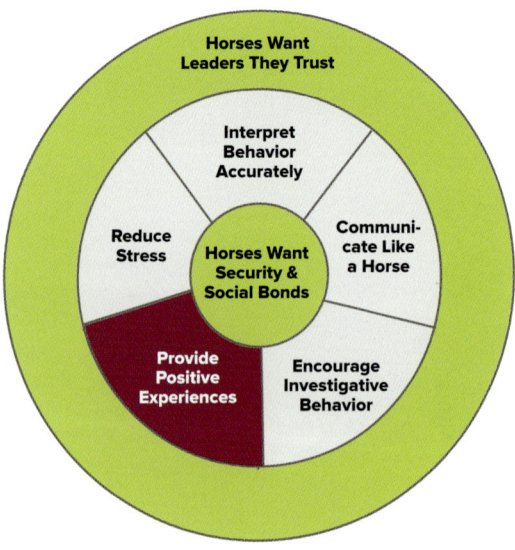

The more reliable a horse's behavior is, the more you can focus on what you want to do, and the less you worry about what he *might* do. Reliability is sometimes perceived as a lack of reactiveness on the horse's part: not spooking, not looking around anxiously. However, nature designed horses to be aware of everything, evaluate potential danger, and react accordingly. Conditioning them not to react is contrary to their survival instincts. No matter how automatically a horse responds to a cue, fear can override habit.

The solution does not lie in what you condition them *not* to do, but in what you show them they *can* do: cope with all sorts of strange and wonderful things, and trust your guidance when they are not sure what to do. Aren't you calmer when you're confident and have a trusted person with you for backup?

Confidence is not a skill; it is a *feeling*. It does not come from training; it comes from lots of little successes that add up to show a horse that he can do whatever you ask of him. Protector Leadership lays the foundation of trust. Friendly Body Language provides communication. Investigative Behavior expands horses' comfort zone. Next, you put these elements together in a systematic Confidence Building program.

Chapter 15 (p. 178) describes the characteristics of a successful Confidence Building program. In chapter 16 (p. 192), Brandy demonstrates some remedial work that she needed in addition to her Confidence Building program with obstacles. Chapter 17 (p. 209) shows how you can allow your horse more freedom without compromising safety, how to use play as a motivator, and how to begin working at liberty.

**Part Six Key Points:**
- Reliability is essential for safety of horse and human, but trying to condition horses not to react to scary things goes against their survival instincts.

- We can work *with* their instincts by providing positive experiences that build their trust in us, and their confidence in their own ability to cope with life.

- People typically exert rigid control over every aspect of their horses' lives; this can be a source of stress, and a barrier to a good working relationship.

**You will learn how to:**
- Improve your horse's reliability with a systematic Confidence Building program that incorporates Investigative Behavior and positive training techniques.

- Strengthen your connection with your horse by allowing him appropriate choices and freedom.

- Work with your horse at liberty using Friendly Body Language.

# chapter 15
# Systematic Confidence Building

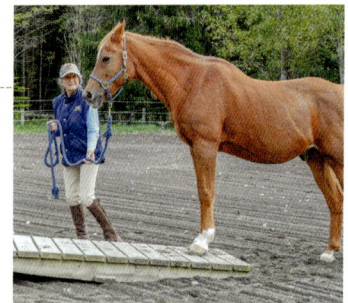

> "I feel it is imperative to develop a bond of trust between myself and my horses before taking them out of their home base for any kind of activity, and that process begins with confidence exercises on the ground."
>
> —Kim Walnes ("Being a Leader/Protector for Your Horse")

Confidence Building is a learning process that works with horses' instincts and innate intelligence. You plan small challenges and make sure the horse feels successful in meeting those challenges. Each success builds more confidence in himself and in you. A planned program gives you flexibility that Investigative Behavior alone does not. Instead of waiting for situations to present themselves, you create them using a variety of obstacles and equipment.

Vanessa Bee's book, *Over, Under, Through: Obstacle Training for Horses* details such a Confidence Building program, the purpose described in her introduction:

"Please note you are not desensitizing the horse (I like my horse sensitive), you are not spook-busting him (I want life in my horse), you are showing him, through a series of exercises, that if he listens to his rider or handler, he will be safe."[98]

In this chapter, I will describe a systematic approach, with special focus on the supportive leadership that helps horses feel safe, successful, and ready for the next challenge. Vanessa's book shows how to go from arena exercises to riding beyond the arena, negotiating all sorts of real world obstacles with confidence in your horse because he has confidence in you.

## A Systematic Confidence Building Program

As the title *Over, Under, Through* indicates, obstacles can be divided loosely into categories.

- **Over:** Poles, tarpaulin, carpet, hula hoop
- **Under:** Umbrellas or flags
- **Through**: Posts, cones, barrels, ribbon curtains

Horses generalize their knowledge and confidence to real world situations, as the jumpers in the Investigative Behavior study generalized different types of jumps. *Over* prepares horses for new footing such as bridges, and step-overs like logs. *Under* might be low branches or doorways, flags, or banners. *Through* includes trees, underbrush, and narrow gaps. Trailers incorporate all three "obstacles" in one: strange flooring, narrow sides, and a roof.

The specific equipment is not important, but variety provides different colors, shapes, textures, smells, sounds, and motions. Balls add motion that can be disturbingly unpredictable to horses. Plastic bags add crinkly noises and flapping. Lawn ornaments might flash and twirl. You can use any items you have around or can lay your hands on cheap. They just need to be safe and either expendable or indestructible no matter how intensely horses investigate them (figs. 15.1 A & B).

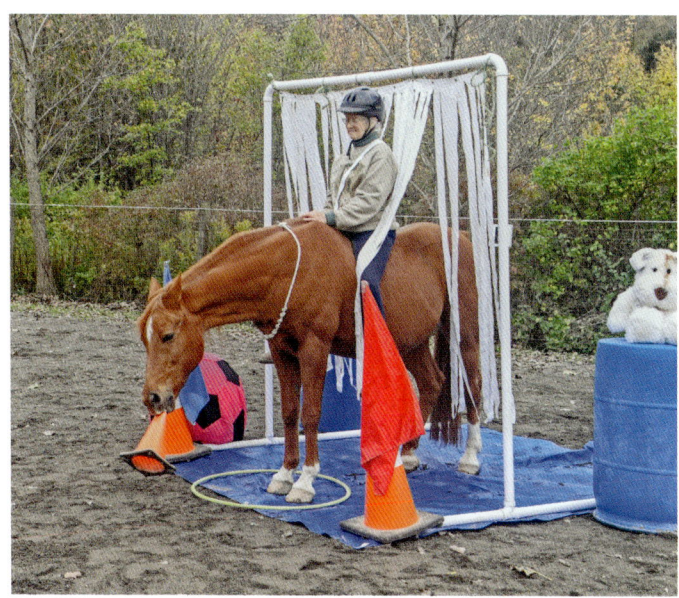

**15.1 A** Bronzz waves a cone amidst some typical Confidence Building equipment. He was comfortable with each piece of it before we put it all together.

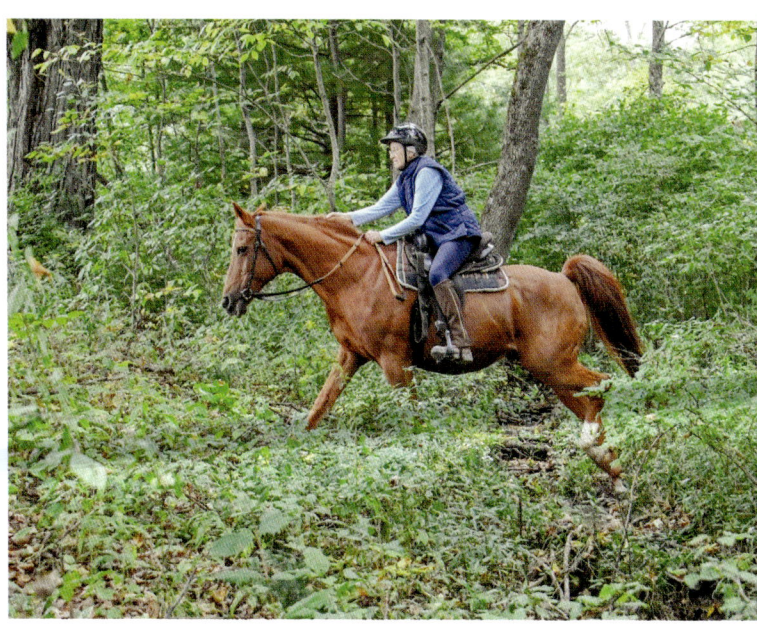

**15.1 B** Horses generalize the information they learn at home to greater confidence in other situations, in this case through underbrush and muddy footing, and over a small creek.

## Steps to Success

Your goal is a confident horse who calmly negotiates each obstacle as directed on a *loose* lead. "As directed" means that you vary what you do with each obstacle at different times so that the horse must watch for your cues.

Successful Confidence Building sessions follow the same principles as any good training or work session. This chapter steps through those principles. I chose a seesaw for Bronzz's demonstration because it is an obstacle that could be frightening and unsafe if not introduced carefully. However, as Brandy will demonstrate in the next chapter, no expensive equipment is required.

**1. Encourage Investigative Behavior, experimenting, and problem-solving.** Horses must be comfortable with new equipment before you ask them to follow your instructions, so you start with Investigative Behavior (fig. 15.2). Allowing them time to experiment and figure things out helps horses make best use of their cognitive abilities.

**2. Start on the ground and demonstrate whenever possible.** When you're

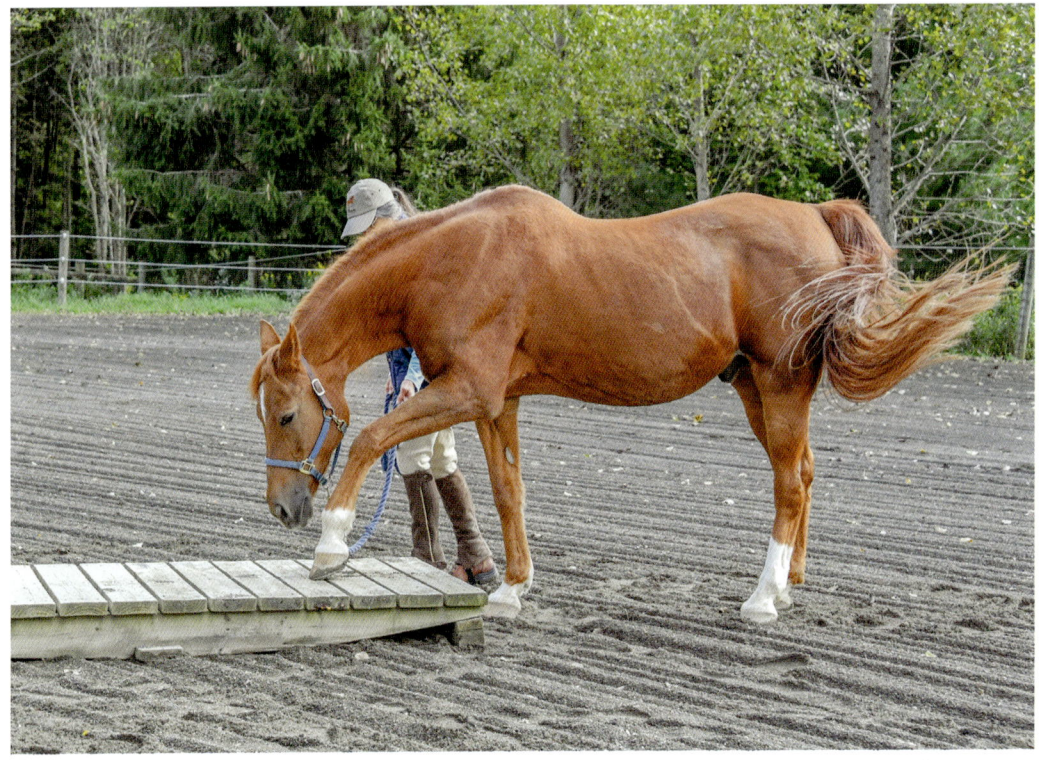

15.2 Bronzz's inspection of the seesaw includes pawing at it. Chocks under each end prevent it from rocking yet.

on the ground, horses can see your instructions, and your own confidence (fig. 15.3). When they are absolutely comfortable with a piece of equipment, then you can mount up and repeat whatever you did on the ground.

3. **Keep a positive attitude.** Laugh a lot, especially when things go wrong. Seriously. Corrections do not build confidence in people or horses. Laughing at mistakes instead dismisses them as unimportant so you can move on in a positive way.

Laughter is also a great stress buster for your horse as well as yourself. I have a friend who giggles when her horse spooks. She trained herself to do that. Her horses go from higher-than-a-kite anxiety to calmly focused faster than any I've ever met. Most of us are not laughing when our horse spooks. That's why we do Confidence Building exercises on the ground where we can laugh.

4. **Start easy and break every task into tiny steps that ensure success.** Since every success builds confidence, baby steps mean faster learning. Watch for Hidden Anxiety, and be sure that the horse stays truly *relaxed*, whether that

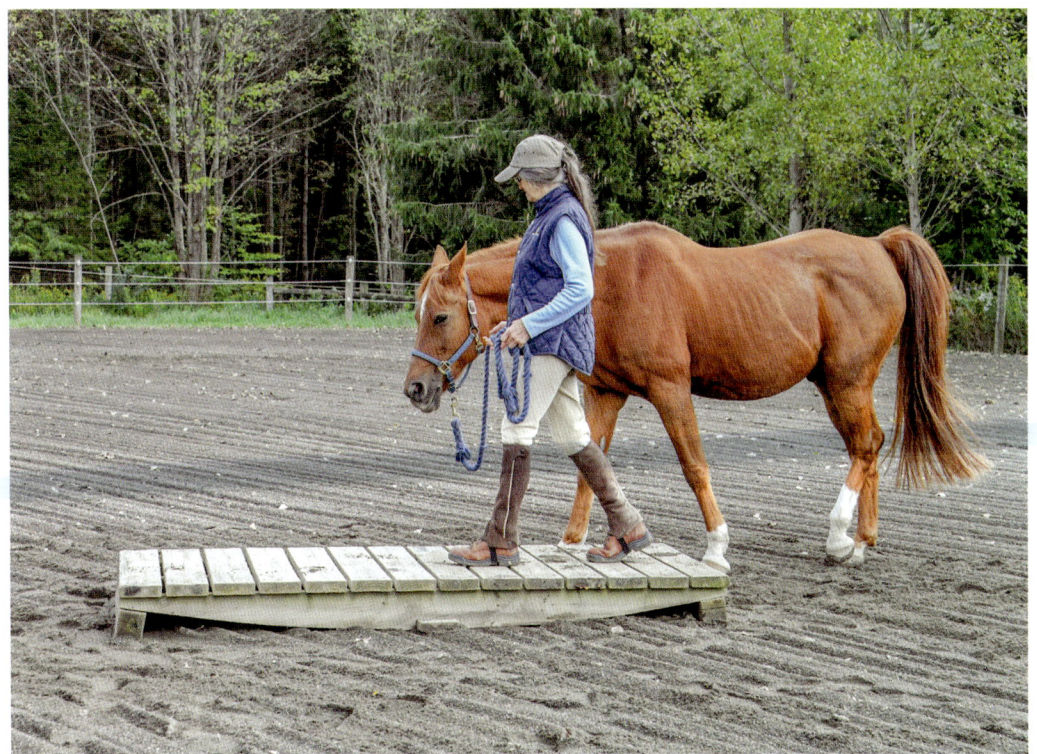

15.3 As Bronzz watches me cross the seesaw, he sees what I will be asking him to do: walk straight from one end to the other, calmly and slowly. Hearing my boots make a different sound on the wood, he can deduce that his hooves will also sound different.

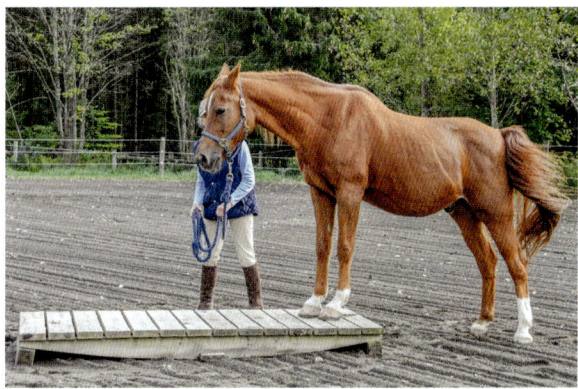

**15.4 A** Bronzz has offered to put both front feet on the seesaw. We pause.

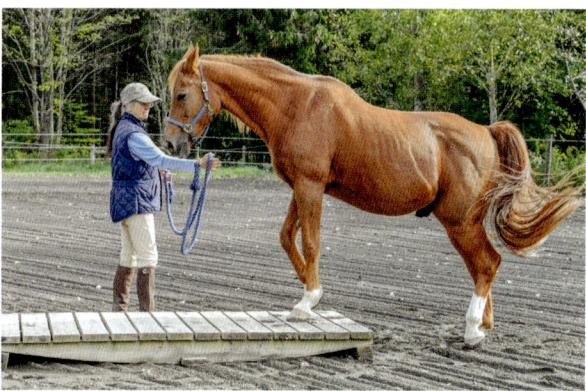

**15.4 B** Then I ask him to back off, calmly and deliberately. I repeat until the horse *offers* to walk all four feet on.

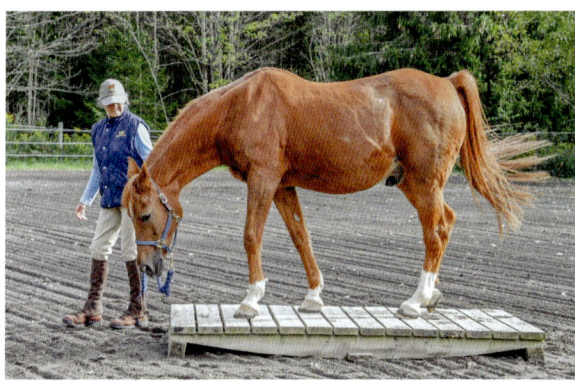

**15.4 C** We pause in the middle to show we do not rush across.

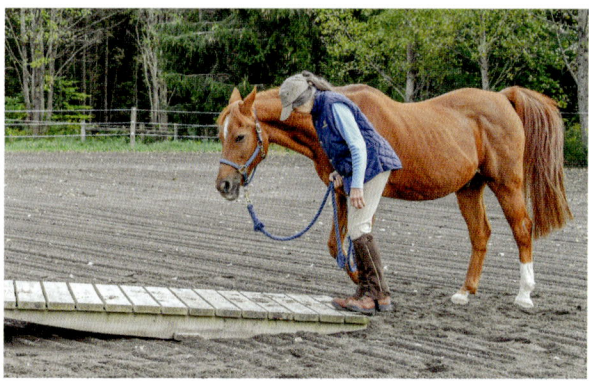

**15.4 D** I demonstrate the bounce when one chock is removed. Bronzz is totally unimpressed. Then I walk across to show him the motion.

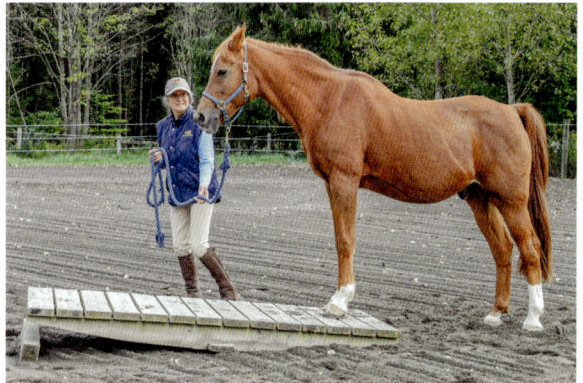

**15.4 E** Bronzz puts two feet on the un-chocked end. Again we back off and repeat until he tells me he is ready to go forward.

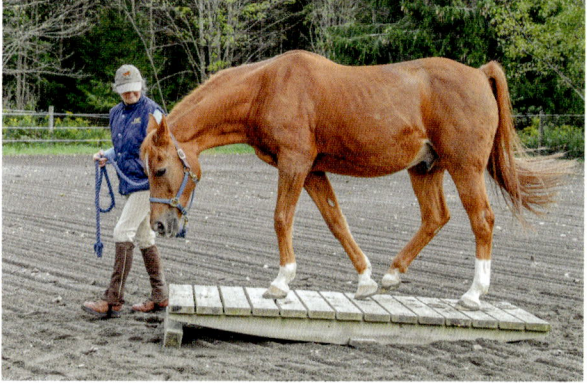

**15.4 F** Bronzz walks across the seesaw with one chock removed. Then we turn around and walk back across it so he could feel the downward motion from the other direction.

takes three minutes or three weeks. You want him to think, "That was so easy, what's next?"

Breaking skills into small enough steps is not as simple as it sounds, especially since many of us have seen more demonstrations that glamorize speedy "training" based on pressure instead of patience. Calm horses making step-by-step progress provide no drama (figs. 15.4 A–G).

I could probably have ridden Bronzz across the seesaw the first time he saw it, but if he'd slipped or stepped off the edge, he would rightfully have seen it as treacherous, and perhaps never trusted it. I was not satisfied to have Bronzz simply cross the obstacle. I wanted him to feel he had *mastered* it, so we repeated the step-by-step introduction, first with chocks and then without (fig. 15.5).

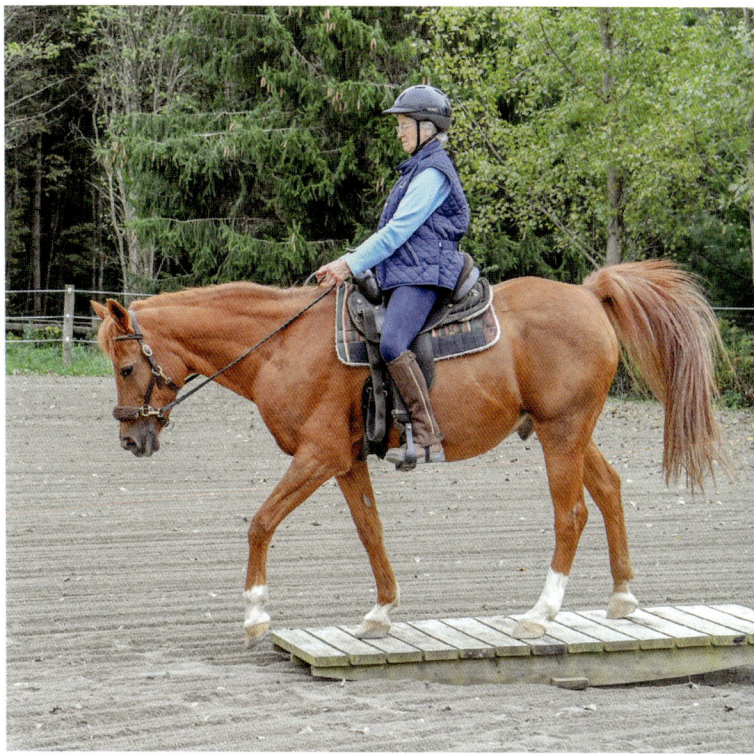

15.5 Now comfortable managing the rocking with my weight on his back, Bronzz has walked calmly across the seesaw, with a pause in the middle to encourage thinking and precision.

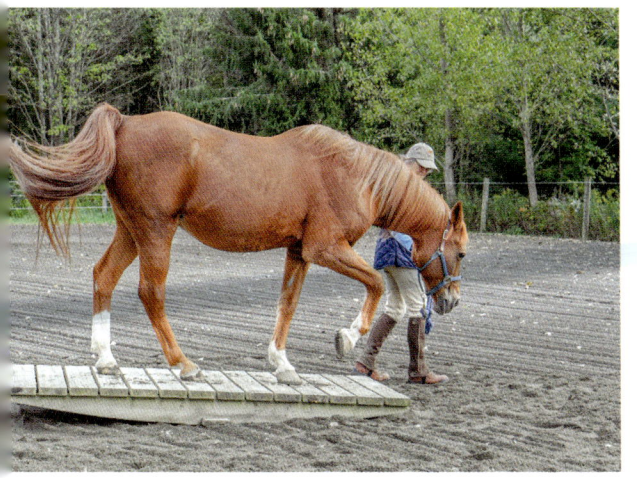

15.4 G With the second chock removed, Bronzz strolls calmly across.

5. **Reward effort.** You do not wait for a task to be completed or perfect. Instead, reward effort and improvement. Low-key rewards such as a stroke on the neck or word of praise can provide encouragement without interrupting what you're doing. A special accomplishment or breakthrough in understanding earns more exciting rewards. The less confident a horse is, the more patience and rewards he needs. Use food judiciously, so it is not a distraction from learning.

6. **Go for precision, not speed.** Do each step slowly and precisely, as dogs are trained in agility—and for the same

reasons. It helps keep everyone safe, and allows you to reward stepwise improvement. If a horse is to negotiate an obstacle at higher speed later, he already has the habit of placing his feet correctly and listening to his handler or rider.

**7. Keep sessions short.** Although the photos of Bronzz demonstrating how he learned to cross the see-saw were taken in one session, his actual introduction was spread out over several days. I spent two or three minutes before our ride, starting each day with a review of the previous step. Short sessions promote efficient, stress-free learning. Both horse and human can maintain focus better, and you prevent boredom. Give the horse processing time in between sessions. You might

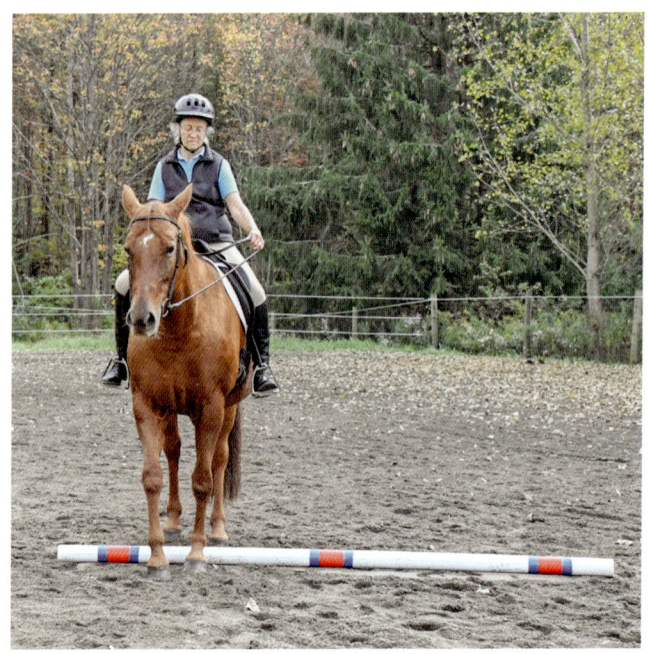

**15.6 A** Although Shiloh already knows how to side-pass, this is the first time I've asked her to do it with front and hind feet on opposite sides of a pole. She is not ignoring me; she's thinking.

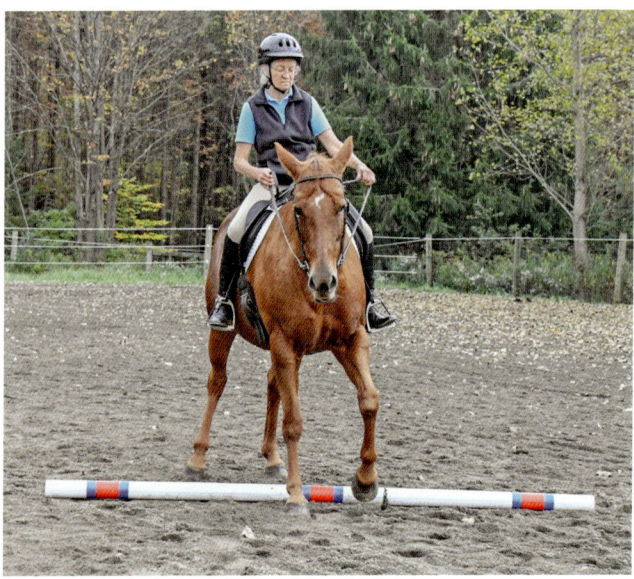

**15.6 B** She experiments. Is backing up the right answer? I quietly reposition her and try again.

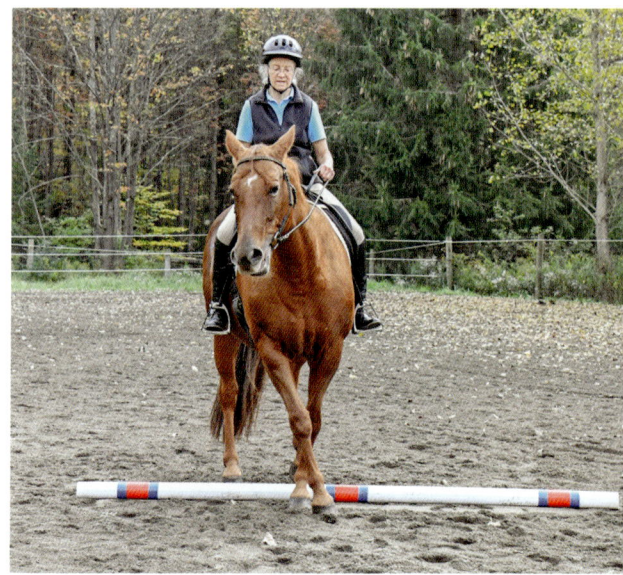

**15.6 C** Now she figures it out.

feel you've accomplished nothing on any given day, but your most important accomplishment is your horse's feeling of, "That was easy. I can do that!" Meanwhile, small layers of progress stack up to reliable skills. These help counterbalance the layers of negative experiences that so many horses have had. As a Tai Chi master once told me, "Once with focus is worth 50 times mindlessly."

8. **Be patient while horses think things through.** Early responses may be slow because horses have to think about what they are doing, just as you have to think when you first practice a new skill. Watch for understanding, ideally with a spark of excitement that says, "I *get* it. I can do it!" Quicker responses come from practice over time. Even familiar cues may need processing time in a new context (figs. 15.6 A–C).

If a horse struggles with something and just does not seem to understand what you want, let it go. Come back to it in five minutes, a day, a week, or a month, and it is amazing how often he will respond more accurately. If not, try a different approach.

Once horses understand what you're asking and are confident doing it, they do not forget. For her first two years with us, Brandy spent winters at the rescue farm with no follow up at all on her training. She forgot *nothing*. Each spring she picked up where we left off as if she'd never been gone.

9. **Incorporate variety.** Practice should be interwoven with other activities or obstacles to prevent boredom. A good rule in all activities is to mix opposites: new skills and old, fast and slow, easy and difficult, mental challenges with harder physical work, and so on. Switch gears often enough to keep the horse interested, but not so quickly he feels pressured or frustrated. Variety is necessary not only for mental health, but to work different muscles for fitness. The longer the session, the more variety is needed.

The "Rule of Three" is a good guide for practicing new skills, as Hertha James describes in *Conversations with Horses*. Three practice repeats in a row *maximum*, then do something else. Return to the new skill no more than three times in a session.[99]

The exception to three repetitions of a new skill is when a horse does something especially well. *Resist the temptation to repeat and "reinforce" it*. Asking him to repeat the new skill immediately can make him think that he got it wrong and should try something different. Instead, reward lavishly; reward is the best reinforcement. Give him a moment to bask in his success and your approval, processing what he just did. Then do something else the horse likes to do, or end the session altogether.

10. **Finish with a success.** Always end with something the horse has done well. Leaving a horse with a positive feeling means he comes back next time with

more confidence, which is your goal in the first place. I like the image Ellen Schuthof-Lesmeister presents in *Horse Training In-Hand*: "You want to finish each session with a proud horse who wants to please you."[100]

## Generalizing the Principles of Success

The same principles apply not only to obstacles but to many new things. I introduced my horses to being vacuumed by letting them watch as my sister vacuumed me. We laughed and talked. The horses craned their necks over their stall partitions to watch. We shut off the vacuum and let them inspect it. Then we moved it far away, turned it on, and let them approach it. By the time we vacuumed them, they were no more concerned than if it were a new curry.

## Flexibility: Six Ways to Introduce Crossing a Tarp

There is not one right way to introduce a new obstacle or skill. If one approach doesn't work, try another. A tarpaulin is a common "over" obstacle because it is a cheap, safe, handy, and versatile way to introduce horses to something underfoot that has an unusual noise, feel, smell, flap, and look to it. A tarp is also an example of an obstacle that can be approached in many ways. These are some possibilities.

**1.** With the tarp spread out fully, walk along an edge, leading the horse beside you with room to stay off the tarp. Walk progressively closer to center as the horse gets comfortable stepping on it.

**2.** Fold the tarp into a narrow strip that the horse can step over. Unfold a bit at a time as the horse begins to step on it.

**3.** Line up two tarps so their corners are just a step apart, and lead the horse through the gap. Gradually close the gap as he gets more comfortable (from *Over, Under, Through* by Vanessa Bee).

**4.** Allow the horse to follow another who crosses a tarp with confidence.

**5.** Place the tarp somewhere the horse passes routinely, but is not forced to cross it. Then ignore it. Familiarity breeds indifference.

**6.** Spread the tarp out in a paddock, safely anchored from any wind. Place hay piles around the edges. Put apples and carrots in the center. Leave the horse alone with it. The horse will not only become comfortable with the tarp but will associate it with good things (from *Horse Agility: Liberty Horse Training* by Koikka Loikka).

When multiple options do not lead to progress, try another obstacle. If a tarp is too anxiety-producing, for instance, try a piece of carpet. You never know what might have happened in a horse's past to persuade him that something is truly unsafe. Drilling horses on obstacles that cause anxiety can escalate anxiety, and undermine trust in you. Instead, focus on what they do well and expand on that.

## Long-Term Benefits of Confidence Building

Research on the long-term benefits of Confidence Building is tricky because researchers would need to be able to retest the same horses years later and know what learning experiences they had in the interim.

Horse owners who keep the same horses have the advantage here. We know what experiences our horses have, and we can observe them over time. Quite by accident, I had a chance to see my horses' reactions to a tarp eight years after they first learned to cross one (using the "familiarity breeds indifference" option), with no practice in between.

They were first introduced to a tarp one hot, buggy summer day when I set up a painting project in my barn aisle. With nothing better to do, the horses hung over their stall doors and watched as I spread out the crinkly blue tarp, hauled out sawhorses, and got busy. No one worried; after all, I was the one walking on the tarp. They soon lost interest, and went to sleep, three-year-old Shiloh flat out and snoring

a few feet from the tarp. That evening at turnout time, I shoved the tarp aside, leaving most of the aisle clear for the horses. I walked on the tarp; they did not.

Coming in the next morning, each horse placed a hoof or two experimentally on the tarp. At turnout time that evening, I arranged it over the center of the aisle, leaving a walkway along the edge. All three chose to walk the full length of the tarp, just slightly alert to it. The next morning they strolled across the tarp as if it wasn't there. My painting project done, I packed away the tarp.

Eight years later, I wanted photos of a horse crossing a tarp for an article (titled

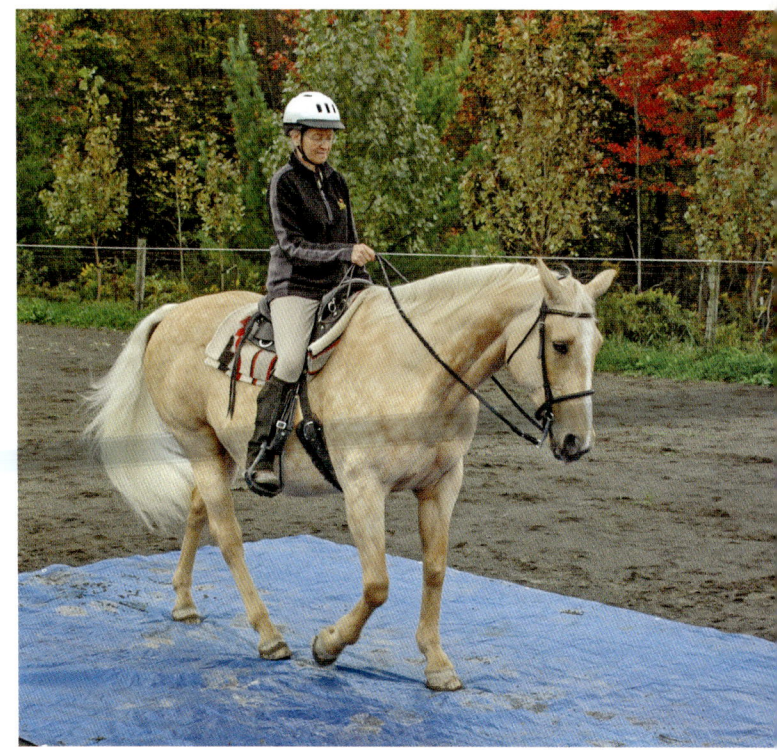

15.7 Sapphire, who normally hated ring work, seemed to find riding across the tarp an entertaining diversion.

PART SIX: POSITIVE EXPERIENCES BUILD CONFIDENCE AND RELIABILITY — 187

"When Horses Train Themselves"). We spread a tarp out in the arena. None of our horses had seen a tarp in the arena before, nor walked on one since my painting project. I saddled Bronzz and Sapphire. Both strolled across the tarp without hesitation, then jogged over it with equal aplomb (fig. 15.7). I declined their offers to canter over it in case it was slippery.

## Obstacle Clinics and Competitions

A clinic can be a confidence booster for you and your horse if you choose carefully. Good clinicians coach riders and handlers on how to help their horses with obstacles, and the reinforcement of a group make horses braver about tackling new things.

Realistic expectations improve the odds of success. Is your horse ready to leave home? Ready for new challenges in a group setting? What level of experience does the clinician assume? Does the program start with people on the ground or riding? What is the clinician's teaching/horse-handling philosophy?

When in doubt, auditing a clinic can provide useful ideas with little expense and no danger of your horse having a traumatic experience. In any case, your horse's most important education happens at home, working at his own pace with you, his trusted leader.

Competitions involving obstacles should also be chosen carefully, especially speed events, as compared to those where horses are judged on precision teamwork with their rider/handler. Pushing horses through obstacles they are not ready for raises anxiety and reduces confidence.

Whatever the setting, you are still your horse's protector. You must never push a horse to do something in order to "prove" to him that he can, or worse, to prove to other people that he will do it if you ask.

I once took Bronzz to an Obstacle Challenge in which the first obstacle was a tarp on a slope with water running over it. It looked slippery, and the horses ahead of us refused it. When our turn came, Bronzz indicated that he wanted to go around it, so I simply directed him on to the next obstacle. I believe he would have tried it if I had asked. But if he slipped, and was hurt or frightened, how could I expect him to trust my judgment in the future? I would rather lose points than my horse's trust.

## Making Progress

Progress depends on many individual variables. Instead of looking for a schedule, write down where your horse is as you start, then compare back to that as you go along. It is easy to focus on what you have not accomplished, and lose sight of how far you have come.

The most important measure of progress is your horse's attitude. If he goes readily to your obstacle "play" area, and

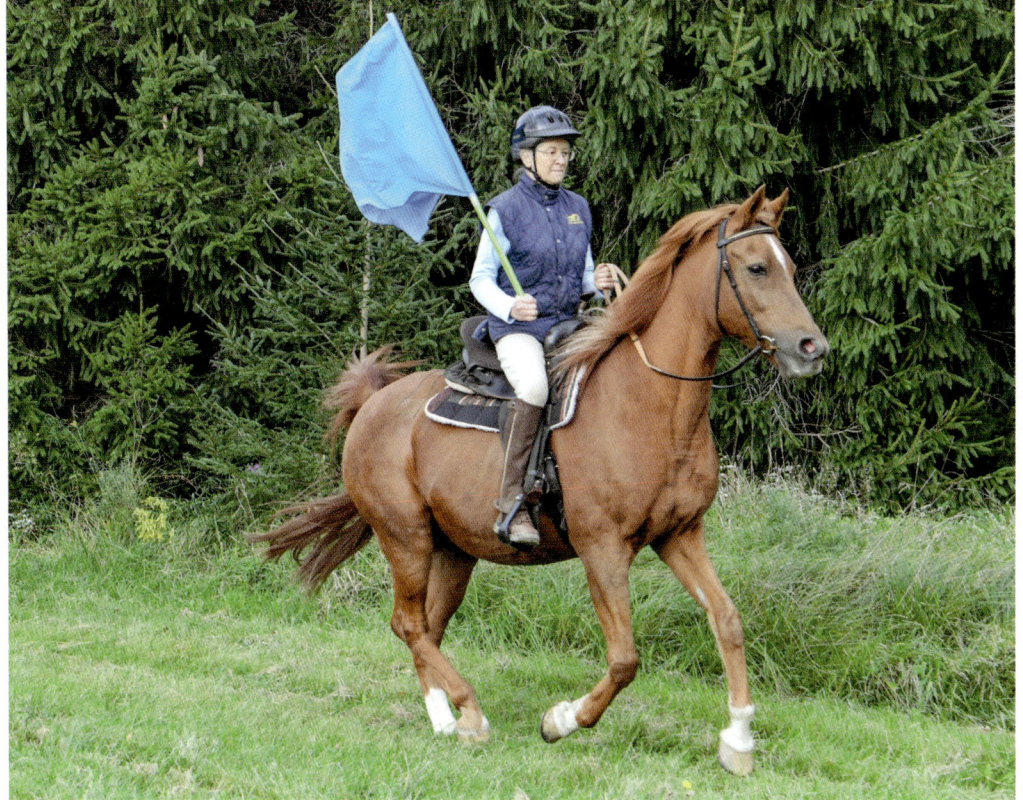

15.8 Bronzz *likes* flags, and cantering with one is even more fun than just waving it.

approaches new things with confidence, congratulate yourself and keep doing whatever you're doing.

If he tries to avoid certain obstacles, resist the temptation to focus on those. Most training programs encourage you to work on what's "wrong" and "fix" it, but that can lead to more frustration and anxiety than progress. Instead, enjoy the things your horse does well, and expand on them (fig. 15.8). Come back to the worrisome things later, or scale back. If he is afraid of big flags, no matter how far away, get tiny flags and work up gradually.

Not every horse will get comfortable with every obstacle. Bronzz still hates stepping in hula hoops no matter what I do.

If your horse tries to avoid the area where you work altogether, watch yourself for any hint of pressure, including a tight lead or coaxing. Try breaking new things into smaller steps. Also notice the attitude you project. Are you cheerful and relaxed or feeling pressured to accomplish something tangible?

If you just sense a general lack of enthusiasm without anxiety, try working for a shorter time and/or less often. The

PART SIX: POSITIVE EXPERIENCES BUILD CONFIDENCE AND RELIABILITY — 189

focus you are asking for is hard work, and cannot be sustained for long spells. Brandy sometimes shows this by yawning profusely when we finish a session.

## The Ultimate Measure of Success

My horses have personalities, thoughts, opinions, and preferences, and a right to express them. I do not expect robot-like obedience to my every whim. My measure of reliability is what they do in situations where cooperation really matters or when someone's safety is at stake. Do they maintain self-control and use good judgment? They do.

Brandy can cut loose with the best of them at playtime, but when a child is handling her, she is a model of decorum. Bronzz ad libs on dressage tests at home, but never at a show. He asks to take favorite trails and move faster when we ride alone, but not when someone else is with us. When we do an obstacle course, he might play silly games with me, but with my grandson, Bronzz is meticulously obedient (fig. 15.9).

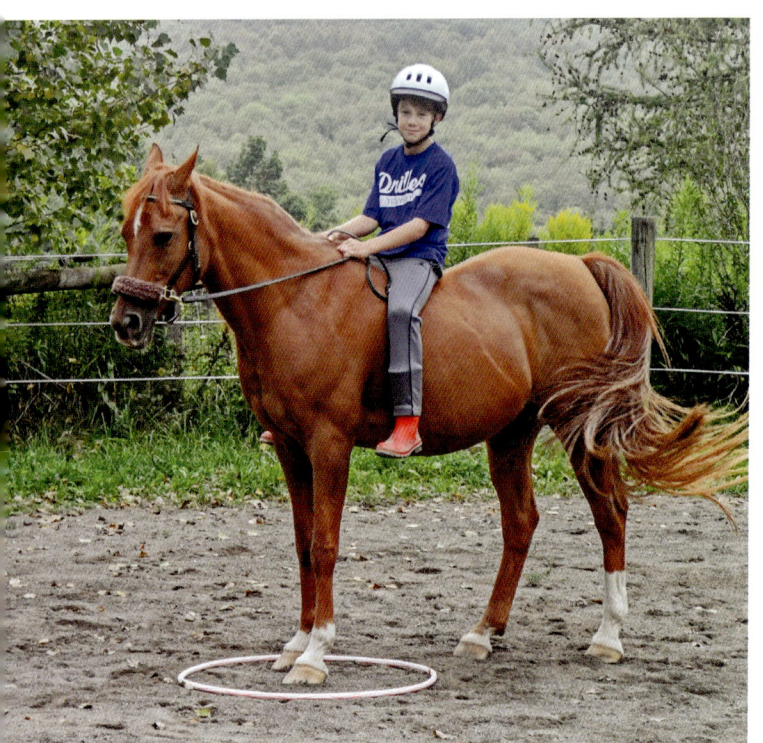

15.9 With me, Bronzz always dodges hoops. For Colin, who rides once a year, Bronzz steps neatly into a hoop every time.

> ### Additional Resources
>
> Hertha James is a whiz at breaking tasks into small steps. Her book *Conversations with Horses* describes the process in detail, including lesson plans. Her free YouTube video series *HorseGym with Boots* provides demonstrations.[122]
>
> *Three-Minute Horsemanship* by Vanessa Bee has 60 lesson plans for practical skills that can be taught a few minutes at a time. It is amazing how much you can accomplish in a short time before or after a ride, or in the barn aisle on a bad weather day. Instead of feeling guilty for not spending more time "working" with my horses, I spend less time, accomplish more, enjoy it more, and leave my horses more eager for next time.

## ❧ Summary

Confidence is the feeling of security a horse has when he believes he can be successful at whatever you ask of him. You cannot measure success by what a horse does, or how many times he does it. You measure success by how *confident* he feels about doing it. Confidence is essential for reliability.

Developing horses' confidence is an educational process that engages their innate learning abilities. You expose them to different circumstances while providing your support, and teaching them what you want them to do. They generalize what they learn and apply it to future situations.

A systematic way to do this is to introduce them to a variety of obstacles representing different categories: *Over, Under,* and *Through.*

The specific activities you do are less important than having a variety of experiences that make the horse feel successful. A successful session ends with a horse who is relaxed, confident, and ready for more.

### THINGS TO TRY

- Think of an obstacle your horse is not familiar with. Before taking him near it, make a game of writing how many steps you could use to introduce him to it, starting with Investigative Behavior. The more steps the better.

- As you introduce your horse to the first step, watch his body language. If he looks calm and confident, go on to your second step. If not, try breaking your first step into more steps.

- End each session at a point where your horse is still curious and confident.

## chapter 16
# Brandy's Confidence Blossoms

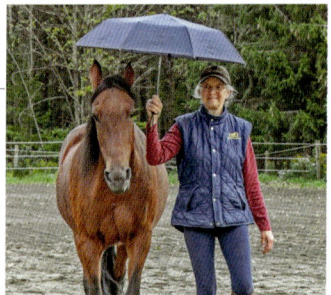

> "Not only have I found that we have been really underestimating the ability of our horses, we've been underestimating ourselves."
>
> —Vanessa Bee *(The Horse Agility Handbook)*

As I've mentioned, Brandy's initial fear of nearly everyone and everything made her unreliable. In addition to Confidence Building exercises with obstacles (the second part of this chapter—p. 196), she needed "remedial" work for confidence and good manners when handled by everyone, including veterinarian, farrier, dentist, or chiropractor.

Preparing for ordinary situations is not glamorous work. Success means events are boringly uneventful. We do not win ribbons, score points, or make the news. But good safe manners grounded in confidence help horses make friends wherever they go. It helps them find and keep good homes, and raises their chances of a nice retirement when they can no longer work. Teaching them good manners is one of the kindest things we can do for our animals. It is a way of giving them our protection even when we are not with them.

### Role Playing for Health Care

I role played each practitioner, using lots of rewards (scratching, praise, and treats) to create positive associations. Brandy was able to learn under the least stressful circumstances because I was the person she knew and trusted most, and I could work in short, casual sessions, starting with her loose in her stall so she did not feel trapped (see chapter 2—p. 26). A lead can be draped over the horse as a safety precaution for the handler (figs. 16.1–16.3). Once Brandy was comfortable with whatever I was doing, she was also comfortable with someone holding her lead at the same time.

Our goal in practice sessions is a relaxed horse who, ideally, thinks this is all a happy game. Real situations might be too stressful for relaxation, but if the horse is not surprised along with other stresses, we have still prepared for good manners.

Even well-behaved horses can be stressed, and appreciate extra patience, TLC, and rewards for good behavior. Bronzz's vet manners are impeccable. His stress is evident only in the fact that when the vet arrives, he retreats to the far corner of his stall and stands facing the wall, head down, as if hoping we'll forget he exists until the vet leaves.

## Farrier

Balancing on three legs is a learned skill. Horses also need to get comfortable having a leg restrained. For a horse who is already anxious, restraint is particularly frightening. Brandy's "Good Farrier Manners" program included overcoming this fear.

To avoid pressure and wrestling matches, I prompted her to lift her leg by squeezing the chestnut. When the hoof popped up, I caught it, and *immediately* set it down gently. Then I gave her a treat or a nice scratch. When this was easy, I started holding the hoof for a second before setting it down. I gradually increased the time I held the hoof, always trying to set it down while her leg was still relaxed in my hand. Hind feet waited until she was comfortable having her front feet handled.

Next, I played with her feet, patting, wiggling, and tapping them with the hoof pick. I gradually lifted each leg forward to the position in which it rests on a hoof stand (fig. 16.1).

At trimming time, my farrier's supremely patient manner reassured Brandy. To reinforce expectations, I held her lead and did Click & Treat (see p. 133) for standing still while holding a foot up. After a couple of visits, Brandy

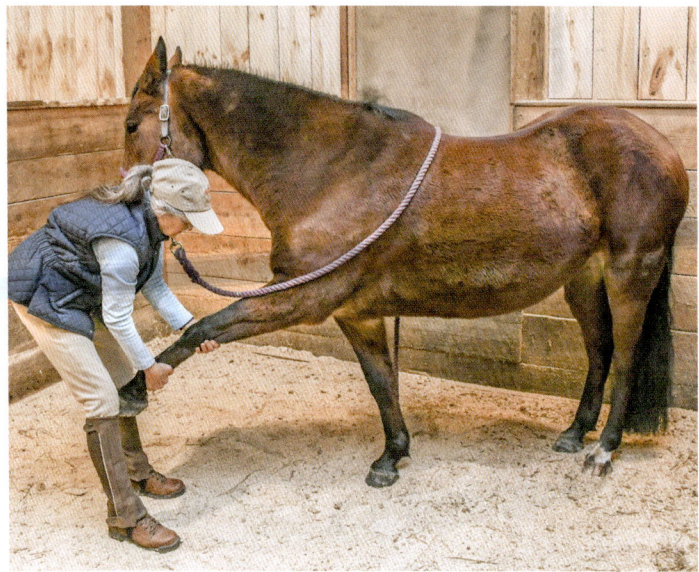

16.1 I pull Brandy's leg forward to hoof stand position.

PART SIX: POSITIVE EXPERIENCES BUILD CONFIDENCE AND RELIABILITY was comfortable with the routine, so I phased out Click & Treat. Soon she was standing tied in the aisle, calmly lifting each foot as needed, while I did chores.

## Veterinarian

Horses can get "white coat syndrome" for the same reason people do; they do not like being poked, prodded, and stabbed. Anxiety can run especially high if an early injury created an association between vets and serious pain.

My goal was for Brandy to enjoy full body touching. Since she loved being scratched on her withers, neck, and shoulders (the mutual grooming area), I started there. I worked my way around to her chest, then up her neck and down her back. I peered closely into her ears and eyes, lifted her tail, and gently touched her udder.

During Brandy's first vet visit, we discovered that she was terrified of shots. The serious consequences of this fear were apparent several months later when she choked. I made an emergency call to our vet who advised we give her Banamine (a painkiller and anti-inflammatory drug). We were not only unable to give Brandy the injection, we stressed her further in the attempt. Fortunately, she recovered without immediate assistance. After that, the vet suggested I desensitize Brandy by mimicking injections.

Nothing was going to convince Brandy that this painful procedure was harmless,

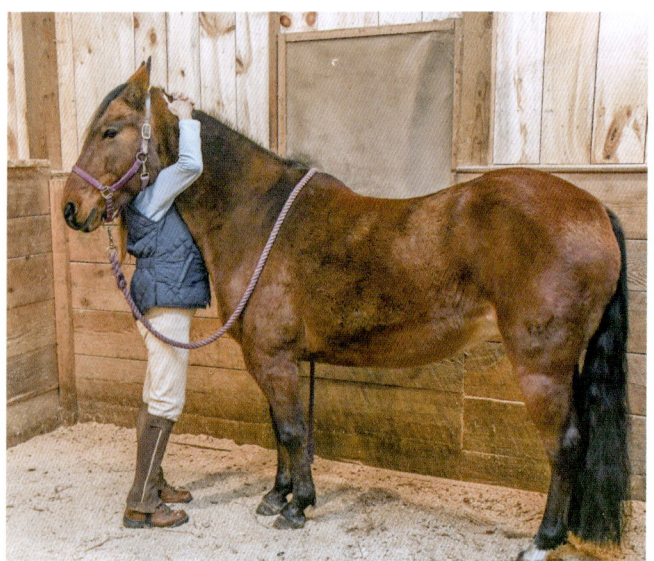

16.2 A  Having someone reach around her neck as a chiropractor might do was a new experience for Brandy.

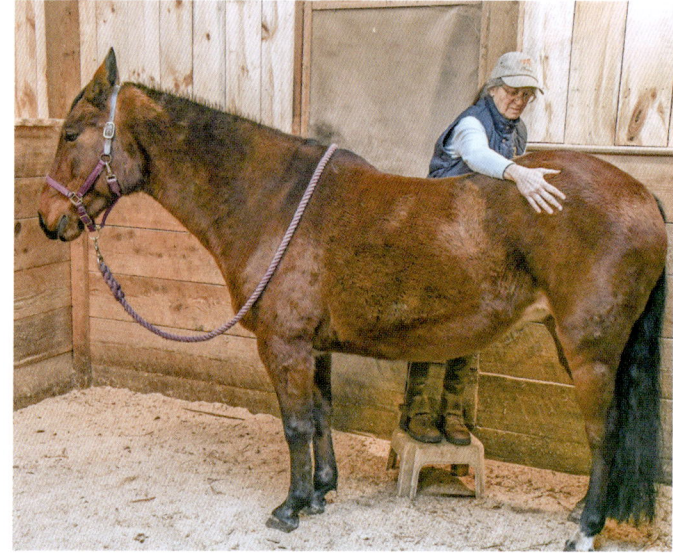

16.2 B  I stand on a stool to reach across her back and gently wiggle her hindquarters side to side.

so I balanced the negative with a reward.

With Brandy loose in her stall, I tapped her neck twice with the side of my hand, then poked her lightly with the tip of a syringe *with the needle removed*. At first this motion sent her scurrying away. When she came back to me, I gave her a treat. After a few sessions she was standing still, looking for the treat. Although she startled the next time the vet hit her with the real thing, her feet did not move. Instead, she looked to me for the praise and treat that she knew she had earned.

## Chiropractor

Chiropractors not only touch horses, but manipulate different body parts. They may also stand on a stool for extra height. The first time I put my hands on Brandy's neck and gently tried to move it, she went wide-eyed and rigid. With rubbing, scratching, and patience, I persuaded her to relax enough that I could move her neck. I stood on a stool and "worked" on her back, lightly rubbing the muscles on either side of her spine. I lifted and manipulated her legs and tail (figs. 16.2 A & B).

When the chiropractor worked on her, Brandy was surprised by the actual adjustments, but since they came in the context of familiar handling, she remained cooperative.

## Dentist

I was most worried about Brandy's first dental visit. I could not imagine a positive

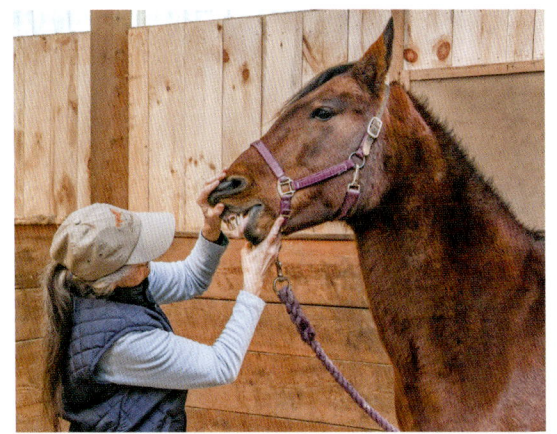

16.3 A I inspect Brandy's teeth so she gets accustomed to having her mouth opened and touched.

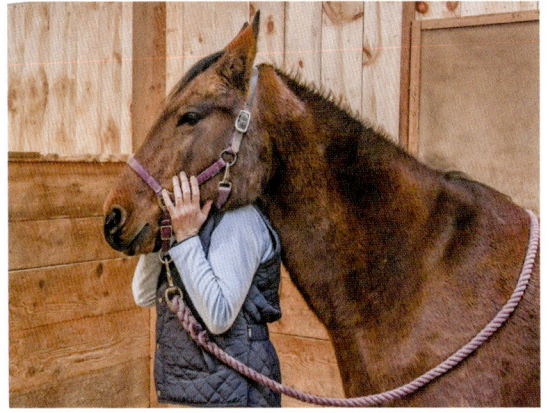

16.3 B I prop her head on my shoulder as my vet's tech does for dental work.

reaction to having two strangers (dentist and assistant) handle her at once, while doing strange things inside her mouth. In preparation, I played with Brandy's lips. I touched and tapped her teeth. I opened her mouth (finger on bars as for bit) and touched her tongue. I lifted her head and propped her lower jaw on my shoulder (figs. 16.3 A & B). All interspersed as usual with praise, treats, and scratching.

When the dentist and her assistant arrived, Brandy backed to the far corner of her stall, eyeing the strangers with suspicion. Observing this, the dentist suggested sedating her, but agreed to my request that we see what she could do without drugs. The dentist introduced herself and her equipment to Brandy in a quiet, matter-of-fact way. To everyone's astonishment, Brandy grew calmer as the dentist proceeded. Brandy was not relaxed; who is *relaxed* for dental work? But she stood still and cooperated.

As we marveled at her good behavior, it occurred to me that I would normally have stood next to Brandy, touching her to offer reassurance. This time, I stood in front of her where she could clearly see me. She watched me for the entire procedure, her eyes never once leaving my face. Apparently that was reassurance enough for her.

## Confidence Building and Horse Agility

I discovered Brandy's Confidence Building program with obstacles mostly by accident. At the time I did not know that any such thing existed. During her first few months with us, we worked on good manners and remedial saddle training, both essential but not exactly fun. I wanted to find some activity that she could actually enjoy doing with me. Thinking that obstacles might be fun, I checked *The Horse Agility Handbook* by Vanessa Bee. In addition to being my reference for body language communication, it provides detailed instructions for introducing obstacles in the context of a supportive relationship. Horse Agility obstacles fit the same categories described in Bee's book *Over, Under, Through: Obstacle Training for Horses.*

I soon discovered that Horse Agility is more than a Confidence Building program. It fine-tunes communication because the horse must watch his handler for precise instructions at each obstacle each time. Many of the obstacles also develop basic training skills such as balance, bending, and body awareness, which are more easily learned in an interesting context where there is a clear purpose for them.

Brandy took to Horse Agility like a duck to water, and her confidence blossomed. I began to suspect that much of her anxiety was an appropriately cautious reaction to her early life experiences, and that underneath the anxiety was a brave pony ready to show what she could do.

### Over

Brandy made short work of the *tarp*. I spread it out in the arena, and walked across it myself to demonstrate. Brandy sniffed it, tasted it, pawed it into a crumpled heap, and then walked right across it. I straightened it out. She pawed it into a mess and walked over it again. After she got tired of playing with it, she just walked over it. Later when I asked her to step on a piece of carpet, a different surface, she needed only a little sniff and

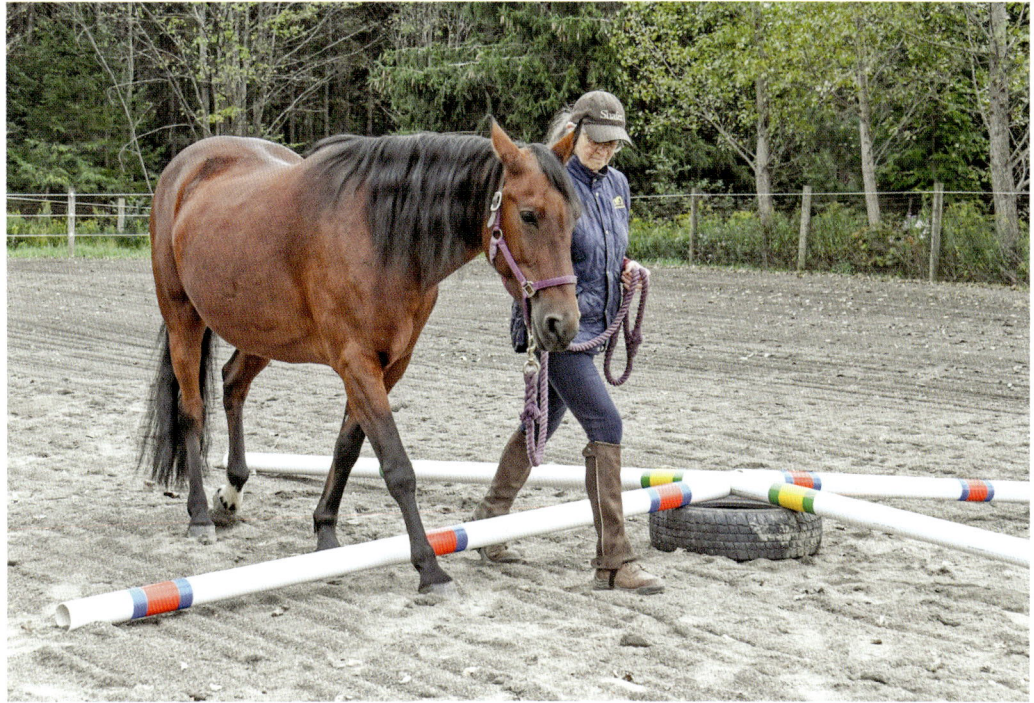

**16.4** Stepping over the pole wheel encourages Brandy to lift her feet and place them precisely.

a couple taps with a hoof to be satisfied.

*Poles* require careful placement of feet (fig. 16.4). Backing over a pole is a special challenge for horses with poor posture such as Brandy's (low back, inverted neck) because they tend to drag their feet. She had to learn to lift her back in order to lift her feet.

A *hula hoop* can look suspiciously like a hole. Many horses resist stepping in it, but Brandy quickly caught on to the game of halt with front feet in the hoop, and later hind feet in it.

The hoop makes a logical place to teach the *stay command* because feet are already parked in a designated place (fig. 16.5). I used the word "stay" along with my palm toward her face, as in dog training. First, I

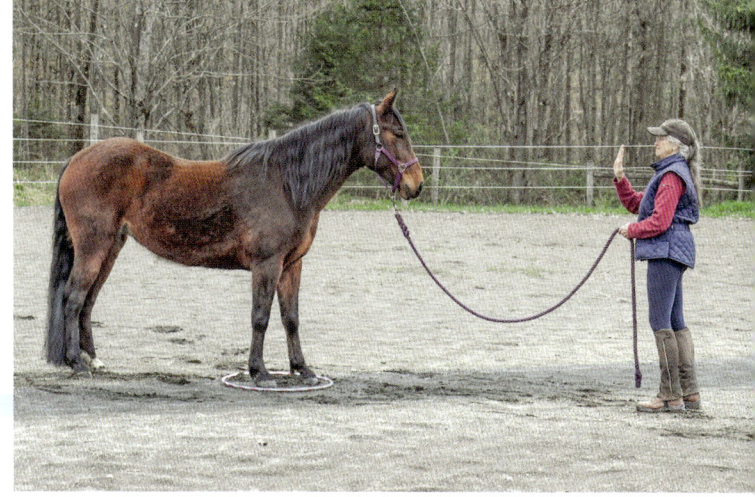

**16.5** A hoop helps a horse understand that front feet stay in place as we practice the *stay command*. I have backed several steps away. I will return to leading position and praise her for standing still before asking her to move.

PART SIX: POSITIVE EXPERIENCES BUILD CONFIDENCE AND RELIABILITY — 197

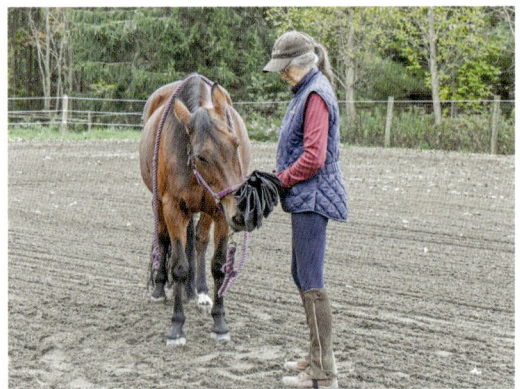

**16.6 A** Brandy's inspection of the closed umbrella includes a serious sniffing.

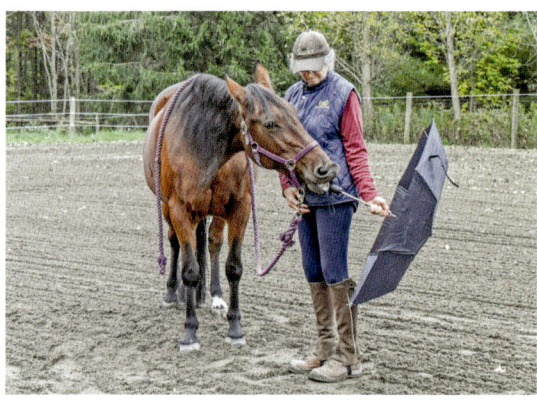

**16.6 B** I have opened it slowly, keeping my body between her and the umbrella. Brandy's inspection now includes a taste.

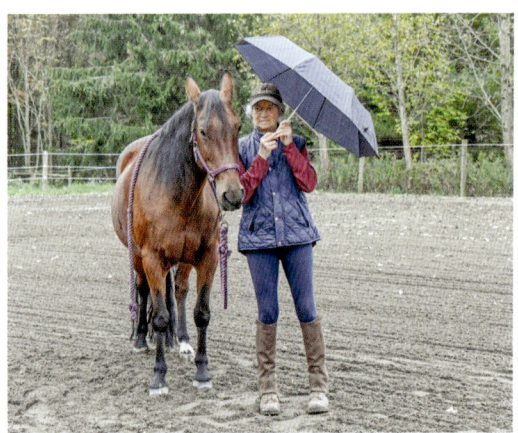

**16.6 C** I raise the umbrella very slowly, ready to lower it if Brandy looks anxious enough to leave.

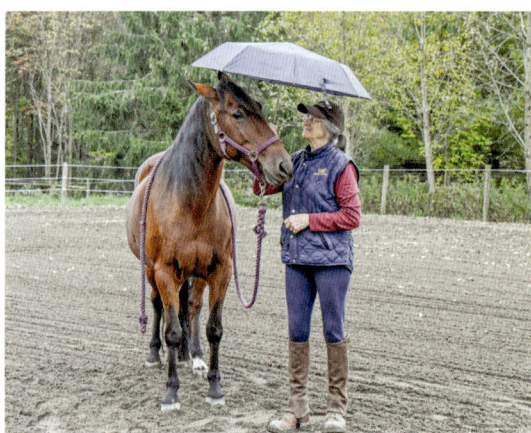

**16.6 D** Brandy looks a little unsure as I move it over her head, so I just wait.

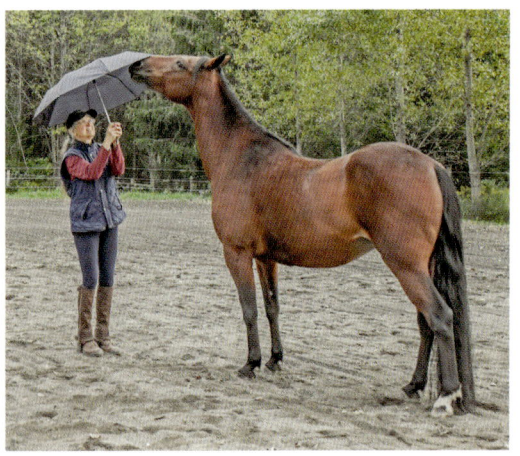

**16.6 E** The next time I bring out the umbrella, it is purely a source of curiosity.

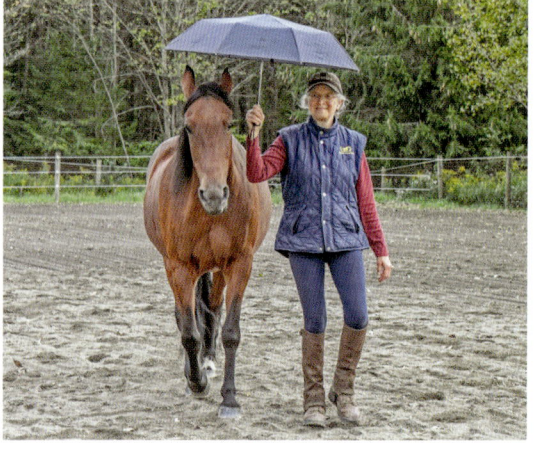

**16.6 F** Brandy is now confident walking under the umbrella with me.

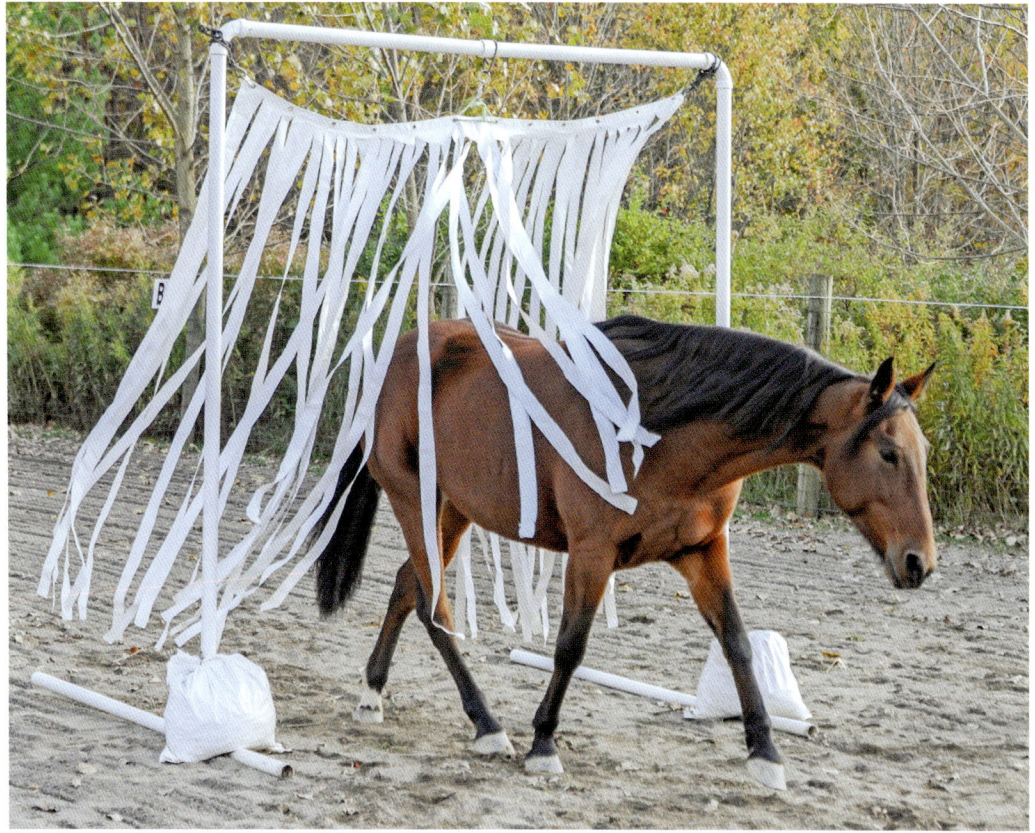

16.7 It would take about 30 pictures to show all the steps that led to this level of confidence: walking through the frame adding one ribbon at a time, then trotting through, then walking and trotting through without me.

just turned to stand in front of her, and returned to the leading position. Then I started backing away one step at a time, always returning to the leading position before asking her to move. Gradually, I backed farther, then walked away frontward until I could flash her a stay signal and jog away.

## Under

An *umbrella* is a simple "under" obstacle. I introduced it to Brandy in small steps, making sure she was relaxed with each step before we moved on. With her lead draped over her back, she was free to leave if she got uncomfortable. It is my job to make sure that curiosity wins out over anxiety (figs. 16.6 A–F).

A *ribbon curtain* is both "under" and "through." I introduced it as described in *The Horse Agility Handbook*: First Brandy walked through the bare frame, then the frame with all the ribbons tied back, then one ribbon hanging down, then one more ribbon at a time. Soon she was strolling through the curtain with confidence, the streamers brushing over her head, between her ears, along her sides and down her back (fig. 16.7).

The ribbon curtain became one of

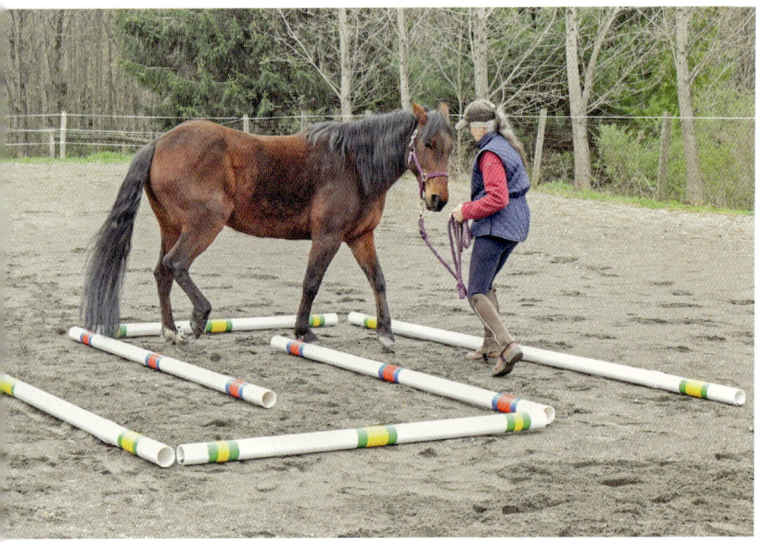

**16.8** The S-bend is 3 feet 3 inches (1 meter) wide. Careful footwork and communication are required to negotiate it when horse and handler must stay inside the poles without touching them. As I back up in front of Brandy, my rounded shoulders invite her to come toward me.

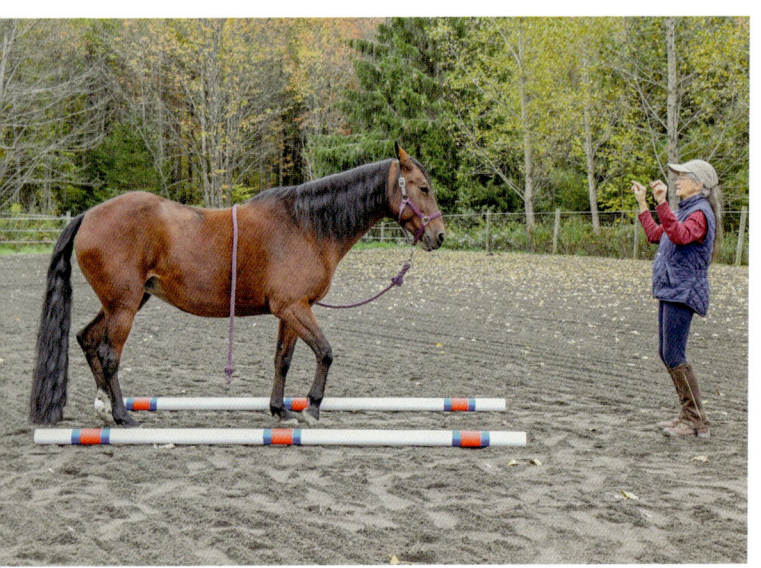

**16.9** After learning to back up beside me, she can now do it with a remote signal. My slight backward lean is part of the signal.

Brandy's favorite obstacles. When I confuse her with something new at liberty, she sometimes trots off and goes through a familiar obstacle on her own. The ribbon curtain is one of them.

## Through

*Weaving around cones* presents two challenges: maintaining leading position on a curve, and bending in the direction of the turn. A correct bend is a foundation skill for any athletic activity a horse may be asked to perform.

*Pole patterns* such as U-turns, L-bends, and S-bends (fig. 16.8) involve more bending, balance, and precision communication.

*Backing* through parallel poles 2 feet (60 centimeters) wide helped Brandy learn to back straight (fig. 16.9).

*Narrow gaps* are a natural source of anxiety. Horses rushing through can crash into handlers and bang rider's knees. We started with barrels 6 feet 6 inches (2 meters) apart. Brandy learned to halt in front of the gap and wait for my cue to proceed through (figs. 16.10 A & B). She also learned to halt *in* the gap and to back through it.

Over time I made the gap narrower, longer, and taller. I made the changes so gradually that she remained unconcerned even when it was a dozen feet long, higher than her withers, only a few inches wider than her sides, and closed at one end. The sides were tarps draped over jump standards, so they moved with each puff of wind.

## Additional Challenges

*Moving objects* show how horses instinctively retreat from something strange that comes *toward* them, yet their curiosity encourages them to follow things that move *away*. They check the thing out as they follow, closing the gap as they get comfortable with it.

This works with any moveable object, such as a ball, bicycle, flag, or something dragged with a rope. If you have an assistant, she can slowly move the object away from the horse while you walk the horse on a loose lead, letting him set the pace and following distance.

Balls are a natural source of concern because they roll around apparently at random or, worse, under their own power. I introduced Brandy to balls by playing quietly with one in the barn aisle until she was reaching over her door, offering to touch it.

Outside, I rolled the ball on the ground ahead of me, letting her see that I controlled its motion. She ignored it. The next time out, she began reaching for it when it stopped, so I clicked and treated increasingly firm touches on the ball. Soon she was pushing it along herself (fig. 16.11).

Horse Agility courses often include a *scary corridor*: two rows of objects that are commonly frightening to a horse. At

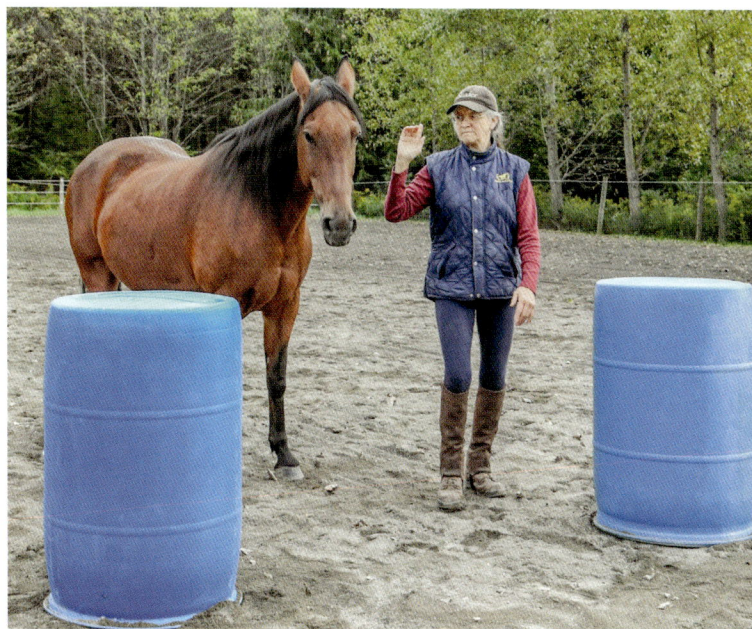

**16.10 A** I signal Brandy to halt in front of the narrow gap. Then I signaled her to stay until I went through *and* asked her to join me. This is just one practical application of the stay command.

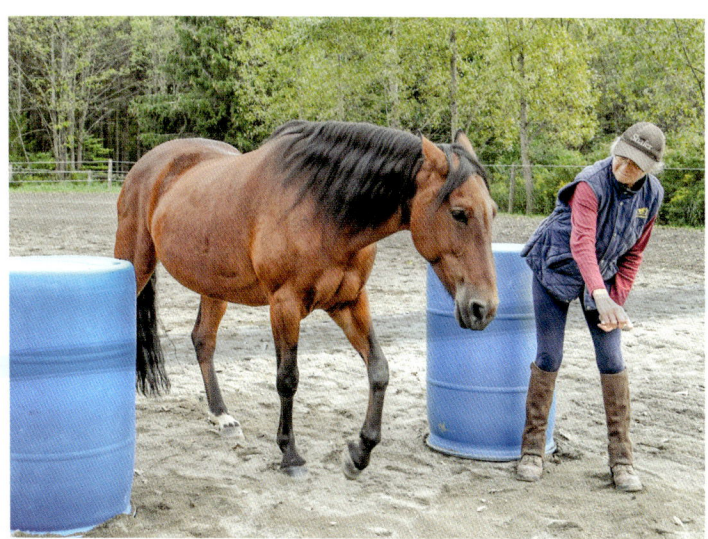

**16.10 B** Brandy's ears always go back as she passes through the narrow gap, then pop up after she exits.

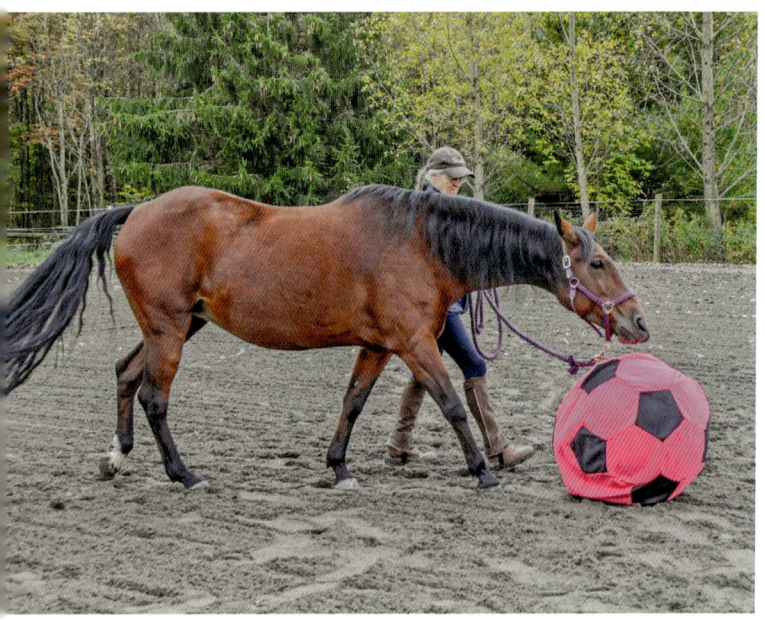

**16.11** Discovering that *she* had the power to make a ball move was a confidence booster that Brandy generalized to other objects that appear to move at random, like lawn ornaments and flags. Dribbling the ball together is now a reward and playtime break.

first, the horse walks between the rows with the handler. Later, he goes through alone, perhaps at a trot or canter (figs. 16.12 A & B).

My "scary" objects have included flags, pennants, old show ribbons, wind chimes, road cones, tires, lawn ornaments, big stuffed animals wearing silly costumes, and a variety of discount store seasonal decorations. Early on, Brandy stopped to inspect new items. As time went on, it became more and more difficult to find anything she even bothered to look at.

The long-term value of the scary corridor is apparent in a recurring question on the Horse Agility website. "What if I can't find any more things that my horse even pays attention to?" That's our measure of success! New and strange items are greeted either with indifference, "Ho hum, I've seen things like that before." Or curiosity, "Oh goodie, a new toy!"

## Practical Application: Brandy Plays Super Pony

Confidence Building exercises are valuable even if a horse never leaves home. One cold, windy afternoon we saw Brandy canter across the pasture, her blanket flying out behind her like a cape. I could guess what happened. I had removed the leg straps from her blanket because it never slipped sideways. What I did not think about was that if the belly straps come undone, the blanket is just hanging around the horse's neck, an accident in the making.

As I threw on boots and coat, Brandy came to a halt, front feet on her blanket, which had twisted around in front of her. I dashed to the barn for halter and lead, then made my way to the pasture as swiftly as I dared. When I reached her, Brandy still had both front feet planted on her blanket. She was tense and concerned, but not ready to panic. I slipped her halter on, then reached up to her withers and unclipped the chest straps of her blanket. As I led her off the fallen blanket, her tension evaporated.

The only casualty in the incident was the blanket. After her work with flags and the ribbon curtain, something flying out behind her did not cause Brandy to panic.

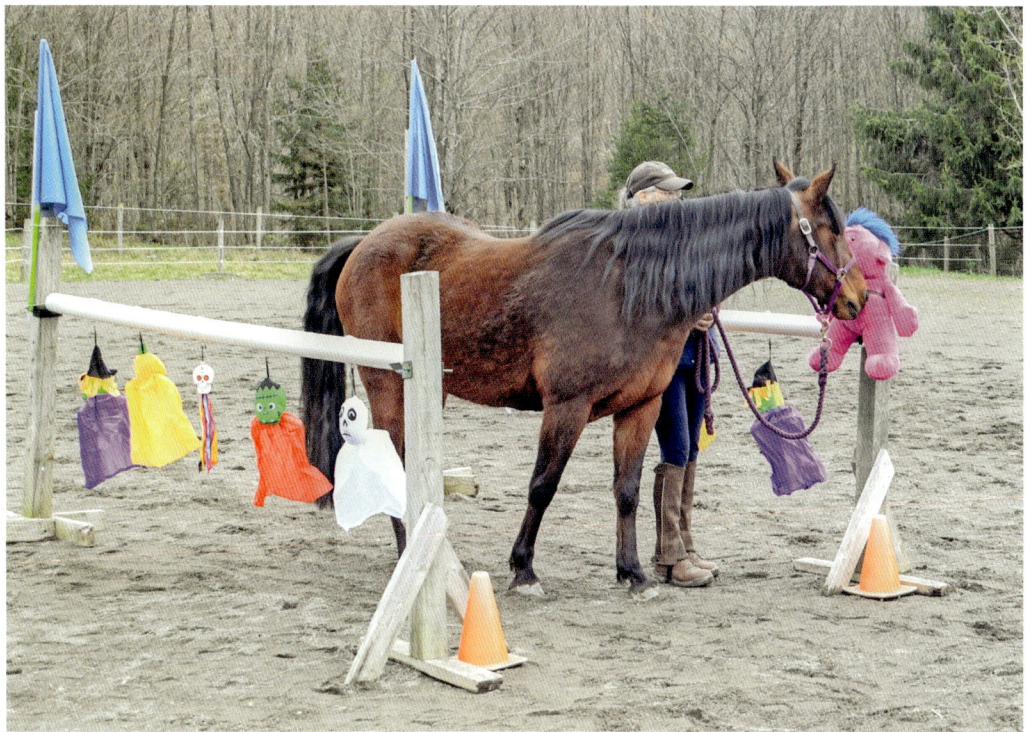

**16.12 A** Brandy has not seen this stuffed critter for a while, so she pauses for a friendly sniff. Stopping to investigate is *always* allowed.

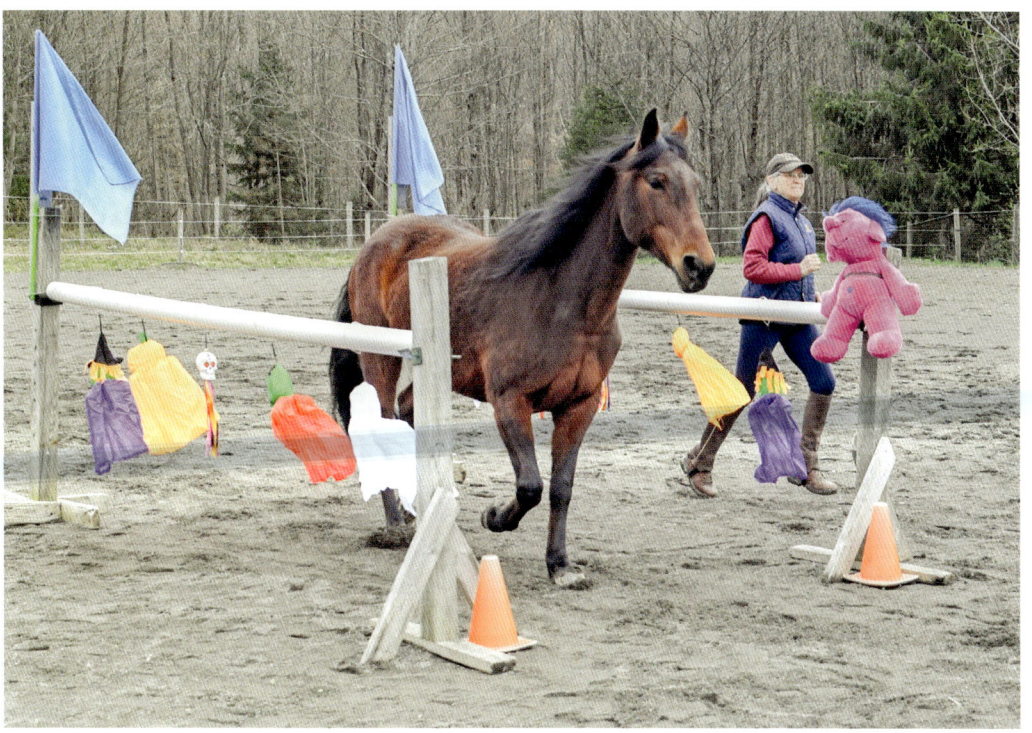

**16.12 B** This is our Halloween-themed version of the scary corridor. Brandy trots through with confidence and enthusiasm, her left ear tuned for my directions.

Nor did she panic when she stepped on the blanket and was trapped. Instead, she waited for me to rescue her.

### Brandy's New Career

By the time Brandy had been with us a few months, I was fretting over the limited prospects of a pony who cannot be ridden or driven. If I actually entered her in an agility competition, I reasoned, I could bill her as an "Agility Pony" in addition to "Pasture Companion." Maybe that would help her find a home. Wishful thinking, I know, but it nudged me in a good direction.

The International Horse Agility Club (www.thehorseagilityclub.com) holds monthly competitions via online videos. The competitions are designed to be educational, with each level including skills that prepare for the next level. The website is also a forum for supportive training discussions among members.

I registered Brandy and myself, downloaded that month's Starter Level course, and set it up in my arena as diagramed. Brandy knew how to negotiate all 10 of the obstacles for that course except the jump. No matter how enthusiastically I demonstrated and encouraged, Brandy would not jump. She just trotted over the pole until I raised it too high, and then she knocked it down. Oh well. The deadline was approaching. It was time to just do the best we could.

The video must be continuous, so you cannot do it piecemeal and splice the good bits together. When we reached the jump, for the very first time, Brandy jumped!

In Horse Agility competitions the horse and handler each earn a maximum of 5 points per obstacle. Although I lost points for inadvertently letting the lead line get tight, Brandy earned a perfect score for her part. The pony who once ran wild had just become one of the first competition agility horses in the United States.

### Brandy *Likes* Her New Career

I spend only 10 or 15 minutes a few times a week on Brandy's agility training, but it adds up. The more relaxed and playful I am, the faster she learns. Once, for an advanced course, she was supposed to halt from a trot with her left front foot on a round marker 12 inches (30 centimeters) in diameter. Impossible, I thought. But I dutifully folded a plastic bedding sack to the appropriate size and demonstrated by placing my own left foot on it. Brandy did not seem to notice, so I got her attention by stamping on it dramatically. She energetically pawed the thing into a heap and looked at me as if to ask, was that really what I meant?

After I stopped laughing, I rearranged the bedding sack, and we went off to play with another obstacle. When we trotted back to the bedding sack a few minutes later, Brandy plopped her left front foot smack in the middle of it and did her little arched neck head shake that seems to say, "I nailed it, I *know* I did!"

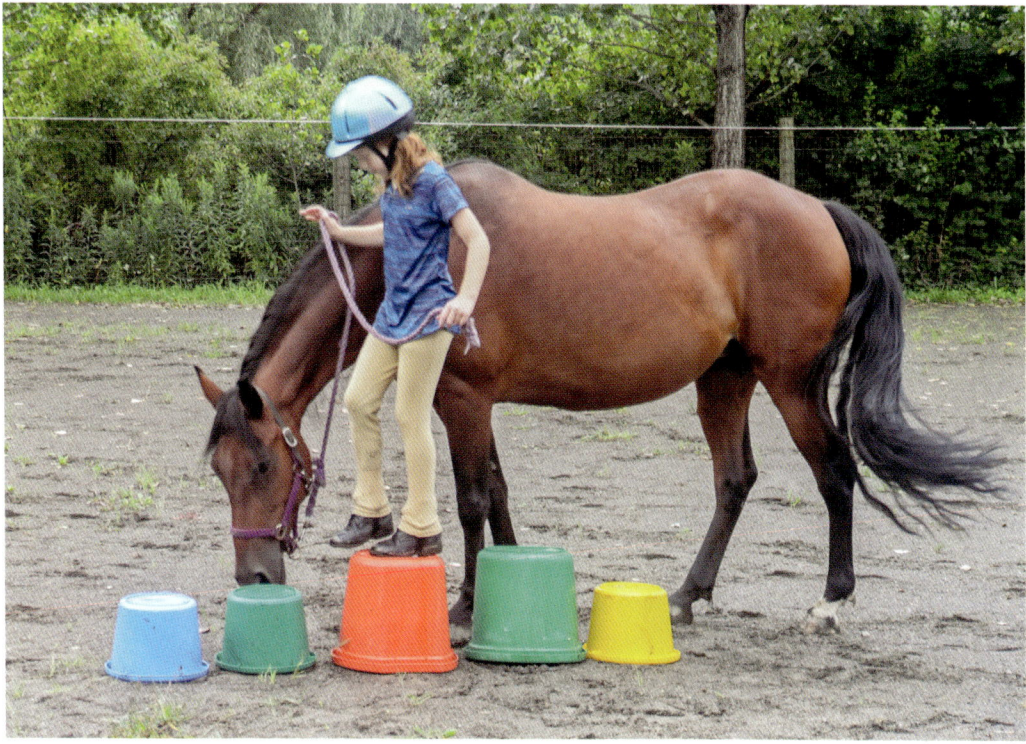

16.13 Brandy tries to decipher what her role is as Camille walks across buckets, an "obstacle" in a summer fun kids' agility course.

Brandy's job expanded to helping me teach Friendly Body Language and Horse Agility to other people. When I hand her lead to another person, she responds to their cues with calm confidence.

Like many horses, she takes special care with children. When young grandchildren visit, she is *their* pony. They lead, feed, groom, and care for her. She has been braided, beribboned, and decorated. Most of all, the children love doing agility courses with her. They learn the body language cues by leading me. Then they practice with Brandy who is not only unfailingly patient, but ready to assist when needed (fig. 16.13).

Horse Agility gives the children a way of interacting with horses that is both challenging and fun. Mistakes are just sources of laughter and reminders to give clearer cues. Meanwhile, the kids are learning about horse behavior and body language, and how to inspire cooperation. The confidence that Colin developed handling Brandy inspired him to do agility courses with Bronzz, and then to mount up for Equagility (fig. 16.14). In Equagility you lead a horse through 5 obstacles, then mount up and repeat the same 5 obstacles. The goal in the mounted portion is to guide your horse with little or no rein pressure. At the basic levels, two reins are used, but points are lost if they go tight. For intermediate courses, one

16.14 Colin guides Bronzz around a U-bend in Equagility. Horse Agility does not require fancy equipment or formal attire. Colin's goal is to communicate with Bronzz using the least possible rein pressure.

lead line is attached to the horse's halter. At the advanced level, no lead or reins are used. A bridle may be worn for safety, but you lose points if you touch the reins. Saddles are optional.

## The Versatility of Horse Agility

A Confidence Building program such as Horse Agility might be just part of a horse's education, preparing him to be more reliable in the career chosen for him.

If Brandy could be ridden, everything she learned in agility would have made her a more confident, precise, focused mount. Instead, it became her career. Brandy has graduated to the most advanced levels of Horse Agility, both on-lead and at liberty. For each of our other horses, Horse Agility became valuable in different ways.

For Sapphire, it provided some of the novelty and stimulation she missed when her trail riding years ended. When you see horses standing around doing nothing,

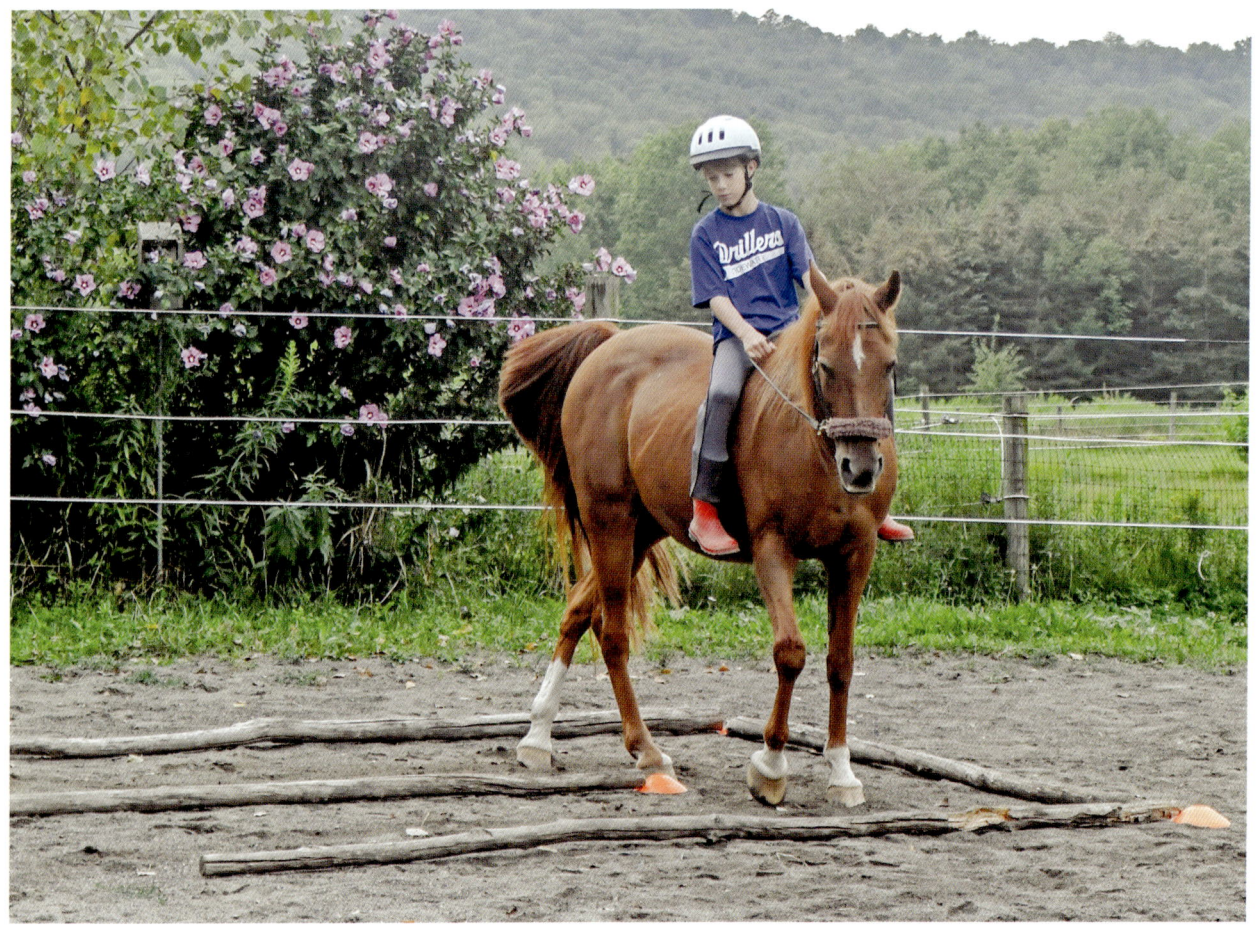

it is easy to overlook the fact that it's because they have nothing to do. Domestic life lacks the interest and challenges that our horses' wild ancestors faced in the course of daily survival. It is up to us to engage their minds when their bodies can no longer do the jobs they once did.

Shiloh enjoys the special time with Jerry since he rarely rides her. She does not seem to care if they do the same things over and over.

Bronzz prefers Equagility, specifically the riding part. To the amusement of everyone who's seen our videos, he trudges through the unmounted part of the course as if he is bored beyond belief. The moment I mount up, his ears come forward, there is a spring in his step, and my biggest challenge is slowing him down.

Equagility is an educational challenge for me. Without reins, I need to use my seat, legs, and weight very precisely. This has significantly improved my riding and my awareness of how minute actions influence my horse.

## More Practical Application: Brandy's Hospital Adventure

A few months ago Brandy developed a persistent cough. Given her previous episode of choke, our vet advised gastroscopy at the equine hospital at Cornell University. Brandy rode in the trailer without a fuss, and walked politely into her assigned stall in the hospital. There she stood trembling in fear. In Brandy's experience trailer trips mean being dropped off and left, often in a strange place. And this place was surely stranger than any she had ever been.

For an hour she shook. Nothing I did calmed her. Then the vet team arrived and she was surrounded by strangers: two veterinarians, a vet tech, and a student. To my amazement, that's when Brandy stopped shaking. A vet exam was something she understood.

The next surprise occurred when I led her into the exam room, already partially sedated. She wobbled into the stocks without hesitation; it was just a narrow gap. Then she headed right for the fascinating piece of (very expensive) equipment that stood at the end of the stocks, ready to investigate and play with it. Apparently neither anxiety nor sedation had squelched her curiosity. I intercepted her in the nick of time.

The scope showed that her cough was caused by mild heaves. We were advised to steam her hay, and keep her out of the barn.

Brandy's anxiety did not fully abate until she was home again, but throughout the day, her behavior was exemplary. I thought of French classical rider Antoine de Pluvinel's observation that when a horse trusts you, he will ask you what to do when he is afraid. Brandy had indeed looked to me for guidance, and had followed my instructions even when she trembled with fear.

### My Pony, My Teacher

Colonel Alois Podhajsky wrote that he learned something from every horse he rode. One of his classic books is titled *My Horses, My Teachers*. I have always thought that if such a humble philosophy was good enough for a horseman of his caliber, it should be good enough for me. Perhaps that's *why* he was such a great horseman.

Brandy has reinforced this principle over and over, and shown me two important variations on it. First, there is much to be learned from a horse you never ride. Everything she teaches me transfers to every horse I ride. In fact, Brandy has clarified and reinforced lessons Bronzz has been trying to teach me for years.

Second, we do not need new horses to learn from if we listen to the horse we are working with. I spent many years riding and learning from different horses, but I knew nothing of where they came from or how well my schooling served them in the future. Longstanding relationships show us the bigger picture of how different things impact our horses' lives and behavior, and how our leadership can make a positive difference.

### Summary

Learning how to behave for anyone who handles him is an important part of a horse's education; it helps him find and keep a good home. Role playing by a trusted caretaker can prepare a horse in advance so that fewer surprises mean less anxiety and better behavior.

Horse Agility is a Confidence Building program that improves communication, balance, bending, and body awareness, all valuable for riding and driving as well as ground work. It also provides challenge, stimulation, and social time for horses who cannot be ridden.

---

**THINGS TO TRY**

- Review your horse's manners for health care practitioners. Could they be better? If so, try role playing the practitioner while showing your horse what he should do. Use lots of patience and positive reinforcement.

- Introduce your horse to one obstacle from each of the three groups: Over, Under, and Through. Notice which ones he seems to enjoy most. Spend extra time on those, expanding from where he is comfortable.

## chapter 17
# Freedom and Liberty

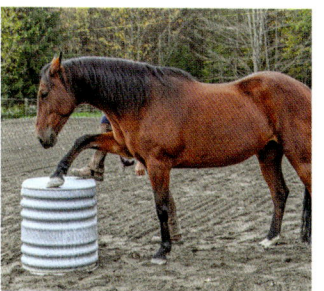

> "Horses do not need 'collars' and 'leads' all the time; they will come when you call them and happily do so if you ask in a language they understand."
>
> —Vanessa Bee *(The Horse Agility Handbook)*

*In riding a horse, we borrow freedom.* This popular quote evokes a lovely image of the power, grace, speed, and agility you can enjoy on a horse's back. The horses' side of this bargain is not always so attractive: *In domesticating horses, we have taken away their freedom.* Humans dictate ownership, jobs, living conditions, diet, turnout, companions, breeding, weaning, and who raises the young.

In addition to this, people often exert such rigid control in everyday interactions that horses have no room to express their individual personalities, no way to tell us when they are uncomfortable, and no incentive to think. Just as with people, this micromanagement undermines self-confidence and trust in leadership, two things we are trying to nurture in our horses. Instead of using their cognitive abilities to figure out what we want, horses "dumb down" and do only what is required.

Rigid control is based on the misconception that if we let a horse "get away" with anything, disobedience will escalate out of control. Once again, herd behavior points to a solution that works because it meets our horses' needs and makes sense to them. Horse herds have clear rules of social behavior, and those rules are respected because conflict among herd mates does not benefit anyone. However, *within those rules* horses have some latitude to suit themselves.

Even without allowing as much latitude as other horses do, you can apply the same principle. By easing unnecessarily narrow restrictions, you can encourage a horse to develop his ability to learn, to use good judgment, and to be a better partner.

You also reduce stress and stress-related problems that result from having too little control over your own life. Each small stress you relieve reduces the odds of stresses piling up until a horse is overwhelmed.

The first part of this chapter describes ways to ease restrictions by giving safe, appropriate choices. The second part shows how play invites initiative, and motivates a horse to engage with you. Finally, I'll show how appropriate freedom of choice and structured play have paved the way to liberty work.

## Four Ways to Give Freedom Safely

For most of us the idea of giving a horse any freedom of choice is radical at first. What if the horse decides he can do things his own way at an inopportune or even dangerous time? My experience is the more appropriate choices I give, the more reliably the horse trusts me when I say, "Not now."

*Sometimes it takes only seconds to make a horse calmer, happier, and more focused.*

Choices are "appropriate" only within the bounds of good safe manners. A savvy 6th grade teacher put into words what horses have shown me over and over. If you start with permissiveness, you struggle forever to set limits. But once you have established good behavior with clear, fair limits, you can relax some rules without losing the good behavior. A simple rule of thumb is: *The more reliably safe a horse's behavior is, the more choices and freedom he earns.*

### Wait a Minute

Sometimes it takes only seconds, literally, to make a horse calmer, happier, and more focused. The horse, as a prey animal, is *supposed* to *monitor his environment*. From his perspective, this is not disobedient or disrespectful. He is looking out for you, too, as herd mates are supposed to do.

Brandy routinely pauses to scan the horizon before going through a gate, even though we're going into her familiar arena or pasture. If I straighten up and ostentatiously scan with her, she takes less time doing it.

Sometimes, Bronzz stops dead on a trail, and stares into the underbrush at something I cannot see, hear, or smell. Occasionally, his head slowly turns as if tracking some creature's progress. When Bronzz is satisfied, he calmly moves on.

When my husband was still riding Sapphire, he made an observation that showed our horses sharing the responsibility for monitoring surroundings. When we rode single file on a trail, the lead horse always had ears forward, while the rear horse rotated ears to the back. When we changed position, the ears reversed at the exact moment that the rear horse overtook the lead horse. We leap-frogged each other many times, and this never varied.

Horses' mental health and their ability to learn are both related to *curiosity*. I indulge my horses' curiosity even when they seem inexplicably nosy about things that they have long since investigated and are not worried about. Brandy routinely checks out everything in the barn aisle. All my horses periodically inspect agility equipment they've long been familiar with.

When we ride in the woods, Bronzz likes to stop and sniff manure piles on the trail. Perhaps he is discovering which of his acquaintances has passed through lately. Our compromise is that Bronzz can sniff all he likes when we're alone, but we do not stop when we're riding with someone else.

Bronzz is adamant about *comfort breaks*. On hot summer days, his face gets itchy and he is desperate to stop and rub it. Allowing him a 5 second rub is more productive than trying to keep him focused while he is shaking his head in irritation. I also let him stop to relieve himself. I once had an instructor who was horrified. "You can't let him do that! What if he stops and poops in front of a judge?" In fact, Bronzz never has. He seems to know it is not the thing to do. At home, however, as we ride past the corner of the arena that he and the mares use for toilet, he knows it is okay to pause and relieve himself. Fine by me; it makes arena cleanup easier.

My horses all know that whatever else we are doing, they may initiate a detour to the water tank for a drink.

Sometimes a pause is an *expression of worry*. An obedient horse who's uncomfortable with trailers, for instance, might pause before loading.

Brandy went through a spell of turning a circle every time I went into her stall with her winter blanket. It started after her blanket shot static electricity sparks, so I suspected it was an expression of concern. If I had scolded or restrained her, I would have added to her anxiety. Instead, I just waited. After the circle she stood still to be blanketed. After a year or so, during which I was more careful not to slide her blanket and produce static, she stopped circling.

The reason for the pause might be a *mystery*. Sammie, my sister's previous horse, always wanted a sip of water before she left her stall. Was this a little power play? Did some instinct tell her to always drink before leaving a water source? Who cares? What's significant is that the more Dani allowed Sammie these small choices, the more cooperative Sammie was in important matters, and the harder she worked when ridden.

None of these pauses are disobedience or disrespect. The horse is not saying, "I won't." He is saying, "Wait a minute." Then he carries right on with whatever we have asked him to do. I would not scold a friend for making me wait 10 seconds. Why scold my horses? They spend plenty of time standing around waiting for me.

## Making Requests

When one partner makes all the decisions, you do not have a partnership, you have a dictatorship. But if you tune into body language, you may notice your horse making subtle requests. I saddle Bronzz, mount up, and as we cross the paddock, he drifts toward the gate that goes to the woods. "Please can we go on a trail ride?"

When we're in the woods, Bronzz may ask to go one gait faster. I feel a little bounce in his walk step, or a single canter step with his hind feet while we're trotting. Sometimes I cue him immediately for the gait he has requested. If I don't, however, he knows his request is duly noted, and I will act on it when I'm ready. Bronzz has opinions on which trails to take, and often it is not the trail toward home. I take this as a huge compliment that he, too, is enjoying our ride.

Bronzz also makes requests when we're in the arena. I ask for shoulder-in, and feel his haunches gravitating toward the center instead. I just gently say with my aids, "No, I'm asking for shoulder-in now." He complies gracefully because he knows that I have noticed, and soon will ask him for haunches-in.

When Brandy and I are working at liberty, her suggestions are not so subtle. If she gets frustrated trying to figure out something new (usually because my signals are not clear enough), she often trots off to another obstacle, like the ribbon curtain or carpet mat, and waits for me there. "Let's play over here instead."

All of these requests are within the bounds of activities we have done together.

## Special Privileges

A well-behaved horse might *earn* privileges that would not otherwise be allowed. He must understand the limits of what you're allowing, and reliably obey when you tell him to do something else. Sometimes I leave Brandy loose in the barn to "do chores" with me. She goes in each of the other horses' stalls to lick out their feed bin, scouts the aisle for dropped hay, sips from the cats' water bowl, sniffs the grazing muzzles in case the food fairy put treats in them, and inspects anything new that is lying around. She earned this privilege because she mills around slowly and carefully, and returns readily to her stall when I point in that direction. Bronzz and Shiloh lost this privilege by heading straight for the hay storage area to make a mess dragging hay bales down.

Bronzz is allowed to rub his itchy face on my back after a ride because he waits until his bridle is off and I've turned my back, and because he never tries to rub on anyone any other time.

## Playtime and Playfulness

The value of play is sadly underestimated in the horse world. It is a huge motivator, morale booster, stress-buster, time to enjoy your relationship with a horse,

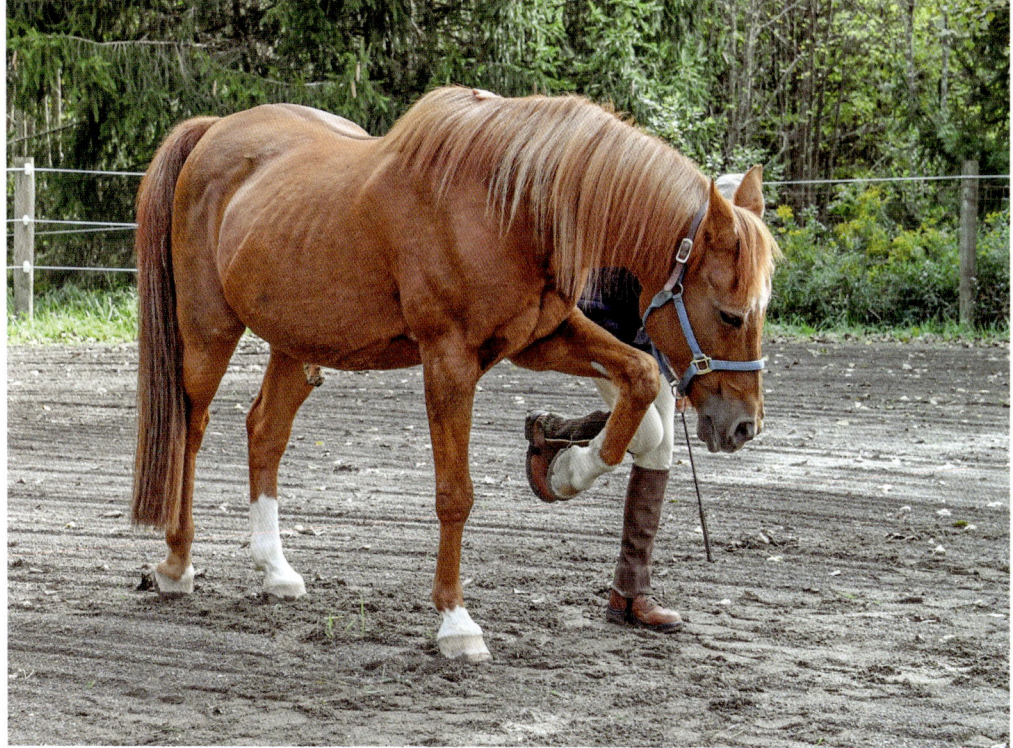

**17.1** Bronzz copies me as I bow and lift one leg. Copying my leg motion is a step toward Spanish Walk.

and an opportunity for horses to take initiative. It should be no surprise to dog people that play can support even the most serious training and competition goals. It is now a well-established part of dog training, even for working dogs with critical jobs.

I find that a playful attitude inspires better focus and more consistent effort. It also keeps my mind open and helps me focus on the positive. As a result I am more often pleasantly surprised by what we accomplish than disappointed by what we do not.

It can be dangerous to turn a horse loose for the kinds of active free-form games you might play with a dog. Horses play rough with each other, and you could easily get hurt. Instead, you can teach specific games with safe rules. Then, within the rules of the game, a horse can take initiative. Games should be played on a lead when there is any danger of a horse becoming too exuberant.

**Friendly Body Language** leads naturally to games based on *copying*. Once a horse understands matching your footfalls at walk and trot, you can suggest other moves. Step sideways, cross your legs over, lift your leg up higher, turn and face the opposite direction, bow and lift a leg at the same time (fig. 17.1). The

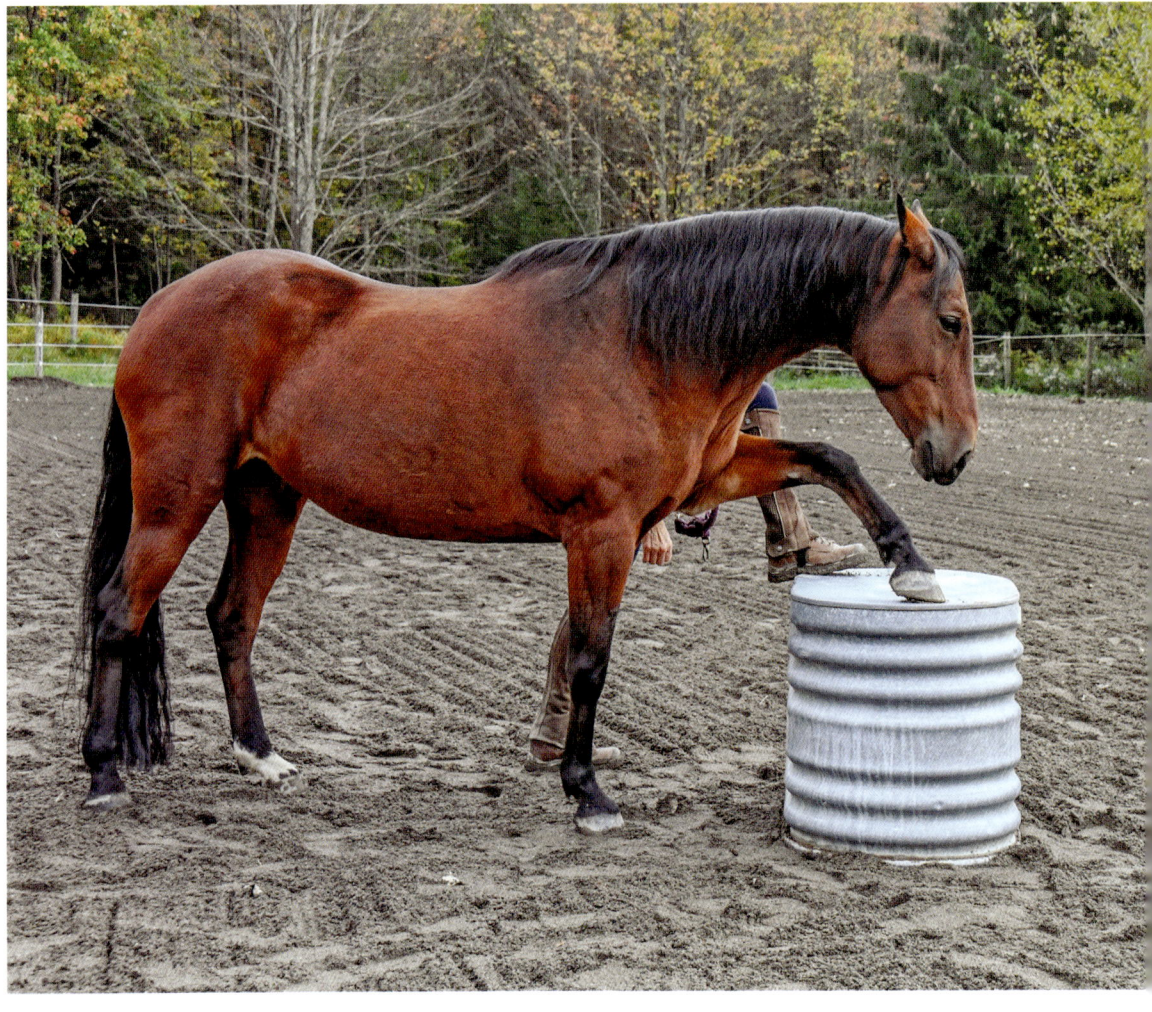

**17.2** It was Brandy's idea to put her foot on the overturned water tank, perhaps because she sees me do it when I mount Bronzz. I copied her.

possibilities and combinations are limitless, and it is an easy way to sneak in training, like "copy my balanced body posture while I halt."

Sometimes Brandy offers to copy, with no encouragement from me. One day as I rolled a barrel across the arena by kicking it, Brandy left her weed nibbling to walk beside me and watch. Then she lifted one front foot and placed it on the barrel. Her hoof slid over the barrel. Standing there with her leg draped over the barrel, she calmly turned to look at me as if to say, "And we're doing this because why?" I laughed and praised her initiative.

If a horse doesn't copy me, I can often get his attention by copying him (fig. 17.2). Horses seem to find that intriguing, and then start watching to see what I will do next. In *Horse Speak,* Sharon Wilsie expands on this idea, showing how you can develop copying and other interactions into conversations.

Bronzz likes to *pick things up*, a game he initiated years ago. I encourage him by laughing and rewarding him. He usually goes for things he has seen me pick up, such as buckets, feed dishes, pitchforks, cones, and poles. Once he seized the top of my winter coat, careful not to grab my shoulder in the process, and attempted to hoist me off the ground.

For years, Sapphire picked up her empty rubber feed tub after every meal, and gave it to me in return for a treat. When her arthritic knees forced her retirement from trail riding, I taught her to pick up a small rubber feed dish and carry it down the barn aisle to a waiting person who then took the dish and placed a peppermint candy in it for her to eat. Guests were charmed, and Sapphire performed the trick with pride for the rest of her life.

Brandy's ball-dribbling game encourages initiative because it is played by a simple rule: we chase the ball and whoever gets to it first pushes it.

Part of the fun of games is discovering and building on what each horse inherently likes to do. Many Clicker Training books describe tricks that can be trained with positive reinforcement; some can also be taught with copying. While "tricks" might sound frivolous or undignified, some are actually valuable skills, such as, "Stand with your front feet on this board," or "Come when I call you." No trick is useless if it promotes positive interaction between horse and human.

## Liberty and Protector Leadership

Working with a horse at liberty is an elusive dream for many people. It doesn't need to be. Being a Protector Leader helps you establish the elements you need for safety and success.

- **The horse feels completely safe with you**. Being impatient, unfair, or placing too much pressure on him at *any* time will undermine the connection needed for liberty.

- **The horse understands your body language.** If he does not respond reliably on a *loose* lead to your cues for walk, trot, turns, halt, and back, more practice is needed with Friendly Body Language as described in chapter 10 (see p. 113).

- **He respects your personal space.** You never know when some unexpected event might overwhelm a horse with excitement. A handler whose horse does not respect her personal space can be in danger.

- **He halts with a remote cue and responds to your recall signal** (see

p. 121), so you can regain the connection if he slips away or gets too excited.

## Liberty and Play

You do not start liberty by playing with a loose horse any more than you'd start jumping by tackling a cross-country course. Liberty absolutely never involves playing with a horse as if you were another horse; this is extremely dangerous. Though skilled liberty handlers often make their interactions look playful, they are built on many hours of slow, careful practice that establishes clear communication and boundaries.

Liberty is the ultimate test of your connection with your horse. Your challenge is to make the experience positive so he *wants* to stay with you.

The horse needs to be *physically comfortable*. Not too stiff, sore, hot, tired, irritated by bugs, or distracted by pent-up energy. If he has too little turnout, or this is the only time he sees grass, you cannot expect to hold his attention.

You need to provide *enough challenge to maintain interest without creating frustration*. This is a delicate balance, and you must continually watch his body language to assess it.

You should be *generous with rewards* even if it is just the positive feedback of a quick stroke or word of praise. They will not keep a horse with you when he is uncomfortable or monumentally bored, but they are ongoing motivators and affirmation of your positive connection. Many people use food; many do not.

We should plan for *progress in tiny steps*. For me, the logical progression goes like this.

First, I place the lead over the horse's neck so I can reach it easily if the horse starts to wander off. We do the same sorts of leading activities described in chapter 10: changing direction, gaits, and speed within walk and trot (see p. 113). Practicing with obstacles helps me hold the horse's interest and fine-tunes our communication. With the safety net of perimeter fencing I can also practice any time I lead a horse anywhere, thus reinforcing the idea of staying with me in a variety of situations.

When the horse consistently stays with me at walk and trot, I try taking the lead off, but leaving the halter on. Next step is halter off, neck rope on. My horses seem to see the halter or neck rope as a signal they are "on duty." The transition to wearing nothing at all was the trickiest for us.

Our other transition was to different leading positions: ahead of the horse, behind, and farther away. We started those on lead in the context of agility courses, which helped Brandy understand what I was asking.

The more patiently and consistently you work the early steps, the faster you will progress, sometimes seeing an exciting leap forward seemingly all at once.

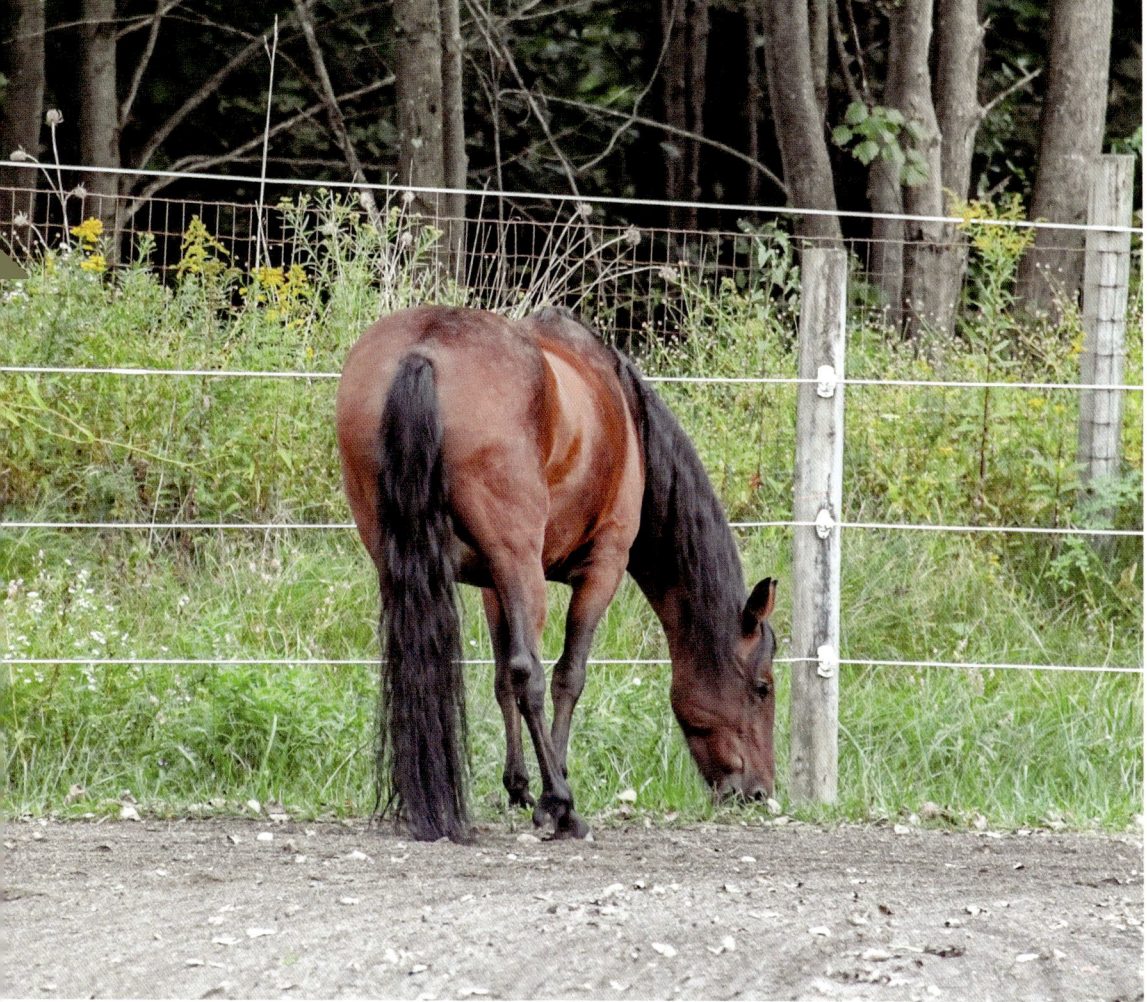

17.3 A horse who is loose in an area larger than a round pen can choose to leave and ignore you. When Brandy is bored, confused, or frustrated, this is the view I get.

Brandy showed me when she was ready to do an agility course at liberty. I had turned her loose in the arena while I did a practice walk through the course, planning where I needed to cue her at each obstacle. Of her own accord, she came over to fall in step beside me, neatly following my directions at each obstacle. For me these are the most exciting moments of horsemanship, when my horse not only shows she understands what I am asking but *offers* to do it of her own free will!

## When They Leave You

When we work at liberty, our horses *will* sometimes leave us (fig. 17.3). This is not disobedience on their part or a failure on ours; it does not mean they

PART SIX: POSITIVE EXPERIENCES BUILD CONFIDENCE AND RELIABILITY — 217

have regressed. This new level of freedom makes our relationship a more equal one. They can now express their feelings and opinions bluntly. We must be willing to listen with a non-judgmental attitude, take the time to figure out what they are trying to tell us, and adjust accordingly. Any attempt to "correct" a horse for leaving ensures that he will leave faster at the next opportunity.

Brandy's reaction to being called back can be enlightening. If she has left because she is bored, she often returns at a trot. When she is anxious or confused, she is more likely to ignore me or walk the other way. If the issue is excess energy, she gallops laps around the arena before returning.

One of Brandy's agility courses had a series of tight turns that I did not think she was ready to do at a trot, so I asked her to walk the course. She wandered off. When I called her back she came at a trot. Suspecting she was bored, I trotted along with her, pointing her toward the first obstacle, the ribbon curtain. She charged through at a brisk trot, and then completed the other obstacles with such enthusiasm I could barely keep up and cue her fast enough!

Even when the reason for leaving is not obvious, you must trust that the horse has one. One day Brandy flatly refused to go through the scary corridor, dodging away at the last moment every time I asked, and running to the opposite side of the arena. Since we happened to catch this on video, I posted the clip on the Horse Agility website, where someone spotted the explanation.

I had set up the scary corridor right next to the woods where deer, turkeys, and other critters hang out. Just before she darted away, Brandy had glanced at the woods. The motion was so quick I had missed it, but clearly something in the woods had worried her and she did not want to be "trapped" in the corridor too close to it.

### Liberty and Round Pen

Working with Bronzz at liberty presented a whole new challenge. Either he passively resisted by walking ever more slowly, or he eased farther away until he was just out of reach, and then trotted off. He often made himself hard to catch, coming right toward me at a prancing trot, then dancing sideways out of reach at the last second. Sometimes, he raced around so frantically I feared he would hurt himself. He has never been hard to catch under any other circumstances.

My current instructor, a whiz at liberty, explained that horses who have had round pen work with too much pressure *for them*, may equate liberty with being chased. This fits the research that shows significant differences in the level of stress horses exhibit in round-pen training

*Any attempt to "correct" a horse for leaving ensures he will leave faster next time.*

depending on how subtle the trainer's cues are, how quickly the trainer recognizes correct responses, releases pressure, and relieves anxiety.[101] The trainer to whom I sent Bronzz for his "bucking problem" (that turned out to be saddle-fit pain) did a lot of work in a round pen. I wondered at the time if he pushed Bronzz too hard, and I now suspect he did.

In order to persuade Bronzz that I was not going to chase him, we did lots of liberty with him right next to me where I could catch his lead. We can now work beyond my arm's reach, but I must be very careful to signal him for the gait I want by moving *ahead* of him and cueing him with my voice and footfalls. If I drop behind him, or even gesture behind him, he takes off and canters along the arena fence in the same posture he used 21 years ago in a round pen: head high and turned to the outside, his body clearly saying, "I do not want to be here."

### Listening and Learning

As you give your horse more choices and freedom, you learn more about him. What makes him anxious, what calms him, what generates enthusiasm, and especially what inspires him to be a partner committed to understanding what you want and doing it to the best of his ability.

## Summary

Domestic horses have very little freedom or control over their own lives, a condition that creates stress in any species. Giving horses appropriate freedom of choice can reduce stress-related problems while strengthening partnerships.

Play is a great motivator and relationship builder. Carefully structured rules help everyone stay safe.

Working with horses at liberty requires a strong connection and clear communication. Protector Leadership provides that foundation.

## THINGS TO TRY

- When your horse says, "Wait a minute," check your watch and see how many seconds elapse before he says, "Okay, I'm ready now."

- Notice when your horse makes any special requests. Keep these in mind to use as rewards or work breaks.

- Think of something fun or funny you might invite your horse to copy (fig. 17.4).

- If you want to venture into really uncharted territory, check out the book *Do As I Do: Using Social Learning to Train Dogs,* by the innovative researcher and dog trainer Claudia Fugazza. She teaches dogs to watch what she does, and *then* copy the action. Can horses do this? Someone needs to find out.

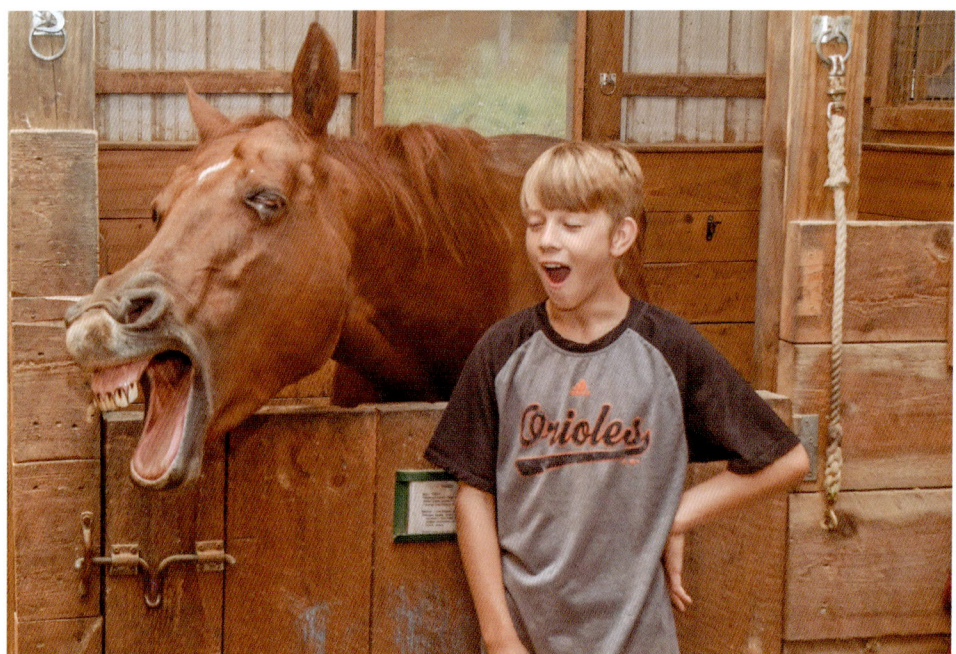

17.4  While hanging out with Shiloh, my grandson discovered that if he yawned, Shiloh yawned too—so extravagantly that her eyeballs rolled.

# PART SEVEN: Reducing Stress

"It is the most natural thing in the world to want the horse to change so he does what we'd like him to do. However, in reality, it is changing what we do that yields the results we want."

—Hertha James *(Conversations with Horses)*

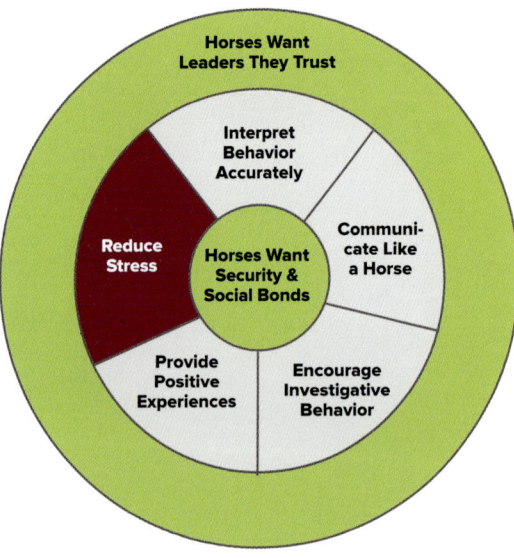

Stress causes or contributes to many of our horses' problem behaviors. Multiple small stresses can pile up for horses just as they do for us, making them less tolerant of each new stressor. Any stress we reduce can have a positive ripple effect on other stresses. Ideally, we address problems quickly, at the source. However, horses are so good at hiding and compensating for problems that the source can be hard to pinpoint. Chapter 18 (p. 224) provides strategies for getting to the root of trouble.

Even better than solving problems is avoiding them in the first place. Many issues are caused by practices that are so widely accepted that people do not typically question them. This seems especially true relative to our riding, and to our horses' living arrangements or lifestyles.

Chapter 19 (p. 236) shows how to lower horses' stress when we ride them by making them more comfortable physically and mentally. These suggestions, not typically included in conventional riding lessons, are based on biomechanics and horse behavior, and apply to riders of all skill levels.

In Chapter 20 (p. 247), I describe what I do to make my horses' daily routines as low stress as possible. Although everyone's circumstances and opportunities differ, I explain why I do what I do in hopes that you will find ideas for lowering stress in your own horse's life, or perhaps recognize that what you are already doing is a good plan.

**Part Seven Key Points:**

- Stress is the cause of many unwanted behaviors, whether it is small stresses piling up or one big stress. Each stress you reduce has a positive effect on your horse.

- Riders often cause their mounts physical and mental stress that is not recognized because horses are very good at compensating for our mistakes.

- A low stress lifestyle helps to improve horses' welfare, behavior, and performance.

**You will learn how to:**

- Use a systematic strategy to identify sources of problems and plan solutions.

- Make your mount more comfortable by implementing suggestions based on biomechanics and horse behavior, but rarely included in conventional riding lessons.

- Identify changes that can reduce causes of stress in your horse's daily life.

# chapter 18
# Problem-Solving Strategies

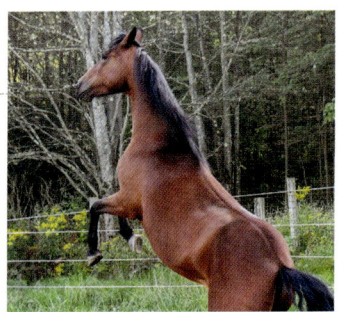

"...the answers will come if you ask the right questions. The hard part is knowing the right questions to ask, and then taking the time to ask them."

—Mark Rashid *(Considering the Horse)*

Problem behavior is a horse telling you something is wrong the only way he knows how: through his body language. Once you know what is wrong, the solution is often obvious. You relieve the pain, confusion, pressure, anxiety, or whatever is distressing the horse. A horse who feels safe and comfortable has no incentive to "misbehave."

Figuring out what's wrong, however, can be tricky. Not only are horses good at hiding and compensating for pain, but each one's personality and history influences how he reacts to different types of stress.[102] [103]

It would be so simple if each behavior had one definitive cause. For instance, barging into your space is always a sign of disrespect. But, it can mean a frightened horse is looking to you for reassurance, just as Brandy did when she first came to us. Or all rearing is aggression. But it is not. Brandy rears when she is playing (fig. 18.1).

You need to look beyond the horse's actions, and ask, *"Why* is he doing that?" When the answer is not obvious, you can be detective, searching out clues, watching for patterns, perhaps enlisting expert help, then testing possible solutions, and watching for your horse to tell you when you've got a good solution. Keep in mind that horses don't *want* to misbehave. They want harmony in their social group, not conflict. No one wants problems solved more than they do.

This chapter looks at three aspects of problem-solving: First, a step-by-step system for deciphering the underlying cause of a problem. Second, how you can address the special needs of a new horse. Finally, what to do when a horse and person are simply not compatible no matter how hard you try.

Remember, if a horse or a situation makes you nervous, take your anxiety seriously, even if you can't articulate what bothers you. Anxiety can be a warning that you are not safe. I know four people who were seriously, and I mean *seriously*, injured by horses. Afterward, each of them said, in almost the same words, "I never really trusted that horse."

And if we could ask the horses, I suspect they would all say that they never really trusted the people.

Confrontations can be dangerous and no one wins. When a situation is headed that way, back off and re-think the problem. Then try a different strategy based on a safe scenario where everyone will win.

## Identifying the Underlying Problem

Sometimes the cause of a problem is obvious, the solution is simple, and all is well. When that is not the case, you can take a systematic approach, one step at a time until you figure out the answer.

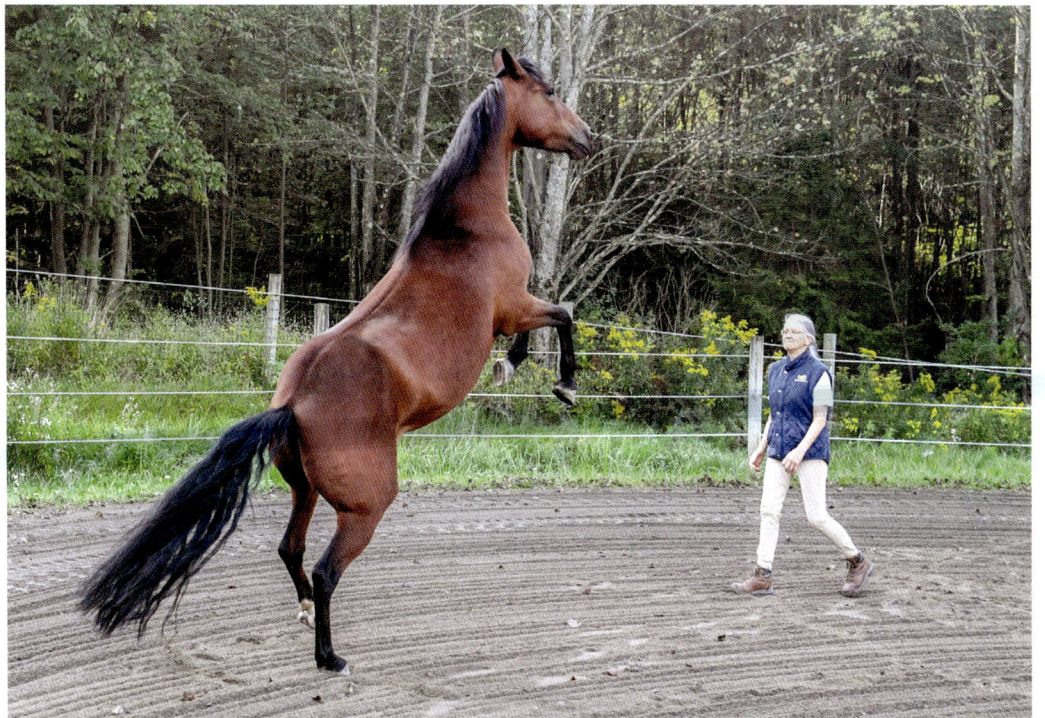

18.1 Brandy has playfully reared, and is carefully pivoting *away* from me. If I lower my head, she immediately comes down and lowers her head. This is not aggression.

PART SEVEN: REDUCING STRESS — 225

## Step 1: Start with the Obvious

If the behavior happened before, what was the explanation then? If it is new, has anything changed? For instance:

- **New tack, rider, feed, turnout situation?** A very sensitive horse I know suddenly started tossing his head. The owner had switched to a new bit. A switch back to the old bit solved the problem.

- **Did he recently have his feet done?** Changes in angles or balance can cause soreness in joints or muscles even if hooves are not sore.

- **Has he gained or lost weight or muscle?** This can change the fit of a saddle. Bronzz is so sensitive he gets cranky when the padding inside his saddle pad shifts the wrong way.

- **Is spring grass coming in or is he suddenly getting more grass?** He could be experiencing inflammation from insulin resistance, pain from laminitis, or a sugar high. Insulin resistance or laminitis require veterinary help. Even if a horse is not insulin resistant, a grazing muzzle may reduce grass intake enough to quell a sugar high.

- **Is he in a stressful situation?** Bronzz has had some spectacular prancing, bucking, screaming, meltdowns at group events that looked chaotic to him.

- **Is this a new home or new owner?** This can cause many issues, addressed later in this chapter (p. 230).

## Step 2: Brainstorm Possible Explanations

When nothing obvious presents itself in Step 1, expand your investigation. Typical reasons for unwanted behaviors (described in chapter 7—p. 77) provide a systematic checklist. Let's suppose a horse is bucking, either while ridden or on a lunge line. Chug through your checklist, considering how each possibility might relate to bucking.

- **Pain:** Your horse's back hurts because of an injury, a badly fitted saddle, a poorly balanced rider, hooves that are not properly balanced, for example.

- **Insecure balance:** Bucking when off-balance is not unusual for horses, even though it seems illogical from our point of view.

- **Confusion and misunderstandings:** No one ever notified him that bucking is not an approved activity.

- **Inconsistent expectations:** A previous rider or handler allowed or even encouraged bucking. I once knew a very sweet Morgan mare who bucked because her rider laughed when she did.

- **Punishment:** He is anticipating punishment, and bucking has been successful at interrupting kicks, swats, or yanks on his bridle.

- **Boredom or fatigue:** He is bored and needs more action or variety.

- **Living conditions and diet:** He is getting too much grain or grass and/or too little exercise so he has more pent-up energy than he can cope with.

- **Pressure the horse cannot relieve:** His rider is failing to release rein pressure or using too much rein and leg at the same time. Or, the handler on the lunge is using too much whip or chasing body language.

- **Stressful situations:** It's show day, and he's stressed because everything is strange and everyone around him is keyed up.

- **Anxiety:** His companions are out of sight and he is afraid of being alone.

## Step 3: Evaluate the Possible Explanations

Now you can home in on the possible explanations that seem most relevant, and ask more questions.

- **When does the behavior happen? All the time or just sometimes?** A horse who pulls on his lead only when he is excited is showing lack of self-control and/or poor focus on his handler. A horse who always pulls on the lead may never have been taught what he should be doing instead.

- **Where does it happen?** When a horse bucks cantering on trails, but not in the arena, I would think of excitement. If it's the other way around, perhaps he is not confident of his balance in the confined space of an arena.

- **Who does it happen with? Everyone or only some people?** A horse who tosses his head with one rider and not with others is saying the first rider is making him uncomfortable, likely with too much rein pressure. When a horse refuses jumps for one person and not others, it is time to evaluate the rider. Is she interfering with the horse's balance, bumping his mouth, landing too hard on his back?

- **What is the horse's emotional state?** A horse who calmly and consistently does the wrong thing probably *thinks* he is doing the right thing. Clearer communication is needed.

  A high level of excitement associated only with the behavior problem suggests pain or anxiety around that location, activity, or person.

> *A horse who calmly and consistently does the wrong thing probably thinks he is doing the right thing.*

A consistently high level of energy points toward a generic issue, like too much concentrated feed, too little turnout, general anxiety, or a high energy horse caught in a job better suited to a slow, quiet horse.

## Step 4: Gather More Information as Needed

By now you might have a good idea what is causing the problem, and be ready to start testing possible solutions (see Step 5). If not, more information is needed.

- **Look for pain first.** Checking for pain is especially crucial when a horse's behavior is aggressive, because of the strong connection between aggression and pain. It is also a high priority if a horse shows the "goat on a rock" posture that Brandy modeled in fig. 7.1: low back and inverted neck, with feet slanted together (see p. 80).

Several factors complicate the assessment of pain.

*Horses anticipate pain,* so the behavior you see might be in advance of the actual situation that causes pain. A horse whose back hurts when he is ridden might resist being caught, pin his ears while being groomed and saddled, and/or refuse to stand for mounting.

*Pain can have multiple causes,* such as poor saddle fit and bad riding, or long toes and dental issues. If you think you've found the cause and resolved it, but the problem persists, it doesn't mean you were wrong. It may mean there was more than one issue all along.

*Pain can come and go,* so it may not be present, or not at the same level, when your practitioner assesses your horse as when you observed the problem.

*The location of the pain does not always point to the root cause*. Bronzz's low back pain was significantly relieved when his farrier adjusted his hoof angles.

- **Engage relevant practitioners.** Every practitioner sees problems from his or her area of expertise. Vets find medical problems. Farriers look at trimming, shoeing, conformation, and hoof health. Chiropractors find pain and imbalances. Dentists address dental and TMJ issues. Trainers see training problems. Instructors see riding problems. Saddle fitters spot abnormalities and asymmetry in backs. Massage therapists home in on stiff and sore muscles. Acupuncturists adjust chi that is blocked or unbalanced.

All may be right as they see different facets of the same issue. It can be especially insightful when two or more team up, as when the sports medicine vet and chiropractor evaluated Brandy together.

Even within their own professions, people have areas of special expertise. A vet might be brilliant at diagnosing lameness, for instance, but not at managing metabolic issues. A farrier might do excellent barefoot trims but not be the best one to shoe a horse with an orthopedic problem. A trainer who excels in competition might not have the patience to teach basic skills or provide confidence-building experiences outside an arena.

- **Be persistent and trust your intuition.** Caring for living creatures is not an exact science. If one practitioner is not helpful, a second or third opinion is called for. It doesn't make the first one incompetent. Each new practitioner has the advantage of a different perspective, and of knowing what the previous one ruled out.

Don't discount your own intuition. Intuition can come from valuable information that is just so subtle you can't define it. Trusting intuition, however, is quite different from jumping to conclusions based on faulty assumptions. Even very experienced horse people can be making faulty assumptions; no one knows everything.

A simple test of the difference is this. People who blame the horse are usually working on faulty assumptions. Good intuition comes from empathy for the horse.

## Step 5: Test Possible Solutions

When you have an idea what the problem might be, it is time to test possible solutions. The more systematically you do this, the more efficiently you can home in on something that works. The motto for this stage is, "If at first you don't succeed, try something else."

- **Change only one thing at a time.** If you change two things at once, you can't assess the impact of either one. For instance, don't use a new saddle the day after your farrier changes your horse's shoeing. If you want someone else to ride your horse to assess whether a problem stems from your riding, then she should ride in your saddle and bridle, preferably in the same place at the same time of day.

- **Trust your horse's feedback**. Only he knows if he is comfortable or not. A saddle might look like a perfect fit. A different bit or bitless option might sound like the perfect solution. A rider's equitation might look perfect. But once everything is in motion, only the horse knows what he *feels*. Just as horses let us know when something is wrong, their behavior will let us know when they're feeling better.

- **Make note of what happens as you try different options.** When I was looking for a saddle for Bronzz, keeping notes not only prevented me from trying the same saddle twice, it helped me see a pattern of what bothered him most, and what looked like better prospects.

- **Recognize the limitations of professional training.** It can be tempting to send the horse to a professional trainer thinking he or she has the expertise to deal better with problems. This depends on the nature of the problem. A good trainer can teach horses to respond reliably to cues, improve their balance, and build confidence with positive experiences. This requires time and patience. Then the owner must have the skills to follow up with consistent handling, and considerate riding.

A trainer cannot be expected to fix problems that stem from pain, too much grain, too little turnout, poor riding, or inconsistent handling.

Legally, anyone can claim to be a horse trainer. Certification only shows the person has attended a course taught by the trainer who issues the certification. It may tell you something of the techniques used, but as Mark Rashid observed, techniques are much less important than the attitude with which they are applied. I have seen more than one horse return from a widely respected but high pressure professional trainer so anxious and reactive that his owner was afraid to ride him.

For your sake and your horse's, select trainers carefully. What other people say about trainers tells us much less than how the horses respond to them. I do not look for robotic obedience. Many horses can be intimidated into compliance quickly. I look for happy, relaxed horses who want to be with their trainer.

If you send a horse to a trainer, stay as actively involved as possible, preferably being present for training sessions. Learn what you need to know to maintain the work the trainer does. Ethical trainers welcome your presence and recognize that long-term success depends on the owner's skills as much as the horse's.

## Step 6: Be Proactive to Head Off Future Problems

Identifying a problem may show that a horse is prone to a particular issue. This can help you prevent future problems or spot them more quickly. If excess energy is a problem, for instance, minimize or eliminate concentrated feed, maximize turnout, and beware of spring grass. If he is prone to boredom, look for constructive new challenges.

## New Horses Need Extra Reassurance that You Will Be a Protector Leader

Special problems can arise with a new horse. A horse who seems calm, tuned in, and polite at the seller's place, may act like a different horse when the buyer gets him home: tense, distracted, spooky, pulling on the lead, crowding the handler, and so on. This is often misinterpreted as disrespectful behavior.

If the new owner is frightened enough, the horse might be sent back. This can result in hard feelings on the part of the buyer, who feels the horse was misrepresented, and/or the seller, who wonders what the buyer did to provoke the horse to behave badly.

From our perspective as Protector Leaders, the problem is obvious. The horse is scared! Let's look at this from his point of view.

One day you are loaded into a trailer and driven away. You might think it is going to be a round trip, but it isn't. Instead, you are unloaded and left in a strange place with new horses, new people, new surroundings, and new expectations. Even the hay and water taste different. How could you *not* be anxious?

So you're on high alert, head up, feet in gear, ready for action. You don't mean to be pushy or intimidating. You're just looking for someone, anyone, two legs, four legs, it doesn't matter, anyone who can help you feel safer. You crowd closer to the person holding your lead, hoping she will be your leader and protect you. Instead, she yells, yanks your lead, and shoves you away. Life just got scarier.

Even when a horse's behavior is good, you can assume there is anxiety underneath. This is the time a horse is most in need of a Protector Leader. Your response defines your new relationship.

You can start by saying with your body language, "You're safe with me. I'm here to protect you, not pressure you" (see p. 23). Quietly use chicken wings or windshield wipers to protect your personal space if needed (see p. 24), or hang out where there is a fence or partition between you. When he is calmly tuned in, start gently directing him with Friendly Body Language: minimum pressure, no punishment; lots of patience and persistence. Reward behaviors you want. Ignore the rest. The better you can apply your Protector Leader skills, the more likely you are to see your new horse's body language shift from, "I'm scared," to "Thank you. You are a leader I want to stay with!"

Your routines, expectations, and cues are probably different from what the horse is accustomed to. Information from previous owners can offer insights into the horse's behavior and the reasons behind it. As long as his behavior isn't dangerous, there's no rush to change it. Once he is settled and feeling safer, you can gradually ask him to do things your way.

Evaluate tack carefully. If he was comfortable in what was used when you test rode him, try to replicate it, at least temporarily. I was concerned about the Tom Thumb bit that Sapphire was accustomed to, because the combination of shanks and joint can act like a nutcracker on a horse's lower jaw. I offered her multiple other choices of bits, but she was tense and less responsive. I conceded to her preference, bought her a Tom Thumb, and she worked happily in that (on a loose rein) for the rest of her riding years.

*This is the time a horse is most in need of a Protector Leader. Your response defines your new relationship.*

Saddle fit is crucial, of course. A poorly fitting saddle can turn a well-behaved horse into a problem real fast.

Meanwhile, every way you can reduce stress in the horse's lifestyle is extra important now: minimum grain, maximum forage, and the maximum turnout that safety allows. A calm friendly companion can help, perhaps at first in an adjacent stall, paddock, or pasture.

## Good Horse and Bad Match

Sometimes problems reflect a fundamental mismatch, a horse in the wrong job or paired with the wrong rider. Even the best leadership is not always enough to make a match work.

- **Anxious horse/anxious rider** is a bad combination. A horse who is in his own comfort zone can stay calm with an anxious rider; school horses do it all the time. A rider who is confident in her skills can steady an anxious horse. When both are anxious, both have just cause for concern. A sensitive horse who works well for one person might become anxious when handled or ridden by multiple people.

- **Green horse/green rider** is another common predicament. We have two individuals with completely different world views, who don't speak the same language or have the same goals in life and, by the way, one of them weighs at least four times what the other one does. It really helps if one of them knows what he or she is doing.

- **Big horse/small rider** (relative to each other, of course) also have a challenge. It requires more skill to follow the motion of a larger horse's stride. A rider who can't do it creates discomfort for herself and her mount. If the horse gets irritated, understandably, there is a bigger buck, and a longer way down. Rule of thumb: the bigger the horse is compared to the rider, the more skilled the rider needs to be. A horse who weighs at least four times the rider plus gear is big enough.

- **Personality mismatches** can also get in the way. Just as there are many nice people in the world you would not choose as close friends, there are many nice horses who would not be good partners. It is valuable to know what sorts of horse personalities you get along with and which you don't. *Ride the Right Horse* by Yvonne Barteau is a thoughtful exploration of this topic. It is also helpful to pay attention to how you feel with different horses you ride or handle, and consider why. This is a good reason to ride as many different horses as you safely can before choosing one.

I chose Bronzz because I liked the way he tuned in to his breeder and took initiative, trotting around the round pen before he was asked. I liked the way he tried to negotiate a change when he was bored. "If I stand still and pretend not to see you, maybe you'll ask me to do something more interesting than going in circles." I liked the calm way he went back to work when Fritz scolded him. This horse, I thought, wants to be a thinking partner, a team player. I didn't care that he ignored me, outright glared in fact when I ran my hands down his legs. He owed me, a stranger, nothing but common courtesy. I was watching how he related to Fritz, the person he'd known and depended on all his life. Bronzz's full sister had better conformation and fabulous gaits, but I wasn't even tempted. She was high strung and over-reactive. I knew we'd be a bad match.

Granted, I was not choosing a horse primarily for performance, but even if you are, you still have to work together. If horse and rider are not comfortable with each other, neither performs their best.

This raises another myth that I think gets a lot of people into no-win situations. Until Bronzz came along I equated feeling safe with being bored. Once Bronzz and I got past his initial green phase, I realized that I felt safe on him anywhere any time. Yet I have never, in our 21 years together, had a boring ride on him. I believe that is because we were a good match from the start and because Fritz's guidance helped me be a leader who met Bronzz's needs, including letting him express his zany personality.

Brandy and I turned out to be a better match than I would have dared to hope, but only because I have been her Protector Leader. Had I maintained my old authoritarian style, ongoing anxiety would have limited her ability to trust me, to learn, and to behave with the reliability that has earned my trust in return.

- **The wrong job** can bring out the worst in the nicest horses. Bronzz, my dream horse, could have been someone else's nightmare. He is not fond of ring work, and though he happily jumps logs on a trail, he always resisted even the tiniest of cross-rails in a ring (probably discomfort from the English saddle, I now realize). If he belonged to someone with her heart set on jumping or a steady diet of ring riding, he would have been a grave disappointment, perhaps labeled lazy, resistant, disobedient, or even dangerous.

Brandy, who hates to leave home, seems quite happy to work in the same arena year in and year out. She could have been a disaster as a driving or trail horse, jobs that by definition would have meant leaving home.

Sometimes compromise resolves the problem. Bronzz does his most earnest arena work when he has recently had a nice ramble in the woods. My sister's previous horse Sammie worked harder at

*If horse and rider are not comfortable with each other, neither performs his best.*

dressage when it was interspersed with jumping, which she loved. Cross-training is good for athletic development as well as mental health.

## When a Match Isn't Working

A good person and a good horse can be a bad match, and it is no one's fault. No amount of trying can salvage a partnership that wasn't meant to be, but reaching this conclusion can be a heart-wrenching process. *Brain Training for Riders* by Andrea Monsarrat Waldo offers compassionate, insightful guidance for making such a decision in the chapter titled "The Right Horse Brings Less Stress."

Your safety is the most important factor in such a decision. Fear is our body's warning that we might be in danger. If you are afraid to ride or handle a horse, take that fear seriously.

Being a good leader does not necessarily mean keeping a horse for the rest of his life. The best leadership might mean making a responsible plan for the horse's future.

That is how Shiloh came to be with us. Her seller, a novice rider, realized that she needed a horse with more training and experience. She described Shiloh to us honestly to the best of her understanding. She also took me up on my invitation to visit our farm and meet our horses so she could see that Shiloh would have a good home with us.

Sapphire's seller, recognizing that Sapphire was never going to be the show horse she wanted, was also scrupulously honest. Reliable on trails but hates ring work, she told us. "No problem," was my husband's response, since he, too, hates ring work. Also, she was too pushy and opinionated for a beginner rider. Though Jerry wasn't much past beginner at that point, he and Sapphire had hit it off on test rides, and he had the support of my experience. A disappointment to her previous owner, Sapphire proved to be a true gem as Jerry's trail horse. In tricky situations when Jerry was unsure what to do, Sapphire's experience and confidence carried them safely through.

## Selling a Horse Ethically

Three simple rules contribute to a responsible plan that serves everyone well. So well, in fact, that we became friends with Sapphire's and Bronzz's previous owners.

**1.** Sell a horse while he is still able to earn himself a retirement home; otherwise, you're it.

**2.** Be honest about the horse.

**3.** Turn away anyone clearly unsuited for this horse in particular—or horse ownership in general.

A friend of mine handled the third point gracefully when someone wanted to buy her rowdy two-year-old Arabian for a child who had never ridden. "Sorry, I've changed my mind," she said politely. "The horse is no longer for sale."

Selling a horse responsibly is not a failure. In Sapphire's case, it was a success story. The time her previous owner spent training her set Sapphire up to be the reliable partner Jerry needed.

If you sell a horse, be sure to give yourself credit for everything you've improved in his time with you, whether it is better nutrition, hoof care, ground manners, training, confidence, or whatever. You've set him up for a better life.

## Summary

- Problem behaviors are signs of distress. Removing the cause of distress is the first step in resolving a problem, often providing a complete and lasting solution very quickly. If the cause is not obvious, you can meet the challenge of deciphering it in a systematic way.

- A horse in a new home is in a very stressful situation. Using Protector Leadership skills to show him he is safe can go a long way to establishing a positive relationship.

- Sometimes a horse and a person are a bad match, through no one's fault. In that case, parting with the horse can be a positive step provided it is done in a way that includes a responsible plan for the horse's future.

### THINGS TO TRY

- What are the earliest warning signs your horse shows when he is anxious, in pain, or otherwise distressed?

- If your horse has a behavior that concerns you, try applying our systematic approach using Steps 1 through 5 to determine the cause(s) and find a solution (see p. 226).

- If you have a new horse, or know another horse who might be in a stressful situation, try standing quietly near him for 5 or 10 minutes doing nothing and asking nothing of him. See what happens.

*chapter 19*
# Being a Considerate Rider

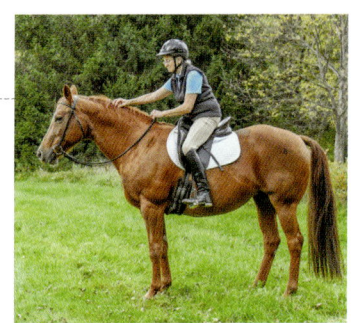

> "So I would like to remind every rider to look to himself for the fault whenever he has any difficulties with his horse."
>
> —Alois Podhajsky *(My Horses, My Teachers)*

It is hard to define a "good" rider because, as Denny Emerson points out in his book *Know Better to Do Better*, many skills are specific to the type of riding you do. In my experience, horses don't care how "good" we are anyway. They care if we are considerate. Not everyone has the opportunity, dedication, and athletic ability to develop a high level of skill, but we can all be considerate.

Considerate riders try to make themselves as comfortable and pleasant as possible for horses to carry. This inspires willing cooperation, and helps our horses perform their best. Many horses have made me look like a better rider than I am because they appreciated my being considerate.

Riders are often unaware when horses are uncomfortable because horses are masters of compensation. Yet the need to compensate takes a toll on a horse. In this chapter, I'll describe some common sources of discomfort for horses that are not necessarily covered in riding lessons. Then I will offer suggestions based on research and biomechanics that can help address these issues, independent of skill level or riding style.[104]

## 13 Ways to Become a Rider Horses Want to Carry

### Groom and Tack Up Tactfully

You can start your ride with a horse who is relaxed and tuned in, or one who is already tense and defensive. In a study where horses and riders were observed during grooming, half of the horses showed pain or aggression. *Half!* This was independent of the rider's skill level.[105] However, if you make grooming a pleasant experience, it can be a social bonding time, as mutual grooming is between horses. You can lower your horse's heart rate and help him feel more secure with you.[106]

Remember that grooming is a significant invasion of a horse's personal space. Tune into his reaction to everything. Notice which curry and brush he likes and how he likes them used, how high he can comfortably lift his feet, what parts of his body he is uneasy having handled, and so on. Is he more relaxed cross-tied, single tied, or in his stall?

I make grooming into social time, talking with my horses and taking their personal preferences and pet peeves into account. Bronzz loves to have his ears curried and his forehead brushed, but doesn't want his tail fussed with. Shiloh likes her body brushed in long hard strokes with a stiff hairbrush. Brandy hates tugs on her mane when it is brushed, so I gently work in lots of detangler first. If a horse nods off while I'm grooming, I consider it a great compliment.

Tacking up deserves the same courtesy as grooming. Set the saddle on gently, like you'd want someone to set a pack on your back. Ease the girth up in at least three stages. Make sure the bridle is straight and adjusted comfortably.

With respectful attention to the horse's feedback, these pre-ride rituals set the stage for cheerful cooperation and good performance.

### Use a Mounting Block or Get a Leg Up

Mounting from the ground is an important skill, but we don't need to prove we can do it every time. It places enormous torque on a horse's spine no matter how smoothly a rider mounts. It also builds one-sided muscles as the horse braces against our weight. People develop one-sided muscles too, quite obvious to most of us when we try mounting from the right.

Reduce stress on your horse's back by using a mounting block, stool, log, or whatever (fig. 19.1). Then hold *mane* and the pommel of your saddle. Hauling yourself up with both hands on the saddle puts maximum stress on your horse's spine. If you're young and agile, consider learning to mount and dismount from both sides so you can alternate.

If your horse doesn't stand at a mounting block, make sure he is relaxed

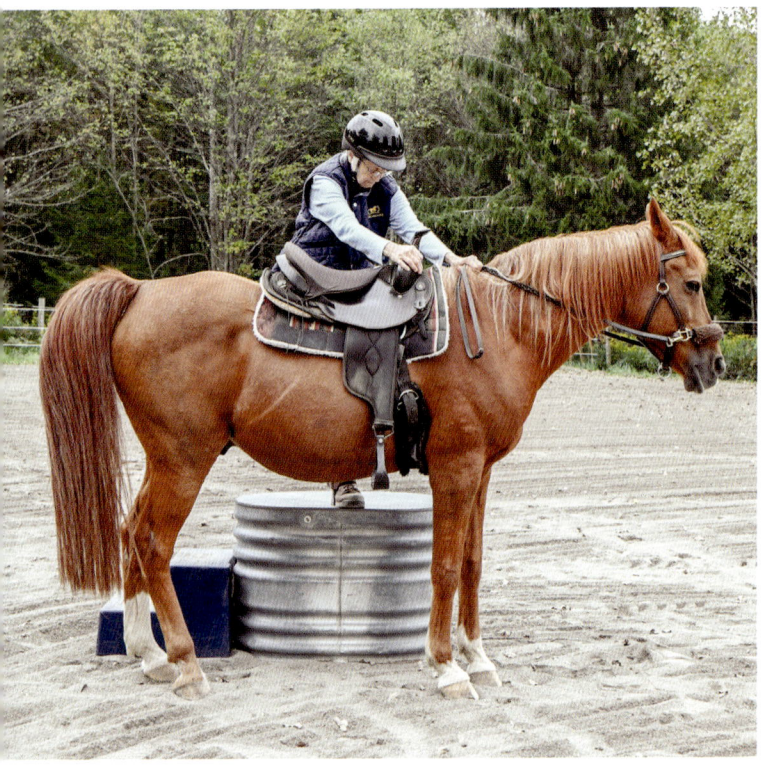

**19.1** Bronzz's and my favorite mounting block is an old overturned stock tank, but Bronzz is accustomed to standing next to any object that I can use for height advantage.

standing still other places first (see "Standing Still," on p. 120). Use lots of rewards, with a primo treat after you mount and before you ask him to move.

Getting a leg up is also a good option. It can be tricky at first, but it is all in the timing and worth the practice.

## Check Your Balance

Poorly balanced riders can cause horses ongoing pain. This was demonstrated clearly in a study comparing two riding schools. At one school, riders had short reins, high hands, and poor leg position, all symptoms of poor balance—and 100 percent of those horses had back pain!

They also showed the high head, inverted neck, and hollow back characteristic of pain (the "goat-on-a-rock" posture—see fig. 7.1, p. 80). At the other school the instructor focused on rider posture and balance. Those riders had better leg position that stabilizes balance, and lower hands. The horses had lower heads, rounder necks, and a smaller percentage of back problems.[107][108]

In *Centered Riding*, Sally Swift described balance as building blocks that must be stacked correctly to minimize muscle tension and strain as we ride.[109] That means ears, shoulders, hips, and feet in alignment (fig. 19.2). To maintain good balance, feet stay under hips even when the upper body adjusts forward and back for speed, hills, or jumping.

Over 2,000 years ago, the Greek cavalry officer Xenophon described this balance as the best way to stay on your horse in battle.[110] It also helps keep you on through spooks, trips, bucks, flying leaps, and other unexpected maneuvers. This applies no matter what your riding style, or whether your horse is gaited. In fact, many riding horses in Xenophon's time were gaited. Equipment, apparel, goals, saddles, stirrup length, and the way you hold the reins may vary, but gravity still works the same.

When your balance is challenged, don't hesitate to grab mane. That is what I did when Bronzz leaped the creek (see fig. 15.1 B, p. 179). It isn't bad form; it is considerate of your horse's mouth. Some people prefer neck straps, but keep in mind that neck straps slip; manes don't.

To check your own balance, get a photo of yourself on your horse from the side; does your body line up like Dani's does? And a photo from the front. Are both sides symmetric with shoulders and stirrups level? Photos at different gaits are helpful because your leg position and balance may shift as you speed up.

## Beware of the Heels-Down Trap

The point of putting your heels down is to anchor your lower leg *under* your body so it provides a solid base of support on which to balance. However, as Wendy Murdoch explains in *50 5-Minute Fixes to Improve Your Riding*, "…most riders are taught to get their heels down incorrectly. Instead of learning to sink their weight into their heels, they typically end up bracing against the stirrups… When they brace the lower leg forward or jam their foot against the stirrup, a tremendous amount of tension is created…"[111] (fig 19.3)

Think of your stirrups as footrests. The weight of your leg holds your foot in the stirrup. When your ankles are

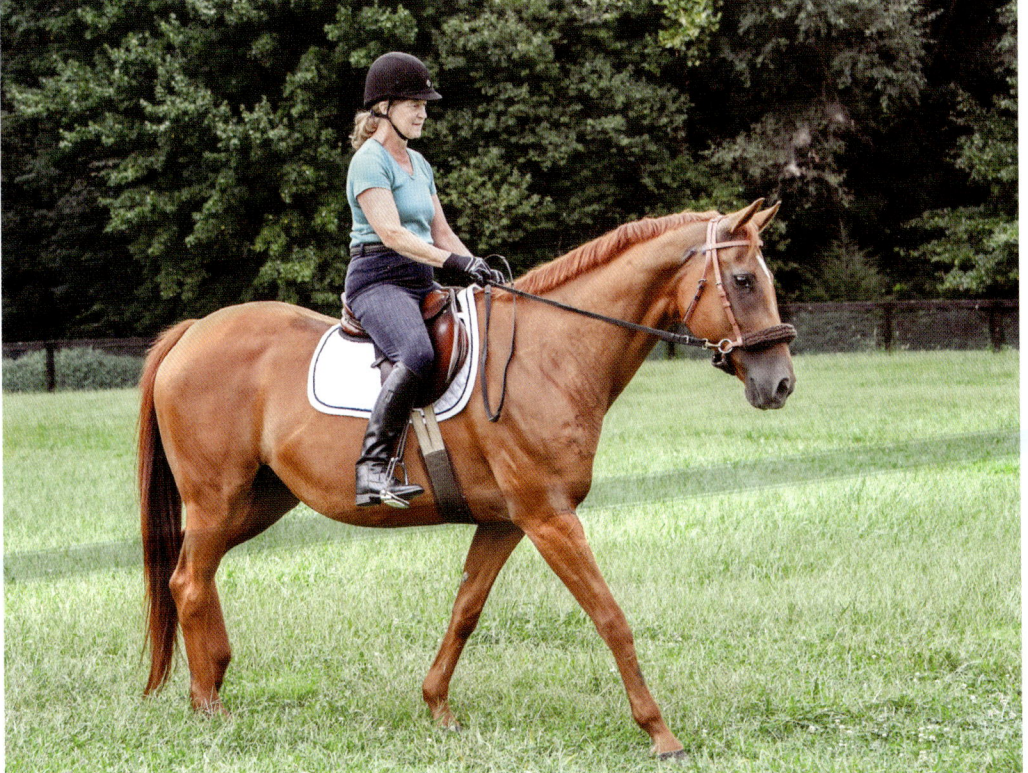

19.2 Good balance works *with* gravity, not against it. A vertical line could pass through Dani's ear, shoulder, hip, and heel. So, if Gracie magically vanished from under her, Dani would land on her feet, not her face or backside.

naturally stiff, like mine, your heels might be level with your toes. That is okay. It is more important to have your legs under you than your heels down. If you can't stand in your stirrups without holding on, check whether you are pushing your heels down too hard or perhaps standing on your toes.

It took me a while to kick the "heels-down" habit, and allow my legs and feet to relax into my stirrups. The payoff is that my leg position is better and my whole body is more relaxed. I can even enjoy winter rides. Instead of getting cold and numb, my happily relaxed feet get warmer as I ride.

## Don't Let Your Saddle Sabotage You

Poorly designed or fitted saddles can wreak havoc with a rider's balance. There is *no* saddle that fits every horse. A saddle that is too narrow for the horse it is on (a common problem) is high in front. This slides the rider's seat toward the cantle, leaving her feet in front of her. Many Western and Australian saddles are designed to do this.

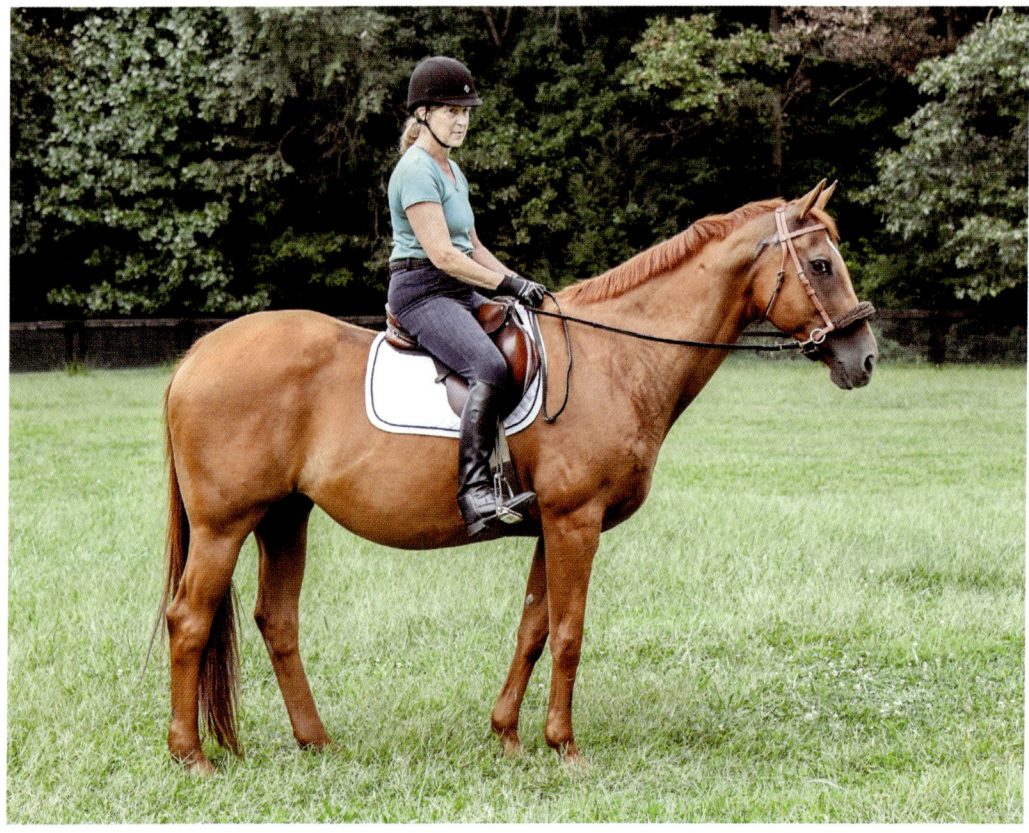

19.3 Dani demonstrates that forcing her heels down moves her leg forward, and her seat back, putting her *out* of balance. Gracie is looking back, wondering what Dani is doing.

If you struggle to keep your feet under you, or a photo shows your feet in front of your body, check your saddle. Your balance might improve dramatically with a properly balanced saddle. If your saddle fits your horse but isn't balanced for you, you might be able to adjust it with a seat saver made of wedge-shaped foam with the thicker end at the cantle, as I have done with Bronzz's saddle.

A saddle with a very deep seat can tip your pelvis and wedge you into a position where it is difficult to move with your horse.

## Beware of Tension

When our horses move, we need to follow their motion at each gait. The more smoothly we can do this, the more comfortable we are to carry. It also helps horses lift their back and engage their hindquarters, which keeps them healthier. This applies equally to gaited horses who, like any other horses, move best when their back is comfortable.

Any stiffness or bracing can cause both discomfort and confusion. Braced legs give an ongoing speed-up cue. Stiff arms or shoulders prevent our hands from gently following the motion of the horse's head, causing bumps on the reins. Stiff hips and back prevent our seat from following the horse's back motion. Riders often find themselves sore after a ride.

Unnecessary tension has many causes: faulty balance; old habits formed when the rider was less secure on a horse; current anxiety about riding; stress in other areas of life; or attempting to hold a position the rider believes is "correct." Too much focus on "correct" equitation can get in our way. Some very effective riders actually look a bit "sloppy" because they are so relaxed.

Riders are often unaware of being stiff or braced. One way to test this is to ask someone to put her hand under your stirrup and lift your leg. Do your hip and knee joints flex, or do you tip to the far side of your horse? If someone wiggles your arm does it yield easily or is it stiff?

## Take Advantage of Posting and Two-Point Position

The bounce of a trot is a challenge. That is why posting was invented. High tech studies using pressure pads show that posting is less stressful on a horse's back than sitting, no matter how skilled the rider.[112] Two-point or jumping position is least stressful on a horse's back.

Western disciplines and higher levels of dressage expect riders to sit the trot, but this assumes the horse's back is strong and the rider is good at sitting trot. Unfortunately, many people attempt to sit before they and their horse are ready. When in doubt, post. It does not make you a less skilled rider; it makes you a more considerate one.

As you post remember that the horse's head remains level in the trot, but now

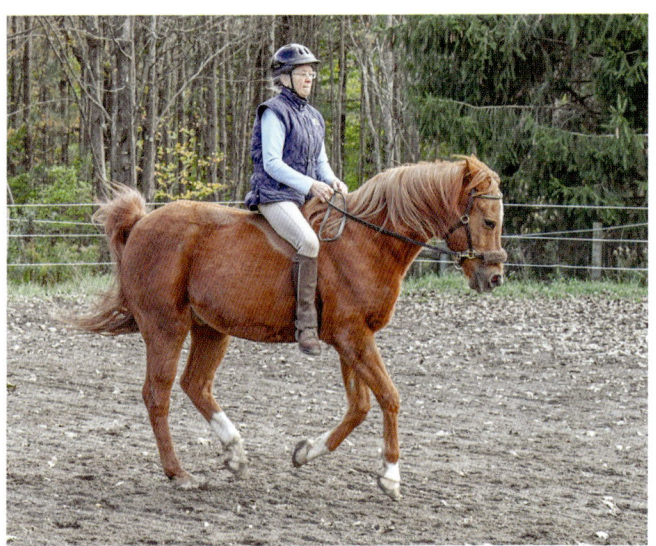

**19.4 A** Bronzz's shoulders come up as he pushes off with his right hind in the first step of a left lead canter. This is the "elegant" phase of the canter stride, most often shown in photographs.

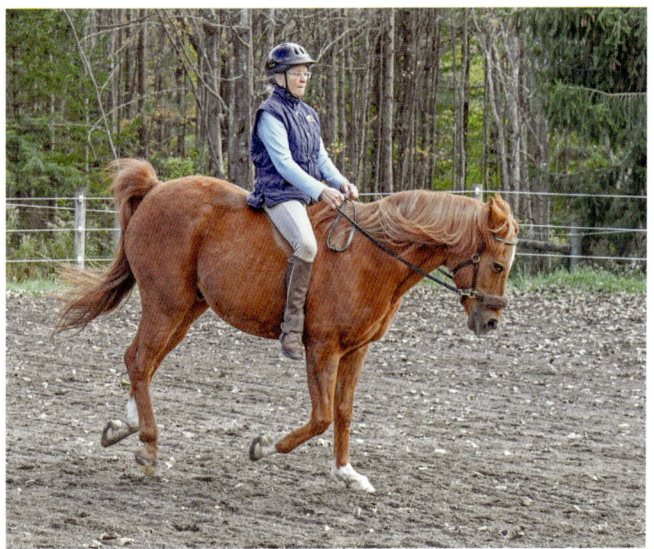

**19.4 B** As Bronzz's hind end comes up at the end of the stride, my body adjusts to the change in his back angle, and my elbow angle opens to follow his head. These photos show one of the challenges of riding bareback; my legs slide forward of Bronzz's ribs, putting me in a "chair" seat.

your body is going up and down. Elbows must open and close in order to keep hands steady *in relation to the horse's mouth*. Try holding a bit of mane with your pinky to make sure your hands are steady.

Sitting a canter is also a challenge especially if a horse has a large back motion (figs. 19.4 A & B). Learning to canter first in two-point position can help a rider get the feel of this motion while stabilizing hands on the horse's neck.

## Use Invisible Cues

When I ride, my goal is to make all my cues so subtle that an observer cannot see what I am doing. This is not only more comfortable for my horse; it helps me focus on being quiet, relaxed, and balanced. The more precise I am, the more precisely my horse responds.

Using invisible cues is a challenge I present to students of all levels. Children are especially intrigued by the idea of making it look like the horse is reading their mind. They are gleeful when I have to ask, "Did you tell your pony to do that?"

If you're thinking, "But my horse won't respond to subtle cues," remember that he can feel a fly land on any part of his body. Try this experiment: always give a whisper-soft cue *first*, and give your horse time to respond. If he doesn't, you can increase the pressure. You will be amazed how quickly he starts responding to the first hint of a cue.

## Maintain Consistent Expectations

We cannot allow a horse to do something one time and scold him for it another. For example, we cannot let him decide to stop trotting even if we were ready to stop anyway; we must ask for at least a couple more steps of trot, and then give the cue to walk. If we train ourselves to be consistent, our horse will be consistent.

There are some things, though, that we might want to allow at some times and not others. To avoid confusion, I establish a cue that gives permission, as I've done with Shiloh about eating grass (figs. 19.5 A–C).

## Stay Tuned-In to Your Horse's Mental State

When I ask students about their mount's mood or feelings, novices are invariably on target with a perceptive answer. More advanced students sometimes seem to view such empathy as childlike or unprofessional, and tend to reply more in terms of how obedient the horse is being. I know some very skilled riders who have been seriously injured because either they did not tune in to their horse's emotional state, or did not take it seriously.

When you make a habit of tuning in to your horse, you'll notice little problems, so you can address them before they become big problems.

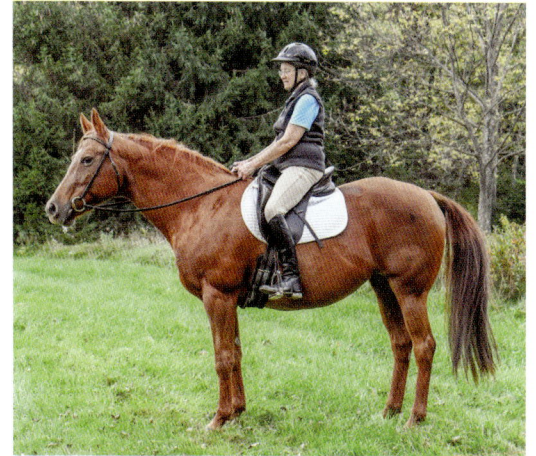

**19.5 A** Though Shiloh is obsessed with eating, she politely waits for permission to eat grass because she knows that during each ride, I will give her permission at least once. No more tug of war.

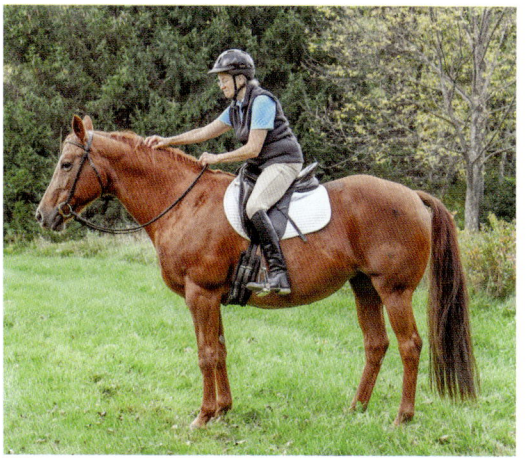

**19.5 B** My hand pressing on her crest is my signal that Shiloh may lower her head and eat. Any "head-down" cue a horse already knows or you want to teach will work. Notice my leg position does not change as I lean forward.

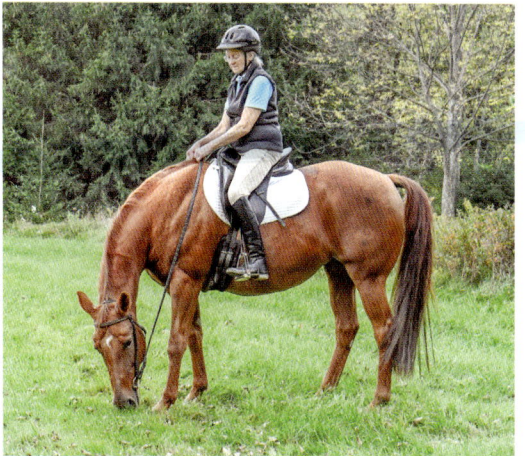

**19.5 C** Now she can enjoy her snack.

You also "catch" your horse doing good things, so you can praise and reinforce them.

## Have a Mental Problem-Solving Checklist

This checklist starts with what *you* might be doing wrong, not the horse. For example, if a horse fails to slow down when you pull the reins, ask: Am I squeezing my legs? Am I leaning forward? Am I pushing on my feet ("putting on the brakes"), which tightens leg muscles? Am I pulling too hard on the reins and creating resistance?

When a horse cuts in on turns, ask: Am I leaning my body into the turn? Am I leaning on my inside stirrup? Am I anticipating the turn and turning my body or pulling the rein too much or too soon? Am I turning my head and looking around the turn before I want the horse to turn?

It helps to be aware of your own riding issues. For instance, I struggle with a tendency to sit more heavily on my right seat bone than my left. This is the first thing I adjust if my horse drifts to the right or takes the left lead when I meant to ask for the right. (Weight on the right seat bone encourages the horse to strike off with the right hind, putting him on the left lead.)

Trust the old saying, "It's never the horse, it's always the rider."

## Learn How to Prevent and Cope with Emergencies

When your horse is frightened, the most reassuring thing you can do is show him that you have a plan. In my experience, it doesn't matter how scared you might be, as long as your cues are clear and decisive, conveying that you are taking responsibility.

Although horse-related emergencies are so varied it is impossible to plan for every eventuality, prior thought and preparation can help you think and act quickly. This is a good reason to learn how to respond to problems like bucking, tripping, spooking, bolting, rearing, or attempts to kick another horse. Think about these and other situations you might possibly face. Plan the best response based on your horse, your skill level, and your circumstances. Rehearse it mentally. Practice the motions while riding, slowly and gently so you don't distress your horse.

If you see a bad situation brewing in time to dismount safely, this is often the best plan. Most horses seem to feel safer with their person on the ground. Consider the horse's level of training and self-control, your skill and confidence, and whether you might actually be safer or better able to control the horse while mounted.

Once a horse is out of control, attempting to dismount is rarely a good idea. The "emergency dismount" (vaulting off a horse) enjoyed a brief wave of popularity until it was observed that it *caused* injuries both in practice and in real emergencies. Realistically, it is nearly impossible to make a controlled dismount when a horse is out of control. From a leadership standpoint, bailing out and letting go of a horse tells him that when he is most frightened and in need of your guidance, you will abandon him.

Good leadership includes knowing when to let someone else take charge. When a horse is already dealing with a situation in an appropriate way, it may be best to sit quietly and stay out of his way. This is often the case with treacherous footing or balance challenges where your interference could make a bad situation worse. Afterward, praise and congratulate the horse on a job well done, so he knows that appropriate initiative is appreciated.

## Choose Riding Instructors Who Understand Horses' Needs

Horses suffer when the focus is only on what the horse is *doing*. This has been the scenario in many clinics I have audited in recent years. Riders want clinicians to help them fix their "horse" problems, and are insulted by any suggestion that this might require adjusting their riding. The result is lots of pressure and repetition. The horse's emotional, and sometimes physical, well-being are overlooked.

Good instructors understand a horse's needs. They help you improve your riding, your communication, and your ability to interpret your horse's responses, so you can help your horse be the best possible partner.

You cannot evaluate an instructor's competence by fame, championships, or how fancy his or her horse is. What matters is being respectfully tuned in to the horses and able to help you work toward your own goals.

### Additional Resources

These are a few resources that can offer valuable help with riding and horsemanship. Their information is based on science and biomechanics, attuned to horses' needs and welfare, and applicable to any type of riding. The websites offer a generous amount of information at no charge.

- Callie R. King's website https://www.crktraining.com/

- Wendy Murdoch's *5-Minute Fixes* books and videos, and online Murdoch Minutes at http://murdoch-method.com/

- Sally Swift's *Centered Riding* books and videos

## ⚞ Summary

If you can stay on our horse and get him to do what you want, it is tempting to think that your riding is just fine. I hope this chapter has persuaded you that your horse's comfort and welfare is sufficient reason to pay attention to your riding. While a horse may be unimpressed with technical skill, he appreciates your attempts to be considerate, and it shows in his performance and behavior.

### THINGS TO TRY

- Imagine yourself in your horse's place. Mentally step through your whole ride from first greeting, through grooming, tacking, mounting, riding, and post-ride activities. Is there anything your horse might like you to change?

- Hold a bit in your hands with your eyes closed. Have someone else slowly pull a rein until you can feel it. Look and see how little pressure it took. Now challenge yourself to a game of, "How little can I do?" and still get a response from your mount. Horses who are accustomed to tuning out extraneous motions may need time to recognize that your subtle motions are actually intentional.

- Have someone video you riding at each gait you do. Watch for three things: Do changes in rein tension show bumps on the bit or bridle? Do you bounce on the saddle? Does your balance stay centered? I give myself a lesson every time I see a video of myself riding.

- Challenge yourself to a ride where you correct only yourself, not your horse (except as safety requires). I have found this so successful that when my mount doesn't do as I thought I asked, my default reaction now is to assess what I just did and adjust myself. It is amazing how often that "fixes" my horse's mistake.

- Choose one topic from this chapter; evaluate your own skills relative to that topic, and what you could do to benefit your horse and yourself.

- Consider lessons in Centered Riding®, or any kind of bodywork, such as yoga, Pilates, Tai Chi, Alexander Technique, Feldenkrais Method®, or martial arts. All are wonderful for developing body awareness, flexibility, and symmetry.

*chapter 20*
# Our Horses' Low-Stress Lifestyle

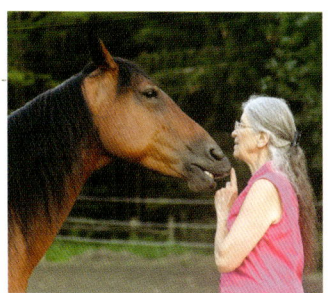

> "If you want the best out of your horse, you'll get the best by first making sure his needs...are met. Good performance is integrally interlinked with good welfare. We need to pay more attention to their social needs and their needs for security and safety."
>
> —Dr. Daniel S. Mills ("Researcher: Prime Equine Performance Linked to Good Welfare")

I'm not sure what my favorite morning view is: My horses in a pasture, calmly munching away (fig. 20.1). Or lined up at the fence that separates their paddock from our backyard, watching through my windows for signs that I'm on my way to serve breakfast. Either way, they've spent the night outside, which means they start the day in a mellow mood.

## Mealtime Routines

Breakfast is somewhere between 7:00 a.m. and 8:00 a.m. I don't feed at a set time, and that is on purpose. I know all the books say we should feed on a schedule because horses have delicate digestive systems and get stressed if we don't stick to a schedule. That is not what I've seen in the real world.

I spent a lot of time in other people's barns before I had my own. Where feeding time was on a reliable schedule, there was much excitement in anticipation. It started 10 or 15 minutes before feeding time, building to a crescendo as food was served. If the server was not in the barn serving up the goods at feeding time sharp, the nickers and door pounding could get frantic. Heaven forbid the food should be *late!* At barns where mealtimes vary I see the opposite. There is little fretting; horses expect the food when it shows up. In my observation it is not a rigid schedule that makes for low stress mealtimes; it's a calm mealtime *routine*.

Details will vary based on facilities and horses, but one important mealtime tradition is clearly supported by research. Hay should be fed 10 to 20 minutes before grain. This is a good practice in general because concentrated feeds are more irritating to equine stomachs than hay is, and because it encourages horses to eat their concentrates more slowly.

Feeding hay first is especially critical for horses with food related issues such as ulcers or choke.[113][114] It also reduces cribbing, apparently because it reduces pain associated with stomach acid.[115]

Our mealtime routine starts with hay served outside. Our paddock is adjacent to the barn, and all pastures open off the paddock, so I don't need to go get horses. They bring themselves to the barn. Since the back of the barn forms a shed, they have a comfortable place to eat their hay, sheltered from wind and rain.

When it is time to come in for their "bucket meals," Brandy is usually first in

**20.1** A favorite morning view from my kitchen window.

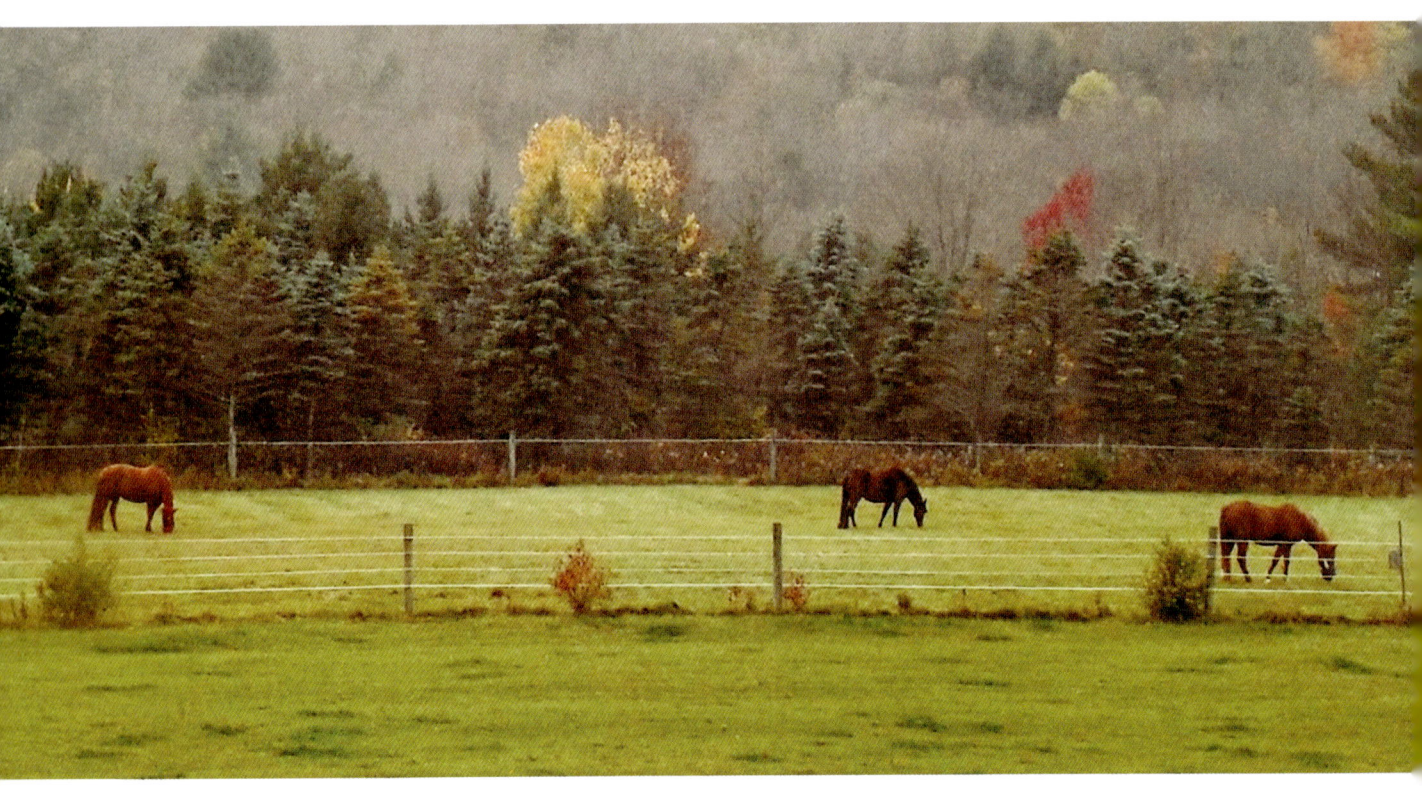

line, but if someone else gets there first, she waits. I open the barn gate, and the horses *walk* to their own stalls. This is non-negotiable. I taught Brandy this by haltering and leading her quietly to her stall for many months. If she tried to jog down the aisle, I quietly took her back outside and reminded her to walk. She discovered that walking was the fastest way to get to her food. Next, I escorted her down the aisle off-lead. Finally, I could just open the gate, and she walked to her stall as the others already did.

Once or twice a year Brandy forgets the walking rule and dashes down the aisle at a trot. I quietly go in her stall, halter her and lead her out of the barn, then escort her down the aisle at a slow walk.

Having the horses come in the barn calmly sets the tone for a relaxed meal. As each horse walks in, I watch for signs of lameness, loose or missing shoes, or any other problems.

Most of the year, the horses will be going back outside after breakfast to have their morning hay and a snooze. While they eat, I put out more hay, attend to the water tank, and scoop manure out of their sheds. Before I let them out, I check Bronzz's hoof temperature, digital pulses, and crest for any sign of trouble related to his insulin resistance.

My horses do not barge out when I open their doors. The rule is feet stay behind the doorsill until invited to come out. I taught this by nicely but relentlessly reminding them that when the door is opened they must stay (the "stay" command described in chapter 16—p. 197) until given permission to leave. When I say, "Go on out," pointing toward the barn door, they walk quietly out of the barn.

I prevent anyone from blocking the exit by sending Shiloh out first, then Bronzz, then Brandy because Shiloh moves for Bronzz who moves for Brandy. Knowing and respecting these herd dynamics goes a long way toward lowering stress.

Dinner is usually between 5:00 p.m. and 7:00 p.m. I try to keep breakfast and dinner at least 10 hours apart and within the same timeframes, so meals don't get too random. The routine is similar to breakfast, except that after dinner, we pick hooves, do the stretches the chiropractor prescribed, and perhaps some grooming. My husband cuts an apple in little pieces so each horse gets exactly 4 bites, a part of the routine they all look forward to.

In addition to breakfast and dinner hay, we serve hay at lunch and bedtime unless the horses are getting enough pasture to compensate. Hay goes on the ground either in sheds or out in the paddock depending on weather and mud.

We do occasionally have an equine rendition of Keystone Cops where the first horse into the barn for a meal ducks into someone else's stall for an extra bite, then the next horse grabs the nearest empty stall, and they're all re-arranged. I've learned the most constructive response is to laugh about it. "Don't be ridiculous, guys," I say, and quietly sort them out. Our calm manner is essential for calm mealtimes.

## The Menu

My menu is non-standard. When I discovered many years ago that Bronzz is insulin resistant, I switched all my horses from sweet feed to unsweetened hay pellets as the basis of their "bucket meals." (I recently switched to chopped forage when I learned that chewing hard pellets is a risk factor for the dental problems Bronzz is now having.)

Brandy was not pleased with the hay pellet-based menu at first. She peered at the meager contents of her feed bin (about one pint's worth), sniffed, and looked at me reproachfully as if to say, "Lynn, this isn't sweet feed. And there's hardly any of it."

"That's right, Brandy," I explained. "Chubby ponies make cute cartoons, but in real life they are not healthy. Grass and hay are all you need to keep in good weight. For your dining pleasure, we have high quality hay pellets with no added sweeteners. And see those little brown pellets? More vitamins in those than in two quarts of sweet feed, and much better for you. All moistened with flax seed oil for healthy omega three fatty acids. Try it. You'll like it."

She looked around and noticed that the other horses were tucking happily into their rations. Sighing, she sampled her new food and found it acceptable.

In addition to vitamins, I supplement my horses' food with minerals that are deficient in our hay, as determined by analysis of our current year's supply.[116] Everyone gets hoof and joint supplements. When Bronzz started losing muscle over his topline, I added extra protein for him. I use some medicinal herbs in consultation with my vet.

I sometimes add healthy garnish like carrot or apple peelings. Their first reaction to parsley was amusingly typical of their individual attitudes about new food. Bronzz glared at me. "This was not served where I grew up." Shiloh made dreadful faces. "Are you trying to poison me?" Brandy dove right in. "Yum. Gourmet food!"

## Turnout

At many barns the default plan is for horses to be in the barn. Turnout happens when humans deem the weather to be nice enough and/or when it fits the human's schedule. Most of the oldest, healthiest horses I've known lived where the default plan is just the opposite. Horses stay outside unless there is a reason for them to come in.

This has been our approach, except on buggy summer days. Our horses

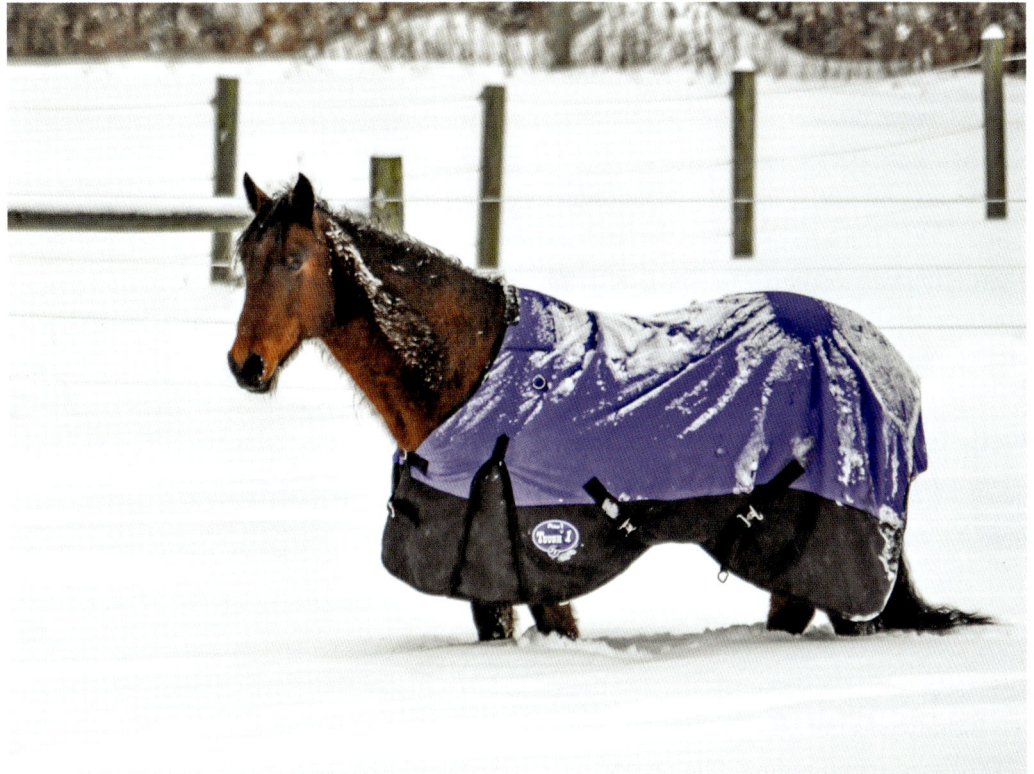

20.2 With two sheds to choose from, a heated water tank, and room to move, Brandy would rather be out in the snow than in the barn. She needs her blanket only in extra cold or windy weather.

always wanted desperately to come in the barn, and their farrier supported them on this. Stamping at flies all day is hard on hooves, he said, so they are better off in their stalls where flies are less bothersome, and bedding cushions any stamping. This seemed like a perfectly reasonable plan until Brandy's recent diagnosis of heaves. This summer our goal is to make our horses comfortable for more hours outside: fly sheets and masks, screens hanging on the front of their turn-out shed, bedding inside it, and whatever else we can come up with.

The rest of the year our horses rarely spend a day in the barn. They come in overnight if it is raining heavily *and* below 45 degrees Fahrenheit, the point at which our vet says wet horses are likely to get chilled. They also stay in for exceptionally cold weather with high winds that swirl into their sheds. Otherwise, they prefer to be outside (fig. 20.2). Bronzz and Sapphire showed us this long ago when they lived at the boarding stable.

We once drove through heavy snow to the stable to bring them in the barn because we knew the owners' policy was, "They're fine outside with a shed and heated water tank." We arrived to

PART SEVEN: REDUCING STRESS — 251

find that not one of the 13 pasture-kept horses was in a shed. Instead, they stood dozing under the stars with snow blanketing their bare backs, snowflakes on their eyelashes, and icicles hanging from their bellies. They blinked blearily at us as if wondering why on earth we were bothering them. Feeling foolish, we wished them good night and went home.

Ice is a dilemma. I worry about injury, yet the longer we keep the horses in the barn, the more likely they are to do something wild and foolish when they get out. When possible I put used bedding as traction on icy spots, especially on their routine pathways. They do seem to be mindful of the ice, and our relatively settled herd dynamics make it less likely that anyone will get chased onto ice.

> *Nothing mellows a horse like moseying and munching forage as nature intended.*

My guide for blanketing is based on my veterinarian's input that a full winter coat is good to about 10 to zero degrees Fahrenheit. I factor in wind chill and adjust for individual variations. Brandy gets cold faster than Shiloh does. Sapphire wore her blanket more as she aged. Bronzz needs his more often because he is partially clipped.

## Pasture Time

Nothing mellows a horse out like moseying and munching forage as nature intended. When my husband and I set up horsekeeping, we dutifully followed advice to improve our pastures by seeding and fertilizing, so our horses could have maximum time enjoying fresh grass. We had no idea that lush pastures could be treacherous for many horses until Bronzz got laminitis. Then we learned that the rich pasture grasses people plant were developed to increase yields in beef and milk cows, the opposite of the marginal vegetation nature adapted horses to eat.

The advice I wish we had is what my sister's veterinarian gives: do *not* seed or fertilize pastures. Just let the native vegetation do its own thing, minus anything toxic, of course. Her pasture is not pretty, but she has healthy horses who graze freely.

The only time we can give our horses 24-hour pasture freedom is when the grass is covered with deep snow and industrious digging is required. Otherwise, Bronzz's glucose goes up (even on frozen winter grass), a warning sign that he is at risk for laminitis. Shiloh gains weight, also a big health hazard.

Everyone with this dilemma needs to find their own solution in consultation with their vet.[117] Ours is a juggling act involving a large paddock with very little vegetation, a sacrifice pasture chewed down to nothing, and grazing muzzles.

Though most horses accept muzzles philosophically, many people resist using them. They are heavy and look uncomfortable. It is tempting to curtail pasture time instead, but that creates a different problem. Knowing their grass time is limited, horses gobble ferociously, raising stress and glucose levels. Grazing muzzles reduce grass intake while allowing lots of healthy heads-down, mosey and munch pasture time.[118] [119] An insert with a smaller hole can be dropped into a muzzle if necessary to further reduce the amount of grass a horse gets.

Our horses' muzzles require lots of padding with halter fleeces to prevent rubs. However, they do not bother our horses nearly as much as they bother us. Our horses see muzzles as their "ticket to graze," because they know that as soon as the muzzles are on, I'm going to open a pasture gate. They eagerly stuff their faces into the muzzles to grab the primo treat in the bottom, then escort me to the gate.

I did not try to muzzle Brandy her first few years with us. I was sure that with her old fears of being trapped, it would not go well. During that time, she noticed that Bronzz and Shiloh got treats in their muzzles. When I took their muzzles out to put them on, Brandy started stuffing her face into their muzzles to eat the treats. I just took extra treats. I started getting the feeling that she expected her very own muzzle.

When I outfitted Brandy with her own muzzle, I included lots of treats. I still expected some negative reaction the first time I left it on her for turnout, but to my delight, she just trooped out to pasture with Bronzz and Shiloh, and started eating as if it was all to her satisfaction.

## Jobs, Responsibilities, and Social Time

Nature did not design horses to stand around all day doing nothing (fig. 20.3). Our horses' wild ancestors had ongoing responsibilities and challenges. They found their own food, water, and shelter, often traveling many miles a day in the process. They maintained social bonds with herdmates. Everyone participated in protecting and socializing the young. Through it all, they were ever vigilant for danger, and ready to move out in an instant. Surely nothing good happens to the physical, mental, or emotional health of a domestic horse who has nothing to do but stand around waiting for the next meal.

When you give a horse a job that suits him mentally and physically, you do him a service. Trail riding is clearly Bronzz's favorite job. He is especially enthusiastic when we explore new trails, have a friend join us, or find an opportunity for a nice, long canter. Brandy likes agility. It's not unusual for her to play with the equipment on her own.

There is one job for which all of my horses are on duty at all times: attend to the safety of any human nearby. That means watching out for personal space, yielding to pressure, and maintaining self-control. No exceptions, no excuses. "I

20.3 When the ground is particularly muddy, I let the horses play in the arena where the footing is safer. Brandy's romps often take her over, under, and through the agility "toys."

spooked," or "She chased me," do not cut any ice with me. Horses manage to avoid bumping into higher ranking horses; they can avoid people just the same. This does not, of course, absolve people of being safe and sensible. Horses are no more perfect than we are. They can be distracted, irritable, make mistakes and bad judgment calls. But the expectation that they take responsibility, too, gives us an extra margin of safety, and makes life calmer and pleasanter for everyone.

Another thing that makes life pleasanter for all of us is lots of social time (fig. 20.4). I take every opportunity for friendly interactions with my horses, so their assumption is that when I show up nice things will happen, and that doesn't always mean food. I greet them with gentle nose touches or neck strokes. I chat with them while I do chores. When I need them to move, I ask politely and touch them gently. I scratch itchy spots. I stand next to them and just hang out.

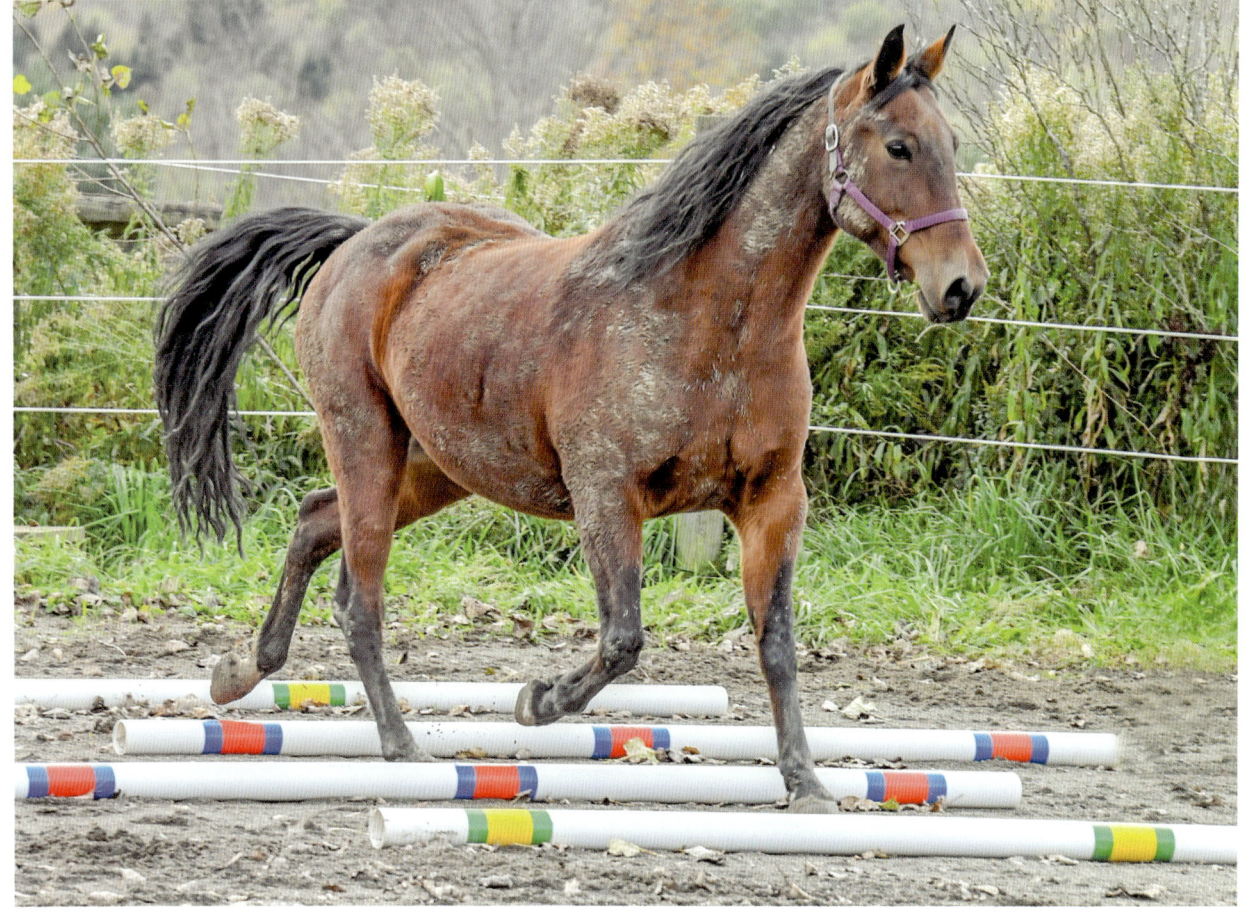

All this positive touching means that when something unexpected happens, like I bump into someone by mistake, they are *not* primed to be defensive. The social time contributes to a positive relationship so that when I want them to focus and work, they are ready.

## ◆ Summary

Low-stress living conditions go a long way toward supporting a horse's physical, mental, and emotional health, which in turn helps make him a better partner. Stress can be reduced with:

- Maximum turnout.
- Compatible companions.
- Maximum forage and minimum concentrated feed.
- Calm mealtime routines.
- Pleasant social time with people without demands to work or perform.

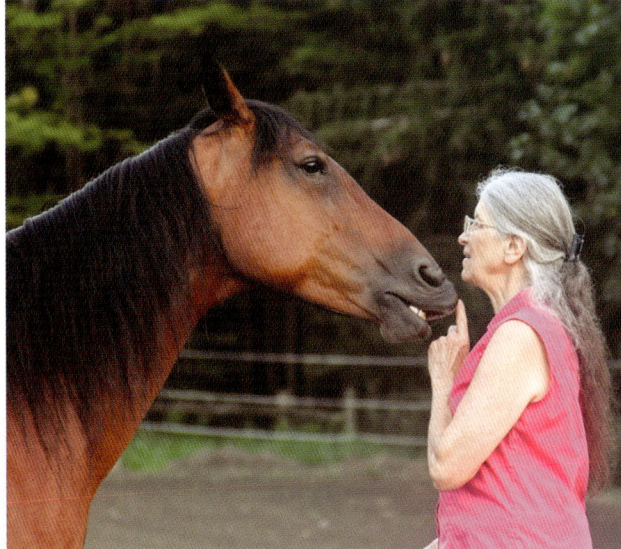

20.4 Brandy takes time out from grazing to come visit with me and nuzzle my finger.

---

### THINGS TO TRY

▶ **Consider what lifestyle stresses your horse might be encountering,** including: too little turnout or too small a turnout space for the number of horses he shares it with, no equine friends to hang out with, too little time eating hay and/or grass, too much concentrated feed, mealtimes that include competition with other horses, or rushed and impatient people, too little undemanding social time with people (see chapter 4, p. 43, for more details).

▶ **Brainstorm what steps you might take to improve on his current circumstances.** If there are concerns you cannot change, often the case at boarding stables, just keep them on your radar to help you understand your horse's behavior better.

# Conclusion

> "If...the rider tries to see in his horse more than some sort of equipment for sport, if he tries to understand his nature and study his character, then the animal will reward his master with willing cooperation and an absolute devotion."
>
> —Alois Podhajsky *(My Horses, My Teachers)*

I once asked a very skilled but rather authoritarian rider what her horse thought his job was. "His job," she replied sternly, "is to do whatever I tell him to." Though this person loved her horse enough to nurse him through an expensive and life-threatening illness, their relationship was a disappointment marred by resistance, bucking, spooking, falls, and well-justified anxiety. No one else even dared ride him. The more diligently she applied all that she had been taught in many years of riding and training horses, the worse matters got. The horse's marvelous athletic talent was going to waste.

When a bad fall landed the owner in the hospital, she had time to ponder the comment a veterinarian had once made about her horse. "He could be a great partner, but *he will be no one's obedient servant*."

Desperate enough now to radically change the way she related to her horse, she tried things she'd been told never to do. She was gentler, more patient, less demanding. She gave the horse latitude to express his personality, and considered his preferences as she planned rides. She did not lower her standards or tolerate bad behavior, but with planning and patience, she became more decision-maker, less disciplinarian. The anxiety behind his "bad" behavior became obvious now that she was willing to see it. She learned when to relieve pressure, back off, or try something different. She found an instructor who showed her how changes in her riding could help her horse do the job she was asking of him, instead of hindering him.

Resistance turned to honest effort. Dramatic spooks became the exceptions instead of daily events. She could enjoy developing his athletic ability instead of managing his behavior.

Having seen these changes as they happened, I accepted the owner's offer to ride her horse. My feelings swiftly went from trepidation to delight. Though I am a less skilled rider than his owner, he earnestly tried to understand and do everything I asked. At the same time, he always had one eye or ear on his owner. When I dismounted, he went straight to her. She was on his radar every minute she was on the farm. His devotion was obvious.

She began taking him to clinics with trainers who were internationally recognized in their discipline *and* respectful of horses. The horse not only worked diligently, he worked with pride. People who hadn't known him in his "wild" past could not believe he had ever been anything but a gentleman with impeccable manners.

The only thing unusual about this story is the happy ending, made possible by his owner's willingness to take a leap of faith and try relating to him differently. He exemplifies many "problem" horses who just want to feel safe and be someone's partner. Many other horses are compliant but stressed underneath because it is their nature to be stoic.

Most novices intuitively want to offer their horses the security and social bonds they need, but for many of us, the more we "learned" about horses, the more faulty assumptions got in our way. As Vanessa Bee observes, "The real challenge is exploding the myths people have long believed about horses."[120]

I hope that with the help of my horses I have succeeded in exploding some myths and replacing them with reality:

- Horses don't care about being dominant; they want security and companionship.

- Horses don't behave "badly" because they want to thwart you; their behavior is their only way of communicating with you.

- Horses don't always need pressure to understand what you want them to do; you can also communicate in very positive ways with your body language and rewards.

- Horses are not naturally "spooky" or "cowardly"; when allowed to investigate new things, they build knowledge and confidence.

- Horses don't learn solely by repetition; they learn more efficiently when you engage their abilities to explore, generalize information, and problem-solve.

- The fact that something is commonly done does not necessarily make it safe, effective, or humane; many common practices are detrimental to horses' welfare and behavior.

One of the most treacherous myths of all is that horses want and need authoritative leadership. If you have any remaining doubts about this, I challenge you to the ultimate test. Give Protector Leadership an honest try, and see what happens. Remember that you may see the difference right away with a new horse, as I did with Brandy, but horses who know you may take time to trust the change.

If you have discovered that you were a Protector Leader all along, I hope you enjoy knowing that you are in the company of great horsemen and horsewomen through the centuries, and that science supports you. Congratulations!

I hope I have also provided ideas and resources that will help you improve your relationship with your horse. For role models and support, look around you for those quiet Protector Leaders whose horses are relaxed, happy, and cooperative. Most of all, trust your horse and your own intuition. When you listen to your horse, and have his best interests at heart, you can be confident you are going in a good direction.

Harry deLeyer, partner of the legendary jumper Snowman, summed it up nicely. "If you take care of your horse, your horse will take care of you."[121]

## About the Author

**Lynn Acton** has a diverse equestrian and academic background that helps her understand horses, relationships, and leadership from an interdisciplinary point of view. Her degrees in sociology and systems science have contributed to her understanding of research studies, the social dynamics of horses, their interactions with people, and how the interconnected parts of complex social systems fit together. After spending time working on a Thoroughbred breeding farm and later retraining off-track Thoroughbreds, Acton became certified by the Certified Horsemanship Association (CHA) to teach both English and Western riding and started a therapeutic riding program for at-risk youth. She currently competes in Horse Agility and Equagility (ridden agility). Find out more about Acton and her horses at LynnActon.com.

# Endnotes

There have been exciting developments in equine behavior research in the last few decades. Researchers are focused more on how horses think and view the world, how they relate to each other and to us, and what changes we as horse people can make to improve our horses' welfare. Ingenious experiments provide insights that are relevant in our everyday interactions with horses. Exploring this research has been part of the fun of writing this book.

Some of the sources cited are scientific papers published by the researchers. Others are articles about research studies, written for magazines such as *The Horse* (www.the-horse.com) or *Equus*. The latter are more fun reading for most of us, and may include additional information from interviews with researchers.

I chose the studies I cited based on their relevance to us as horse people. I did not include "studies" where the researcher had a financial interest in the outcome.

[1] Kim Walnes, "Being a Leader/Protector for Your Horse" http://www.thewayofthehorse.com/images/WalnesLeadership.pdf (accessed 3/24/19)

[2] Magali Delgado & Frédéric Pignon with David Walser, *Gallop to Freedom: Training Horses with the Founding Stars of Cavalia* (Trafalgar Square Books, 2009) p. 32

[3] Vanessa Bee, *The Horse Agility Handbook* (Trafalgar Square Books, 2012) p. 40

[4] Xenophon, *The Art of Horsemanship,* translated by Morris H. Morgan (Dover Publications, Inc., 2006)

[5] Elizabeth Letts, *The Eighty-Dollar Champion: Snowman, The Horse That Inspired a Nation* (Ballantine Books, 2011)

[6] Cathrynne Henshall & Paul D. McGreevy, "The role of ethology in round pen horse training—A review," *Applied Animal Behavior Science,* 2 April 2014 http://www.appliedanimalbehaviour.com/artic le/S0168-1591(14)00081-1/fulltext (accessed 3/24/19)

[7] Christa Leste-Lasserre, "Excitement, Feeling, and Attachment's Impact on Training," *The Horse,* 2 Aug 2013 http://www.thehorse.com/articles/32311/excitement-feeling-and-attachments-impact-on-training (accessed 3/24/19)

(9th International Society for Equitation Science Conference, held July 17-19 at the University of Delaware, Newark).

[8] Carrie Ijichi, et al, "Harnessing the power of personality assessment: subjective assessment predicts behaviour in horses," Behavioural Processes, Volume 9, June 2013, pages 47-52 http://www.sciencedirect.com/science/article/pii/S0376635713000399 (accessed 3/24/19)

[9] Elke Hartmann, Janne W. Christensen, Paul D. McGreevy, "Dominance and Leadership: Useful

Concepts in Human–Horse Interactions?", *Journal of Equine Veterinary Science,* Volume 52, May 2017, pages 1-9 https://www.sciencedirect.com/science/article/pii/S0737080617300059 (accessed 1/31/19)

[10] Mark Rashid, "Passive Leadership," http://www.markrashid.com/docs/leadership.pdf (accessed 3/24/19)

[11] Kim Walnes, "Being a Leader/Protector for Your Horse," http://www.thewayofthehorse.com/images/WalnesLeadership.pdf (accessed 3/24/19)

[12] Mark Rashid, *Horses Never Lie: The Heart of Passive Leadership* (Skyhorse Publishing, 2011) pages xiv-xv

[13] Margie Goldstein, "Empathy: The Secret Ingredient for Success," *HorsePlay Magazine,* Nov 1993

[14] Mark Rashid, *Considering the Horse: Tales of Problems Solved and Lessons Learned* (Johnson Books, 1993) p. 123

[15] Jane Goodall, *Hope for Animals and Their World* (Grand Central Publishing, 2009)

[16] Highland ponies (Scotland), Icelandic horses (Iceland), Camargue horses (France), Jeju ponies (South Korea), Hokkaido ponies (Japan), Kaimanawa horses (New Zealand), Grand Canyon mustangs, Pryor Mountain mustangs, and Assateague ponies on Assateague Island. A herd of semi-feral ponies is kept at New Bolton Center (University of Pennsylvania) specifically for research.

[17] RIRDC Equine Research News, "Dr. Paul McGreevy on Horse Behavior" March 1996 http://www.equusite.com/articles/behavior/behaviorDrMcGreevy.shtml (accessed 12/16/17)

[18] F. Heitor, M. do Mar Oom, L. Vicente, "Social relationships in a herd of Sorraia horses Part I. Correlates of social dominance and contexts of aggression," *Behavioural Processes,* Sept 2006. http://www.ncbi.nlm.nih.gov/pubmed/16815645?dopt=Abstract (accessed 3/24/19)

[19] Rikako Kimura, "Mutual grooming and preferred associate relationships in a band of free-ranging horses," *Applied Animal Behaviour Science,* Sept 1998. http://www.appliedanimalbehaviour.com/article/S0168-1591(97)00129-9/abstract (accessed 3/24/19)

[20] S. M. McDonnell, J.C.S. Haviland, "Agonistic ethogram of the equid bachelor band," *Applied Animal Behaviour Science* 43 (1995) 147-188 http://research.vet.upenn.edu/Portals/49/95Agonis.pdf) (accessed 12/16/17)

[21] Cathrynne Henshall, Paul D. McGreevy, "The role of ethology in round pen horse training – A review", *Applied Animal Behaviour Science,* June 2014, pages 1-11. https://www.sciencedirect.com/science/article/pii/S0168159114000811 (accessed 12/16/17)

[22] Hrefna Sigurjónsdóttir; Machteld C. van Dierendonck; Sigurdur Snorrason and Anna G. Thórhallsdóttir, "Social relationships in a group of horses without a mature stallion," *Behaviour,* Volume 140, Issue 6, pages 783 – 804, 2003. http://booksandjournals.brillonline.com/content/journals/10.1163/156853903322370670 (accessed 12/16/17)

[23] Sue McDonnell, PhD, *Understanding Horse Behavior* (The Blood-Horse, Inc, 1999) p. 13

[24] Cathrynne Henshall, Paul D. McGreevy, "The role of ethology in round pen horse training – A review," *Applied Animal Behaviour Science* June 2014, pages 1-11. https://www.sciencedirect.com/science/article/pii/S0168159114000811 (accessed 12/16/17)

[25] Konstanze Krueger a, Birgit Flauger a, 1, Kate Farmer b, Charlotte Hemelrijk c "Movement initiation in groups of feral horses," *Behavioural Processes* Volume 103, March 2014, pages 91-101. http://www.sciencedirect.com/science/article/pii/S0376635713002222 (accessed 12/16/17)

[26] Lea Briard, Camille Dorn, Odile Petit, "Personality and Affinities Play a Key Role in the Organization of Collective Movements in a

Group of Domestic Horses," *Ethology:* International Journal of Behavioural Biology, June 16, 2015. http://onlinelibrary.wiley.com/doi/10.1111/eth.12402/abstract (accessed 12/16/17)

[27] Robin Foster, "When the Herd Moves, Who Leads and Who Follows?," *The Horse,* July 20, 2017 https://thehorse.com/110684/when-the-herd-moves-who-leads-and-who-follows/ (accessed 1/31/19)

[28] Briard L, Deneubourg JL, Petit O., "How stallions influence the dynamic of collective movements in two groups of domestic horses, from departure to arrival," *Behavioural Processes,* 2017 Sept https://www.ncbi.nlm.nih.gov/pubmed/28549567 (accessed 1/31/19)

[29] Sue McDonnell, PhD, *Understanding Horse Behavior* (The Blood-Horse, Inc, 1999) p. 23

[30] Will James, *Smoky The Cowhorse,* (Aladdin Books, 1993) Chapters I – IV

[31] Cathrynne Henshall, Paul D. McGreevy "The role of ethology in round pen horse training—A review", *Applied Animal Behaviour Science,* June 2014 Volume 1555, Pages 1-11. http://www.appliedanimalbehaviour.com/article/S0168-1591(14)00081-1/fulltext (accessed 3/24/19)

[32] Christa Leste-Lasserre, "Study: Human Interaction Shapes Horses' Negative Emotions," *The Horse,* May 22, 2014 http://www.thehorse.com/articles/33927/study-human-interaction-shapes-horses-negative-emotions (accessed 12/18/17)

[33] Cathrynne Henshall, Paul D. McGreevy "The role of ethology in round pen horse training—A review", *Applied Animal Behaviour Science,* June 2014 Volume 1555, Pages 1-11. http://www.appliedanimalbehaviour.com/article/S0168-1591(14)00081-1/fulltext (accessed 3/24/19)

[34] Christa Leste-Lasserre, "Study: Human Interaction Shapes Horses' Negative Emotions," *The Horse,* May 22, 2014 http://www.thehorse.com/articles/33927/study-human-interaction-shapes-horses-negative-emotions (accessed 12/18/17)

[35] Janne Winther Christensen, "Early-life object exposure with a habituated mother reduces fear reactions in foals," *Animal Cognition,* January 2016, Volume 19, Issue 1, pp 171–179. https://rd.springer.com/article/10.1007/s10071-015-0924-7?no-access=true (accessed 3/24/19)

[36] Christa Leste-Lasserre, "Foals Follow Dams' Leads When Dealing With Scary Objects," *The Horse* Nov 1, 2014 http://www.thehorse.com/articles/34801/foals-follow-dams-leads-when-dealing-with-scary-objects?utm_source=Newsletter&utm_medium=behavior&utm_campaign=11-02-2014 (accessed 12/18/17)

[37] Christa Leste-Lasserre, "Study: Human Interaction Shapes Horses' Negative Emotions," *The Horse,* May 22, 2014 http://www.thehorse.com/articles/33927/study-human-interaction-shapes-horses-negative-emotions (accessed 12/18/17)

[38] S. Henry, M. Bourjade, M. Hausberger, "Impact of unrelated adults on the behavior of weanlings & young horses," Ethologie Animale et Humaine. European Federation of Animal Science Annual Meeting 2011 http://www.eaap.org/Previous_Annual_Meetings/2011Stavanger/Papers/Published/S15_Henry.pdf (accessed 2015, no longer available online)

[39] Camie Heleksi, "Studying Animal Behavior," PowerPoint Slideshow presentation. https://www.slideserve.com/consuela-arcelia/studying-animal-behavior

[40] AJ Waters, CJ Nicol, NP French, "Factors influencing the development of stereotypic and redirected behaviours in young horses: findings of a four year prospective epidemiological study", *Equine Veterinary Journal,* Sept 2002. http://www.ncbi.nlm.nih.gov/pubmed/12357996 (accessed 12/20/17)

[41] Sue McDonnell, *Understanding Horse Behavior: Your Guide to Horse Health Care and Management,* (The Blood-Horse, Inc., 1999) p. 61.

[42] Martine Hausberger, Emmanuel Gautier, Christine Müller, Patrick Jego, "Lower learning abilities in stereotypic horses," *Applied Animal Behaviour Science,* Volume 107, Issues 3–4, November 2007, Pages 299–306. https://www.researchgate.net/publication/248335951_Lower_learning_abilities_in_stereotypic_horses (accessed 12/31/17)

[43] Charlene Strickland, "Stereotypic Behaviors," *The Horse,* Apr 1, 1997. http://www.thehorse.com/articles/10676/stereotypic-behaviors (accessed 12/31/17)

[44] C Nicol, "Understanding equine stereotypies," *Equine Veterinary Journal,* Apr 1999. https://www.ncbi.nlm.nih.gov/pubmed/11314230 (accessed 12/20/17)

[45] Christa Lesté-Lasserre, "Equine Stereotypies: Vice or Coping Mechanism?" *The Horse,* Oct 11, 2016 http://www.thehorse.com/articles/38285/equine-stereotypies-vice-or-coping-mechanism?utm_source=Newsletter&utm_medium=health-news&utm_campaign=10-11-2016 (accessed 1/11/16)

[46] Thierry Steimer, PhD, "The biology of fear- and anxiety-related behaviors." Dialogues in clinical neuroscience, 2002 Sep; 4(3): 231–249 http://www.ncbi.nlm.nih.gov/pmc/articles/PMC3181681/ (accessed 4/7/2016)

[47] Martine Hausberger, Emmanuel Gautier, Christine Müller, Patrick Jego, "Lower learning abilities in stereotypic horses," *Applied Animal Behaviour Science,* Volume 107, Issues 3–4, November 2007, Pages 299–306. https://www.researchgate.net/publication/248335951_Lower_learning_abilities_in_stereotypic_horses (accessed 12/31/17)

[48] R. Malavasi, L Huber, "Evidence of heterospecific referential communication from domestic horses (Equus caballus) to humans," *Animal Cognition,* Sept 19, 2016. http://www.ncbi.nlm.nih.gov/pubmed/27098164 (accessed 12/16/17)

[49] Christa Leste-Lasserre, MA, "Study Confirms Horses 'Talk' to Human Handlers," *The Horse,* Jun 9, 2016 http://www.thehorse.com/articles/37681/study-confirms-horses-talk-to-human-handlers?utm_source=Newsletter&utm_medium=health-news&utm_campaign=06-14-2016 (accessed 12/16/17)

[50] Monamie Ringhofer, Shinya Yamamoto, "Domestic horses send signals to humans when they face with an unsolvable task," *Animal Cognition,* May 2017 http://link.springer.com/article/10.1007/s10071-016-1056-4 (accessed 12/16/17)

[51] Christa Leste-Lasserre, "Excitement, Feeling, and Attachment's Impact on Training," *The Horse,* 2 Aug 2013 http://www.thehorse.com/articles/32311/excitement-feeling-and-attachments-impact-on-training (accessed 12/16/17)

(Paper presented at the 9th International Society for Equitation Science Conference, July 17-19 at the University of Delaware, in Newark.)

[52] Carrie Ijichi, et al, "Harnessing the power of personality assessment: subjective assessment predicts behaviour in horses," *Behavioural Processes,* Volume 9, June 2013, pages 47-52. http://www.sciencedirect.com/science/article/pii/S0376635713000399 (accessed 12/19/17)

[53] Sue McDonnell, PhD, "Detecting Discomfort," *The Horse,* Dec 1, 2011 http://www.thehorse.com/articles/28496/detecting-discomfort (accessed Nov 27, 2017)

[54] Clemence Lesimple, Carole Fureix, Veronique Biquard, and Martine Hausberger, "Comparison of clinical examinations of back disorders and humans' evaluation of back pain in riding school horses," BioMed Central Veterinary Research, 2012 Oct 15. http://www.ncbi.nlm.nih.gov/pmc/articles/PMC4015870/ (accessed 12/31/17)

[55] Sue Dyson, Jeannine Berger, Andrea D. Ellis, Jessica Mullard, "Development of an ethogram for a pain scoring system in ridden horses and its application to determine the presence of musculoskeletal pain," *Journal of Veterinary Behavior:* Clinical Applications and Research, Volume 23, January–February 2018, pages

47-57. https://www.sciencedirect.com/science/article/pii/S1558787817301727 (accessed 12/7/17)

56 Press release, "Research on Pain Scoring System for Ridden Horses Continues," *The Horse,* Dec 5, 2017. http://www.thehorse.com/articles/40005/research-on-pain-scoring-system-for-ridden-horses-continues?utm_source=Newsletter&utm_medium=lameness&utm_campaign=12-06-2017 (accessed 12/31/17)

57 Clémence Lesimple, Carole Fureix, Emmanuel De Margerie, Emilie Sénèque, Hervé Menguy, and Martine Hausberger, "Toward a Postural Indicator of Back Pain in Horses (Equus caballus)," PLOS ONE, published online 2012 Sept 7  http://www.ncbi.nlm.nih.gov/pmc/articles/PMC3436792/  (accessed 1/16/18)

58 Joyce Harman DVM, MRCVS, *The Horse's Pain-Free Back and Saddle-Fit Book* (Trafalgar Square Books, 2004) pages 9-11

59  Karen Gellman, DVM, PhD and Judith Shoemaker, DVM "Standing up for Success" http://www.yourbalancedhorse.com/pdf/PosturalRehabEquusArticle.pdf (accessed 3/23/17)

60  Carole Fureix, Herve Menguy, Martine Hausberger, "Partners with Bad Temper: Reject of Cure? A Study of Chronic Pain and Aggression in Horses," PLOS ONE published online August 26, 2010 http://journals.plos.org/plosone/article?id=10.1371/journal.pone.0012434  (accessed 3/23/17)

61  Sue Dyson, Jeannine Berger, Andrea D. Ellis, Jessica Mullard, "Development of an ethogram for a pain scoring system in ridden horses and its application to determine the presence of musculoskeletal pain," *Journal of Veterinary Behavior:* Clinical Applications and Research, Volume 23, January–February 2018, pages 47-57. https://www.sciencedirect.com/science/article/pii/S1558787817301727 (accessed 12/7/17)

62 Press release, "Research on Pain Scoring System for Ridden Horses Continues," *The Horse,* Dec 5, 2017. http://www.thehorse.com/articles/40005/research-on-pain-scoring-system-for-ridden-horses-continues?utm_source=Newsletter&utm_medium=lameness&utm_campaign=12-06-2017 (accessed 12/31/17)

63 Clémence Lesimple, Carole Fureix, Emmanuel De Margerie, Emilie Sénèque, Hervé Menguy, and Martine Hausberger, "Toward a Postural Indicator of Back Pain in Horses (Equus caballus)," PLOS ONE published online 2012 Sept 7  http://www.ncbi.nlm.nih.gov/pmc/articles/PMC3436792/  (accessed 1/16/18)

64 Joyce Harman DVM, MRCVS, *The Horse's Pain-Free Back and Saddle-Fit Book* (Trafalgar Square Books, 2004) page 207

65 Amanda Sutton, *The Injury-Free Horse* (Trafalgar Square Books, 2001), p 55

66 Amanda Sutton, *The Injury-Free Horse* (Trafalgar Square Books, 2001), p 50

67 Susan Harris, *Horse Gaits, Balance, and Movement* (Howell Book House, 1993) p. 80.

68 AVSAB Position Statement, "The Use of Punishment for Behavior Modification in Animals," The American Veterinary Society of Animal Behavior website.  https://avsab.org/wp-content/uploads/2016/08/Punishment_Position_Statement-download_-_10-6-14.pdf (accessed 12/31/17)

69 Sue McDonnell, PhD, "Horse Behavior: War on Punishment," *The Horse,* Jun 20, 2008. http://www.thehorse.com/articles/21325/horse-behavior-war-on-punishment (accessed 12/31/17)

70 Carol Sankey, Marie-Annick Richard-Yris, Séverine Henry, Carole Fureix, Fouad Nassur, Martine Hausberger, "Reinforcement as a mediator of the perception of humans by horses (Equus caballus)," *Animal Cognition,* September 2010  https://link.springer.com/article/10.1007/s10071-010-0326-9 (accessed 4/11/19)

71 Michelle, N. Anderson, "Managing the Anxious Horse," *The Horse,* Feb 5, 2016 http://www.thehorse.com/articles/37095/managing-the-anxious-horse?utm_source=Newsletter&utm_medium=behavior&utm_campaign=02-07-2016 (accessed 3/23/17)

72 Amy Victoria Smith, Leanne Proops, Kate Grounds, Jennifer Wathan, Karen McComb, "Functionally relevant responses to human facial expressions of emotion in the domestic horse (Equus caballus)," Biology Letters, February 2016.  http://rsbl.royalsocietypublishing.org/content/12/2/20150907 (accessed 12/1/18)

73 Press Release, "Horses Can Read Human Emotions, Study Shows," *The Horse,* Feb 11, 2016  http://www.thehorse.com/articles/37128/horses-can-read-human-emotions-study-shows (accessed 12/1/18)

74 Katrina Merkies et al. "Does the Human Voice Have a Calming Effect on Horses?", *Journal of Equine Veterinary Science* 33(5):368 · April 2013  https://www.researchgate.net/publication/257243334_Does_the_human_voice_have_a_calming_effect_on_horses  (accessed 3/29/16)

75 Emerson, Denny. *Know Better to Do Better* (Trafalgar Square Books, 2018) p. 205

76 Christa Lesté-Lasserre, MA. "Study: Human Interaction Shapes Horses' Negative Emotions," *The Horse,* May 22, 2014  http://www.thehorse.com/articles/33927/study-human-interaction-shapes-horses-negative-emotions

77 Carol Sankey, Marie-Annick Richard-Yris, Séverine Henry, Carole Fureix, Fouad Nassur, Martine Hausberger, "Reinforcement as a mediator of the perception of humans by horses (Equus caballus)," *Animal Cognition,* September 2010  https://link.springer.com/article/10.1007/s10071-010-0326-9 (accessed 4/11/19)

78 Kathleen Lindley Beckham, "Learned Helplessness," https://greyhorsellc.wordpress.com/2018/11/09/learned-helplessness/?fbclid=IwAR0d6z9bi-T7o8k2ij4u3cU9krL1lqI56tC0gfXIO4a4P-fbSnAnT_wLyxdxQ  (accessed 12/24/18)

79 McDonnell, Sue. *A Practical Field Guild to Horse Behavior* (Eclipse Press) p. 314

80 Magali Delgado & Frédéric Pignon, *Gallop to Freedom: Training Horses with the Founding Stars of Cavalia* (Trafalgar Square Books, 2009) p. 31

81 Xenophon, *The Art of Horsemanship,* translated by Morris H. Morgan (Dover Publications, Inc., 2006) p. 35

82 Konstanze Krueger, "Behaviour of horses in the "round pen technique," *Applied Animal Behaviour Science,* April 2007 Volume 104, Issues 1-2, Pages 162-170. http://www.appliedanimalbehaviour.com/article/S0168-1591(06)00137-7/abstract (accessed 12/24/18)

83 Cathrynne Henshall, Paul Damien McGreevy, Barbara Padalino, "The radio-controlled car as a herd leader?  A preliminary study of escape and avoidance learning in the roundpen," Conference Paper, Proceedings of the 8th International Equitation Science Conference (Edinburgh) January 2012. https://www.researchgate.net/publication/289530907_The_radio-controlled_car_as_a_herd_leader_A_preliminary_study_of_escape_and_avoidance_learning_in_the_roundpen (accessed 12/24/18)

84 Carol Sankey, Marie-Annick Richard-Yris, Séverine Henry, Carole Fureix, Fouad Nassur, Martine Hausberger, "Reinforcement as a mediator of the perception of humans by horses (Equus caballus)," *Animal Cognition,* September 2010  https://link.springer.com/article/10.1007/s10071-010-0326-9 (accessed 4/11/19)

85 Peter F. Cook, Ashley Prichard, Mark Spivak, Gregory S. Berns, "Awake canine fMRI predicts dogs' preference for praise vs food," Social Cognitive and Affective Neuroscience Advance Access, September 1, 2016. http://media.wix.com/ugd/58d36a_d2c0b05ac3dd474087acda3cb7092d2a.pdf (accessed 3/7/17)

[86] Zoë W. Thorbergson, Sharon G. Nielsen, Rodney J. Beaulieu & Rebecca E. Doyle, "Physiological and Behavioral Responses of Horses to Wither Scratching and Patting the Neck When Under Saddle," *Journal of Applied Animal Welfare Science,* Volume 19, 2016 – Issue 3. http://www.tandfonline.com/doi/abs/10.1080/10888705.2015.1130630?journalCode=haaw20 (accessed 1/10/18)

[87] Christa Lesté-Lasserre, "Do Horses Prefer Patting or Scratching?", *The Horse,* Nov 12, 2014. http://www.thehorse.com/articles/34855/do-horses-prefer-patting-or-scratching (accessed 1/10/18)

[88] Temple Grandin and Catherine Johnson, *Animals Make Us Human: Creating the Best Life for Animals* (Mariner Books, 2010)

[89] Sue DcDonnell, Ph.D., *A Practical Field Guide to Horse Behavior: The Equid Ethogram* (Eclipse Press, 2003) pages 84-85.

[90] Dr. Stephen Peters & Martin Black, *Evidence-Based Horsemanship* (Wasteland Press, 2012) pages 43-45.

[91] Jack Murphy, Carol Hall, Sean Arkins, "What Horses and Humans See: A Comparative Review," *International Journal of Zoology* Volume 2009 (2009), Article ID 721798 http://www.hindawi.com/journals/ijz/2009/721798/ (accessed10/12/14)

[92] EB Hanggi, JF Ingersoll, TL Waggoner, "Color vision in horses (Equus caballus): deficiencies identified using a pseudoisochromatic plate test," *Journal of Comparative Psychology.* 2007 Feb;121(1):65-72 http://www.ncbi.nlm.nih.gov/pubmed/17324076 (accessed 1/8/18)

[93] M. J. Morgan, A. Adam, and J. D. Mollon, "Dichromats detect colour-camouflaged objects that are not detected by trichromats," Proceedings of the Royal Society of London, 22 June 1992. Series B, vol. 248, no. 1323, pages 291–295 http://rspb.royalsocietypublishing.org/content/248/1323/291 (accessed 1/1/18)

[94] Evelyn Hanggi, "The Thinking Horse: Cognition and Perception Reviewed," AAEP Proceedings, 2005 http://www.equineresearch.org/support-files/hanggi-thinkinghorse.pdf (accessed 1/8/18)

[95] A. Telatin, "The use of the investigative behavior to improve the training of the jumping horse," *Journal of Veterinary Behavior,* April, 2013 Volume 8, Iss2, Page e21. http://www.journalvetbehavior.com/article/S1558-7878(12)00264-X/fulltext (accessed 1/11/18)

Angelo Telatin, "The use of the investigative behavior to improve the training of the jumping horse," Presented at the International Society of Equitation Science annual conference (Holland 2011) http://www.angelotelatin.com/en/horse-training-methods/investigative-behavior-pkv1/ (accessed 1/1/18)

[96] Sue McDonnell, PhD, "Habituation vs. Learned Helplessness in Horses," *The Horse,* Nov 29, 2018. https://thehorse.com/110232/habituation-vs-learned-helplessness-in-horses/ (accessed 12/16/18)

[97] Konstanze Krüger, Kate Farmer, & Jurgen Heinze, "The effects of age, rank and neophobia on social learning in horses," *Animal Cognition,* May 2014 http://link.springer.com/article/10.1007/s10071-013-0696-x (accessed 10/28/15)

[98] Vanessa Bee, *Over, Under, Through: Obstacle Training for Horses* (Trafalgar Square Books, 2015) p. 4

[99] Hertha James, *Conversations with Horses: An In-Depth Look at Signals & Cues Between Horses and Their Handlers* (Powerword Publications) p. 165

[100] Ellen Schuthof-Lesmeister and Kip Mistral, *Horse Training in-Hand: A Modern Guide to Working from the Ground* (Trafalgar Square Books, 2009)

[101] Alexandra Beckstett, "Professional vs. Amateur Round Pen Training Techniques,"

*The Horse,* Dec 3, 2015 http://www.thehorse.com/articles/36795/professional-vs-amateur-round-pen-training-techniques?utm_source=Newsletter&utm_medium=health-news&utm_campaign=12-08-2015 (accessed 1/10/18)

[102] Carrie Ijichi, Lisa M. Collins, Emma Creighton, Robert W. Elwood, "Harnessing the power of personality assessment: subjective assessment predicts behaviour in horses," *Behavioural Processes* Volume 96, June 2013, pages 47-52 http://www.sciencedirect.com/science/article/pii/S0376635713000399 (accessed 2/10/19)

[103] Christa Leste-Lasserre, "Researchers Develop Subjective Equine Personality Test," *The Horse,* June 13, 2013 http://www.thehorse.com/articles/32036/researchers-develop-subjective-equine-personality-test (accessed 2/10/19)

[104] Much of the information in this chapter comes from Centered Riding, developed by Sally Swift who detailed the ways that riders influence their mounts with their bodies, for better and for worse. I have also learned from lessons with three of Sally Swift's apprentices who have expanded on her work: Wendy Murdoch, known for her innovative teaching techniques, on-line Murdoch Minutes, and excellent books and DVDs (http://murdochmethod.com/); Susan Harris, author of *Horse Gaits, Balance and Movement* and co-creator of Anatomy in Motion (http://www.anatomyinmotion.com/); and Mitzi Summers, internationally known Centered Riding and Certified Horsemanship Association clinician. My current instructor, Melani Alexander Fuchs, is a former event rider and life-long teacher who incorporates classical dressage, Centered Riding, and movement-based learning into her riding instruction.

[105] Christa Leste-Lasserre, "Study: Many Riders Don't Groom Horses Properly or Safely," *The Horse* (on-line) Nov 3, 2017 http://www.thehorse.com/articles/39871/study-many-riders-dont-groom-horses-properly-or-safely?utm_source=Newsletter&utm_medium=health-news&utm_campaign=11-07-2017 (accessed 3/26/19)

[106] Christa Leste-Lasserre, "Excitement, Feeling, and Attachment's Impact on Training," *The Horse* Aug 2, 2013 http://www.thehorse.com/articles/32311/excitement-feeling-and-attachments-impact-on-training (accessed 3/16/19)

Paper presented by Dr. Paul McGreevy and Andrew McLean, PhD at the 9th International Society for Equitation Science Conference, 2013 University of Delaware.

[107] Christa Lesté-Lasserre, "Posture of Rider and Rider Linked, Study Shows," *The Horse,* Jun 10, 2010 http://www.thehorse.com/articles/25677/posture-of-rider-and-rider-linked-study-shows (accessed 3/26/19)

[108] Clémence Lesimple, Carole Fureix, Hervé Menguy, Martine Hausberger, "Human Direct Actions May Alter Animal Welfare, a Study on Horses (Equus caballus)," PLoS ONE, April 28, 2010. http://journals.plos.org/plosone/article?id=10.1371/journal.pone.0010257 (accessed 1/13/18)

[109] Sally Swift, *Centered Riding* (Trafalgar Square Books, 1985) p. 19

[110] Xenophon, *The Art of Horsemanship,* translated by Morris H. Morgan (Dover Publications, Inc., 2006) p. 41

[111] Wendy Murdoch, *50 5-Minute Fixes to Improve Your Riding: Simple Solutions for Better Position and Performance in No Time* (Trafalgar Square Books, 2010), p 52

[112] Peham C1, Kotschwar AB, Borkenhagen B, Kuhnke S, Molsner J, Baltacis A., "A comparison of forces acting on the horses back and the stability of the rider's seat in different positions at the trot," *The Veterinary Journal,* Volume 184, Issue 1, April 2010, pages 56-59 https://www.sciencedirect.com/science/article/pii/S1090023309001488 (accessed 1/13/18)

[113] Kristen M. Janicki, "Feeding Choke-Prone Horses," *The Horse* Sept. 24, 2018 https://thehorse.com/136619/feeding-choke-prone-horses/ (accessed 4/2/19)

114 Erica Larson, "Gastric Ulcers in Horses: 30 Years of Research," *The Horse* Nov 30, 2018 https://thehorse.com/163371/gastric-ulcers-in-horses-30-years-of-research/ (accessed 4/2/19)

115 Christa Leste-Lasserre, "Does Feeding Hay Before Grain Reduce Cribbing?" *The Horse* Sept. 19, 2013  https://thehorse.com/116775/does-feeding-hay-before-grain-reduce-cribbing/ (accessed 4/2/19)

116 I base this supplementation on articles by Dr. Eleanor Kellon and information from the Equine Cushings and Insulin Resistance Group on the internet and facebook.

117 The ECIR (Equine Cushings and Insulin Resistant) website (https://www.ecirhorse.org/) and facebook group provide excellent in-depth resources for managing horses with laminitis or at risk for it. They have no products to sell, and skilled assistance is available at no charge. Research is extensive and current.

118 Kentucy Equine Research Staff, "Grazing Muzzles for Horses: How Effective Are They?", Equinews Nutrition & Health Daily May 16, 2013 https://ker.com/equinews/grazing-muzzles-horses-how-effective-are-they/ (accessed 4/20/19)

119 A.C. Longland, C. Barfoot, P.A. Harris, "The effect of wearing a grazing muzzle vs. not wearing a grazing muzzle on intakes of spring, summer and autumn pastures by ponies," Part of the Forages and grazing in horse nutrition book series (EAAP, volume 132), pp 185-6, https://link.springer.com/chapter/10.3920/978-90-8686-755-4_20  (accessed 4/2/19)

120 Vanessa Bee, *The Horse Agility Handbook* (Trafalgar Square Books, 2012) page xii

121 Elizabeth Letts, *The Eighty-Dollar Champion: Snowman, The Horse That Inspired a Nation* (Ballantine Books, 2011)

122 Hertha James, Horse Gym with Boots educational video series https://herthamuddyhorse.com/2014/12/27/horsegym-with-boots-video-clip-series-on-youtube/

# Reading and References

Barteau, Yvonne, *Ride the Right Horse: Understanding the Core Equine Personalities and How to Work with Them* (Storey Publishing, 2007).

Bee, Vanessa, *3-Minute Horsemanship: 60 Amazingly Achievable Lessons to Improve Your Horse When Time Is Short* (Trafalgar Square Books, 2013).

— *The Horse Agility Handbook: A Step-by-Step Introduction to the Sport* (Trafalgar Square Books, 2012).

— *Over, Under, Through: Obstacle Training for Horses* (Trafalgar Square Books, 2015).

Delgado, Magali & Pignon, Frédéric, *Gallop to Freedom: Training Horses with the Founding Stars of Cavalia* (Trafalgar Square Books, 2015).

— *Building a Life Together: You and Your Horse* (Trafalgar Square Books, 2014).

Dorrance, Tom, *True Unity* (Word Dancer Press, 1994).

Emerson, Denny, *Know Better to Do Better: Mistakes I Made (So You Don't Have To)* (Trafalgar Square Books, 2018).

Fugazza, Claudia, *Do As I Do: Using Social Learning to Train Dogs* (Direct Book Service, 2014).

Goodall, Jane, *Hope for Animals and Their World* (Grand Central Publishing, 2011).

Harman, Joyce, *The Horse's Pain-Free Back and Saddle-Fit Book* (Trafalgar Square Books, 2004).

Harris, Susan E., *Horse Gaits, Balance and Movement* (Turner, 2016).

Heuschmann, Gerd, *Tug of War: Classical versus "Modern" Dressage* (Trafalgar Square Books, 2018).

Hill, Cherry, *How to Think Like a Horse* (Storey Publishing, 2006).

McDonnell, Sue, *A Practical Field Guide to Horse Behavior* (Eclipse Press, 2003).

— *Understanding Horse Behavior* (Eclipse Press, 1999).

James, Hertha, *Conversations with Horses* (CreateSpace, 2015).

James, Will, *Smoky the Cowhorse* (Aladdin, 2008).

Letts, Elizabeth, *The Eighty-Dollar Champion: Snowman, The Horse That Inspired a Nation* (Ballantine Books, 2012).

Murdoch, Wendy, *50 5-Minute Fixes to Improve Your Riding* (Trafalgar Square Books, 2010).

— *40 5-Minute Jumping Fixes* (Trafalgar Square Books, 2011).

Peters, Stephen & Black, Martin, *Evidence-Based Horsemanship* (Wasteland Press, 2018).

Podhajsky, Alois, *My Horses, My Teachers* (Trafalgar Square Books, 1997).

Rashid, Mark, *Considering the Horse* (Skyhorse Publishing, 2014).

— *Finding the Missed Path: The Art of Restarting Horses* (Trafalgar Square Books, 2017).

— *Horses Never Lie* (Skyhorse Publishing, 2015).

Schuthof-Lesmeister, Ellen, and Mistral, Kip, *Horse Training In-Hand* (Trafalgar Square Books, 2009).

Sutton, Amanda, *The Injury-Free Horse* (David & Charles, 2006).

Swift, Sally. *Centered Riding* (Trafalgar Square Books, 1985).

— *Centered Riding 2: Further Exploration* (Trafalgar Square Books, 2002).

Wilsie, Sharon, and Vogel, Gretchen, *Horse Speak: The Equine-Human Translation Guide* (Trafalgar Square Books, 2016).

Xenophon, *The Art of Horsemanship* (Dover Publications, 2006).

# Index

Page numbers in *italics* indicate illustrations.

Aggression
    causes of, 53, 57, 78, 80, 84, 228
    in domestic vs. free-roaming horses, 37, 44
    as learned behavior, 40
    warning signs, 84
Agility training. *See* Horse Agility
Aids. *See* Cues
American Veterinarian Society of Animal Behavior, 84
Angelou, Maya, 175
*Animals Make Us Human* (Grandin), 140
Anthropomorphism, 13
Anticipation, 70–71
Anxiety
    causes of, 7–8, 45, 79, 86–87, 93
    "hidden," 87–88, 95, 181
    in investigative behavior, 164
    prevalence of, 11
    in rider/handler, 88, 92, 225
    in unwanted behaviors, 23–24, 53, 57, 78, 146, 227
Approach and retreat, 155
Assateague Island, free-roaming horses on, 34–42, 141, *142*
At liberty. *See* Liberty work
Attachment, signs of, 74–76
Attention-seeking behavior, *72*, 75
Authoritarian leadership, 14, 28, 42, 92–93, 233, 258
Avoidance, 79

Bachelor bands, 35, 37
Backing up, 118, *118*, 200, *200*
Balance
    of horse, 81–83, 226
    of rider, 9, 238–39, *239*
Balking, 160
Balls, 161–64, *162–63*, 201, *202*
Bareback riding, 207, *242*
Barrels, 200–201, *201*
Barteau, Yvonne, 232
Bee, Vanessa, 10, 126, 178, 186, 190, 209, 257
Behavior. *See also* Unwanted behaviors
    overview, 64–65, 76, 89, 98
    atypical, 80
    "bad," reinterpretation of, 90–98
    as communication, 64
    in free-roaming herds, 34–42
    positive, misinterpretation of, 66–76
    Protector Leadership based on, 11
    substitution of, 71–72
Behind the vertical, 82, *83*
"Being a Leader/Protector for Your Horse" (Walnes), 7, 10, 12
Bella, 161–64, *162–63*
Bits, 80, 226, 231
Blankets/blanket safety, 202, 211, *251*, 252
Body language, of horse, 14–15, 64, 100, 224
Body language, of rider/handler. *See also* Friendly Body Language
    guidelines for, *18*, 90–91, 106, 113, 115, 126
    in leadership, 16
    in liberty work, 215
    with new horses, 231
Bomb-proofing. *See* Desensitization
Boredom, 84, *85*, 227, 233
*Brain Training for Riders* (Waldo), 234
Brandy
    author's relationship with, 28, 208, 233
    background, 3, 11–12, 18–21, 25–28
    communication and, 115–122, 125
    confidence building, 192–96, *193–95*, 210, 212, 214, *214*, *217*
    in herd dynamics, 53–59
    interpreting behavior of, 67–68, 75, 85, 94–98
    investigative behavior, 143–46, *143–45*, *156–57*, *157–160*, *159*, 170–73
    personality, 190, *225*, 233
    training considerations, 185, 204–8, *205*, 216–18, 248–49
Breaking lessons down, 26, 168, 181, 183, 189–190, 216
Breeding, selective, 93
Bribes, vs. rewards, 129
Bronzz
    author's relationship with, 28, 60–61, 232–33
    background, 3, 90–91
    communication and, 123, *131*, 133, *136*
    confidence building, *179*, 181–84, 183, *189–190*, 210–11, *213*, 215
    in herd dynamics, 51–54, 57–59
    interpreting behavior of, 67–68, 70, 72–73, *72*, *74*, 75, 85, *85*, 90–92
    investigative behavior, 151–52, 166–170
    personality, 233, 253
    training considerations, 205–7, *206*, 218–19
Bucking, 91–92, 94–98, 226–28

Calming supplements, 45, 78, 86
Canter, 119, 242
Carbohydrates, 45, 86, 248

Catching horses, 18–19, 21–22, 121–22, *122*
*Centered Riding* (Swift), 238, 246
"Chicken wing" exercise, 24, *24*, 120
Children
    horse's manners around, 97, 120, *124*, 125
    introducing horses to, 172–73, *172*, 232
    as Protector Leaders, 98
    teaching considerations, 205, *205*, 242
Chiropractors, 228, 195
Clicker training, 133–35, *134*, *136*, 215
Color camouflage, 147, *147*
Communicate Like a Horse, overview, 100–101, 112, 127, 138. *See also* Communication; Pressure; *body language entries*
Communication
    in agility training, 196
    body language as, 64
    in building horse's confidence, 176
    clarity of, 113
    by horse, 64, 66–69, 210–12, 229
    horse's generalization of, 120
    pressure in, 7–8, 86, 109–12, *111*
    as source of unwanted behaviors, 89
    things to try, 112, 127, 138
    two-way, 126
Compensatory behaviors, 79, 81, 236
Competitions, 204, 233
Concentrates, 45, 86, 248
Conditioned responses, 122–23, 164, 176
Confidence, of rider/handler, 205
Confidence building
    overview, 191, 208, 219
    benefits of, 89, 187–88, 202
    case histories, 192–204
    copying in, *213*
    exercises for, 179–186, 196–208, *197–203*
    flexibility in, 186–87
    pressure/release and, 8
    things to try, 191, 208, 220
    vs. training, 141–42, 176
Confinement/confined spaces, 44, 45, 46, 201–2, *203*
Considerate riding, 236–246
*Considering the Horse* (Rashid), 26–27, 224
Consistency, 13, 83–84, 137, 226–27, 230, 243
Control issues, 174, 177, 209–10
*Conversations with Horses* (James), 126, 141, 154, 185, 190, 221
Copying, 40, 47–48, 213–15, *213–14*. *See also* Synchronizing
Corrections, 8, 84, 91, 181
Corridors, in agility training, 201–2, *203*
Creek crossings, 168–69, *169*
Cribbing, 46, 47

Crowding, 23–24, 120, 134–35, 224
Cues. *See also* Body language, of rider/handler
    horse's response to, 71, 112, 125
    use of, 104, 106–7, 110, 242, 246
    verbal, 115, 118
Curiosity, 45–46, 161, 164, 173–74, 201, 211. *See also* Investigative Behavior

Death, horses' response to, 56
deLeyer, Harry, 10, 258
Delgado, Magali, 1, 10, 16, 108, 113
Dental care, 81, 195–96, *195*, 228
Desensitization, 45, 161–64, 170, 178, 194–95
Diet
    of domestic vs. free-roaming horses, 38, *39*, 45
    guidelines for, 85–86, 227, 247–250
Dismounting, 160–61, 244–45
Disobedience, 72–74, 92–93. *See also* Unwanted behaviors
Ditch crossings, 158–160, *159*
*Do As I Do* (Fugazza), 220
Dog training, insights from, 6, 18, 73, 129, 132, 213, 220
Domestic horses
    dependence on people, 207
    freedom to learn, 209–10
    herd dynamics, 11, 32–33, 43–45, 49
    investigative behavior in, 141
Dominance structures
    in domestic vs. free-roaming horses, 11, 43, 49
    leading position and, 22–23
    rider/handler assumptions about, 28, 51, 58–59, 92–93
Downward Dog yoga stretch, 135, *136*
Drilling, 84–85, 185, 187
Driving position, 22–23, 116

Emergencies, 9, 244–45
Emerson, Denny, 107, 236
Emerson, Ralph Waldo, 51
Emotions, in horses
    assessment of, 14–15, 227
    behavior and, 12–13
    learned helplessness, 109, 163–64, 209–10
    respect for, 16–18
"Empathy, the Secret Ingredient for Success" (Goldstein Engle), 13
Endorphins, 46
Energy, of rider/handler, 104, 106, 120, *120*
Equagility, 205, *206*
Equipment, 80–81, 125, 231. *See also* Obstacles; Saddles/saddle fit
Eye contact, 67, 106

Farriers/farriery, 193–94, *193*, 228
Fatigue, 84, 227
Fear, in horses
    behavior in, 76, 164
    case histories, 18–21, 25–28
    investigative behavior and, 155
    sources of, 45, 47, 84, 102, 231
Feedback, from horse, 229
Feelings. *See* Emotions, in horses
Feet, movement/control of, 120–21
Feral horses. *See* Free-roaming horses
Fidgeting, 87
*50 5-Minute Fixes* (Murdoch), 239
Fight/flight response, 19–20, 47, 87
Flooding, 163–64
Foals
    domestic, 45–48
    in free-roaming herds, 34–40, *37, 41*
    learning by, 91, *114*, 151
Food. *See* Diet; Treats
Footing, 252, *254*
Forage. *See* Grass, access to
Forehand, falling onto, 82
Freedom of choice, 209–10, 217–18
Free-roaming horses
    herd dynamics, 34–35, *35*, 49
    investigative behavior in, 141, *142*
    social bonds among, 11, 32–33, 35–40, *35–37, 39*
Freeze response, 87, *88*
Friendly Body Language
    overview, 113, 126–27
    benefits of, 124–25, 176
    clarity in, 123
    demonstrations of, 115–124, *115–121*
    with new horses, 231
    practicing, 125–26, 127, 205
    synchronizing in, 114–15, 213–15
    using rewards with, 137
Friendships, among horses, 38, 54–56, *55*, 58, 61, 146. *See also* Horse/human relationships
Fritz (breeder/trainer), 75, 90–91, 96, 123, 233
Fugazza, Claudia, 220
Fun breaks, as reward, 131, *131*

*Gallop to Freedom* (Pignon and Delgado), 1, 10, 16, 108, 113
Games, 117, 121, 213–15
Gap obstacles, 200, *201*
Gates, 70, *70*
Geldings, 37–38, 43
Generalization, by horse, 120, 125, 179, 186, *202*
Goldstein Engle, Margie, 13
Gracie, *83, 111, 150*

Grain, 45, 86, 248
Grandin, Temple, 139, 140
Grass, access to, 45, 226, 243, *243*, 252–53
Grazing muzzles, 133, 226, 252–53
Greetings, 16–18, *17, 36*
Grief, 56
Grooming
    consideration during, 237
    mutual, 35, 37, *55*
Groundwork. *See* Leading/groundwork
Guarding behavior, *60*, 61

Halters/haltering, 19
Halts, 117–18, *118*, 215–16
Hand signals, 115
Hanging out, 22, 29
Harem bands, 34–35
Harris, Susan, 82
Hay, feeding of, 248, 249
Head
    balance role, 81–82, *82*
    rubbing of, 211, 212
Head-down position, 119–120, *119, 243*
Heels-down position, 239–240, *240*
Helmets, 156
Herd bound behavior, 61
Herd dynamics, 34–35, 43–45, 49, 51–59. *See also* Dominance structures; Social bonds
Hill, Cherry, 99
Hoof care, 81, *81*, 93, 250
Horse Agility. *See also* Liberty work
    benefits of, 196–208, *197–203*, 208
    case histories, 204–8, *205*
    communication in, 126, 196
    competitions/clinics, 188, 204
    introducing obstacles, 179–186
*The Horse Agility Handbook* (Bee), 10, 126, 209
*Horse Agility* (Loikka), 186
*Horse Gaits, Balance, and Movement* (Harris), 82
*Horse Speak* (Wilsie), 63, 110, 126, 215
Horse/human relationships. *See also* Protector Leaders
    attachment in, 74–76
    case histories, 60–61, 256–58
    children and, 98
    mismatches in, 234
    ownership considerations, 44, 230–35
    as partnership, 2, 12–13, 66, 67
    riding and, 243–44
    as social bond, 22, 29, 254–55, *255*
Horsemanship, resources regarding, 245. *See also* Protector Leaders
Horses. *See* Domestic horses; Free-roaming horses; Horse/human relationships

*How to Think Like a Horse* (Hill), 99
Hula hoops, *72, 190,* 197, *197*

Ijichi, Carrie, 77
Imitation. *See* Synchronizing
Initiative. *See* Motivation, of horse
Injections, 194–95
Instructors, choosing, 245
Insulin resistance, monitoring, 249, 250
International Horse Agility Club, 204
Interpreting Behavior, overview, 64–65, 76, 89, 98. *See also* Behavior
Introductions, 16–18, *17*
Investigative Behavior
    overview, 140, 152, 165, 174
    benefits of, 151–52
    case histories, 166–173
    downsides, 173–74
    examples of, 161–64, *162–63,* 180
    guidelines for, 155, 164, 168
    as horses training themselves, 141, 160, 165
    on the lead, 155–58, *156–57*
    as learning process, 141
    Protector Leaders in, 154–55, 160, 168–69
    retraining jumpers with, 149–151, *150*
    under saddle, 158–161, *162–63*
    sequence of, 143–46, *143–45*
    things to try, 153, 165, 174
Isolation, effects of, 44, 46

James, Hertha, 126, 141, 154, 185, 190, 221
James, Will, 40
Job, of horse, 233–34, 253–55, 256
Jumping, 83, 149–151, *150,* 152, 233

King, Callie R., 245
*Know Better to Do Better* (Emerson), 107, 236

Lameness, 80, 81
Laughter, *131,* 181
Lazy horses, 92–94
Leadership. *See also* Protector Leaders
    authoritarian, 14, 28, 42, 92–93, 233, 258
    communication in, 114
    in domestic vs. free-roaming horses, 32, 38, 40, 45
    myths about, 257–58
    responsibilities of, 61
Leading/groundwork
    avoiding tension in, 26–27
    confidence-building exercises, 181–83, *181–84*
    early training, 91
    handler position in, 22–23, 116, *116,* 158, 216
    in introducing liberty work, 216–17
    investigative behavior exercises, 155–58, *156–57*
    synchronizing in, 115–120
Learned helplessness, 109, 163–64, 209–10
Learning, by horses. *See also* Investigative Behavior; Training
    vs. conditioned response, 123
    in domestic vs. free-roaming horses, 40, *41,* 47–48, *48*
    encouraging, 209–10
    investigative behavior in, 164
    vs. obedience, 146
    of unwanted behaviors, 84–85
Leg position, of rider, 239–240
Leg up, for mounting, 237–38
Liberty work
    overview, 219
    guidelines for, 126, 215–19
    horse leaving during, 217–18
    play and, 216–17
    Protector Leaders and, 215
    synchronizing in, 120
    things to try, 220
Listening, to horses, 13, 64, 219
Living conditions
    of free-roaming herds, 38
    mealtime routines, 247–250
    new horses and, 232
    as source of unwanted behaviors, 85–86, 227
    turnout, 250–53
Loikka, Koikka, 186
Looking away, 161, 210–11
Loose horses, 118, 121, 122, 216–18
Lungeing, *82,* 119
Lyme disease, 93

Mane, grasping for rider support, 237, 238
Manners
    confidence building for, 192–96, 208
    expectation of, 13–14, 132, 190, 210, 248–49, 253–54
    Friendly Body Language and, 124
    retraining for, 8
Mares, 34–35, 37–38, 43, *114*
Maternal deprivation stress, 46
McDonnell, Sue
    on behavior, 31, 34, 40, 43, 51, 109
    on habituation, 162
    on pain, 78
    on punishment, 84
Memory, 148, 185
Mentors, 14
Misbehavior. *See* Unwanted behaviors

Mistakes
   ignoring, 8, 69, 91, 128, 181, 205
   learning from, 4, 205
Modeling behavior, 47–48. *See also*
   Synchronizing
Motivation, of horse, 71, 135, 211–15
Mounting, 237–38, *238*
Murdoch, Wendy, 239, 245
*My Horses, My Teachers* (Podhajsky), 66, 128,
   166, 208, 236, 256

Neck, of horse, 81–82, *83*
Neck straps, 239
Negative reinforcement, 107, 108
Neutral actions, 23–25
Note-taking, 229

Obedience, 73, 146, 256
Obstacles, training with, 178–191, 202–8. *See
   also* Horse Agility
*Over, Under, Through* (Bee), 178, 186
"Over" obstacles, 196–99, *198*
Ownership considerations, 44, 230–35

Pace, 117, 183–84
Pain
   assessing for, 25, 97, 228
   causes of, 80–81
   mistaken for aggression, 97
   signs of, 79–80
   in of unwanted behaviors, 77–81, 91, 93,
      151, 226
Pasture time, 252–53
Patience, importance of, 110, 155, 185, 220
Pausing to think, 69, *69*, 211
Pecking orders. *See* Dominance structures;
   Rank
Perceptual abilities, of horses, 146–49
Permissiveness, 13–14. *See also* Manners
Personal space
   of horse, 37, 52–54, 106
   of rider/handler, 23–25, 76, 120, 134–35,
      215, 224, 253–54
Personality mismatches, 232–33
Physical issues, in unwanted behavior, 89
Pignon, Frédéric, 1, 10, 12, 16, 108, 113
Play, 38, 211–15, 216–17
Pluvinel, Antoine de, 102, 207
Podhajsky, Alois, 66, 128, 166, 208, 236, 256
Poles/pole patterns, 197, *197*, 200
Positive Experiences, overview, 176–77. *See also*
   Confidence building; Horse Agility
Posting trot, 241–42

Posture
   of horse, 79, *80*, *94*, 228, 238
   of rider/handler, *18*, 104
*A Practical Field Guide to Horse Behavior*
   (McDonnell), 31, 34, 43
Practice, 121, 193
Praise, 129, 131, 216
Pressure
   overview, 112
   alternatives to, *111*, 114–15
   in communication, 7–8, 86, 100, 103, 108,
      109–12, *111*
   consistent use of, 107
   meaning of, 106–7
   pitfalls of, 21, 107–9, 146, 152
   release of, 107, 110, 112, 219
   as source of stress, 104–7
   strength/intensity of, 104–6, *105*, 109–10,
      218–19
   things to try, 112
   timing in, 107
   training methods using, 108, 122
   in unwanted behaviors, 86–87, 93, 227
   used among horses, 102–3, *103*
   yielding to, 106
Prey animals, horses as, 146–49
Privileges, earned by horse, 212
Problem horses, 256–58. *See also* Unwanted
   behaviors
Progress, defining, 188–190
Protector Leaders
   overview, 2–6, 15
   benefits of, 4, 12–13, 32–65, 148–49, 176, 258
   case histories, 7–15
   defined, 2
   guidelines for, 4–6, 10, 12–14, 188
   horses as, 11, 42
   investigative behavior role, 144, 146, 154–
      55, 160, 168–69
   in liberty work, 215–16
   for new horses, 230–35
   responsibilities of, 13–14
   things to try, 15
   trust in, 16–29
Punishment, 6, 71, 84, 109, 227

Rank, 37, 44, 45, 51–59
Rashid, Mark, 12, 26–27, 224, 230
Rearing, 224, *225*
Recall, 121–22, *122*, 215–16, 218
Reduce Stress
   overview, 222–23, 235, 246, 255
   considerate riding, 236–246
   lifestyle considerations, 247–255

problem-solving strategies, 224–235
  things to try, 235, 246, 255
Refusals, in jumping, 149, *150*, 151
Relationships. *See* Horse/human relationships
Repetition, 84–85, 185, 187
Requests, made by horses, 212, 220
"Researchers Develop Subjective Equine Personality Test" (Ijichi), 77
Resistance, 79, 93, 110, *111*
Resource guarding, 44, 51, 57
Respect, 2, 16–18, 93
Rest breaks, *130*, 131, 210, 211
Restrictive equipment, 80–81, 125. *See also* Trapped sensation
Rewards
  overview, 129–131, 138
  benefits of, 128–29, 185
  in clicker training, 133–35, *134*, *136*
  as earned, 129, 132
  with Friendly Body Language, 137
  in liberty work, 216
  limitations of, 137
  things to try, 138
  timing of, 130–31, 132
  types of, 72, 129, 131–32
  uses of, 58, 135, 137, 167–68, 183
Ribbon curtains, 199–200, *199*
*Ride the Right Horse* (Barteau), 232
Rider position, 238–242, *239–240*, *242*
Riders/handlers. *See also* Horse/human relationships
  expectations of, 83–84, 226–27
  insecurity in, 73
  mental checklist for, 244
  responsibilities of, 258
  as source of problems, 80, 227, 236, 244
Riding disciplines, 233–34, 241–42. *See also* Under saddle work
Role models, 14
Round pens, working in, 21, 25–26, 122, 218–19
Routines, 132–33, 226, 247–250
**Rude horses.** *See* Manners
"Rule of Three," 185
Rushing, 83

Saddles/saddle fit
  case histories, 25–28, 91–92, 94–98
  pain and, 80
  for riders, 240–41
  in troubleshooting unwanted behaviors, 226, 228, 232
Safety considerations, 14–15, 160–61, 202, 225, 234, 244–45. *See also* Manners; Security

Sapphire
  author's relationship with, 3, 28, 52, 53, 55–56, 61, 234
  communication and, 112, 133
  confidence building, *187*, 210, 215
  in herd dynamics, 51–59
  interpreting behavior of, 68, 72–74, 75
  investigative behavior, 144, 146, *153*
  training considerations, 206–7, 231
Scary objects, 166–173. *See also* Obstacles
Schedule, vs. routine, 247–48
Security
  overview, 11, 32–33, 42, 49–50
  case histories, 20–21, 51–62
  in domestic vs. free-roaming horses, 34–42, 43–50
  horse's feeling of, 16, 26, 64, 122, 124–25
  rider/handler as source of, 78–79
See-saw obstacles, 180–86, *180–84*
Shiloh
  author's relationship with, 3, 28, 60–61, 234
  communication and, 133–35, *134*
  confidence building, 220
  in herd dynamics, 51–54, 56–59
  interpreting behavior of, 67–68, *82*, 88, 92–94, 98
  training considerations, 207, *243*
Sitting trot, 241–42
*Smoky the Cowhorse* (James), 40
Snickers, 7–10, 19–20, 52–53, 71, 129
Social bonds
  overview, 32–33, 42, 49–50, 61–62
  case histories, 51–62
  in domestic vs. free-roaming horses, 11, 34–42, 44–48
  foals and, 46–47
  between horse and rider/handler, 22, 29, 254–55, *255*
  things to try, 42, 50, 62
Speaking, to horses, 18, 22
Speed, 117, 183–84
**Spooking, 68–69, 87, 161–64.** *See also* Investigative Behavior
Stall confinement, 44, 46–47, 86
Stallions, 34–35, 37–38, 40, 46
Stamping, of feet, 106, 251
Standing still, 26, 120–21, *120*, 237–38, 249
"Stay" command, 197, *197*, 199, *201*, 249
Stepping back, 18–19
Stereotypies, 46–47
Stirrups, use of, 239–240
Stoicism, 79–80, 222
Stress. *See also* Anxiety; Reduce Stress
  in horse, 77, 87, 223, 227

on horse's back, 237
in rider/handler, 210
Studies and experiments cited
   overview, 258
   communication, 67, 68
   facial expressions, 106
   rider balance, 238
   training approaches, 86–87, 108, 149–151
   visual perception, 148
Success, finishing with, 185–86
Supplements, 86, 250
Swift, Sally, 238, 245
Synchronizing
   benefits of, 114–15
   in confidence-building exercises, 180–81
   demonstrations of, 115–124, *115–121*
   vs. pressure/release, 114–15

Tacking up, 237
Talking, to horses, 18, 22
Tarps, 186–87, *187*, 188, 196
Telatin, Angelo, 149, 151
Tension, 79, 241
"Thinking the Way Animals Do" (Grandin), 139
Thistle, 20
*Three-Minute Horsemanship* (Bee), 190
"Through" obstacles, 200–201, *200*
Trail riding, 142–43, 166–170, 233
Trailers and trailering, 173
Trainers, professional, 228, 229–230, 245
Training
   vs. confidence, 141–42
   marketing of, 108
   Protector Leadership as, 12–13
   repetition in, 84–85, 185, 187
   session duration, 184–85, 189–190
   as source of unwanted behaviors, 89
Trapped sensation, 106, 107, 155, 161
Treats
   behavior issues around, 25, 57, 88
   in clicker training, 133–35, *134*, *136*
   structured routines for, 132–33
   uses of, 132, 167–68
Trick training, benefits, 215
Trot, 119, 125, 241–42
Trust
   overview, 29
   case histories, 19–28, 92
   in catching horses, 18–19
   cultivating, 2, 16–18, 114, 155, 176
   as earned, 6, 233
   preserving, 188

of rider in horse, 73–74, 123–24, 225
signs of, 74–76
things to try, 29
Tuning in/tuning out, 75, 91, 107, 243–44
Turnout, 250–53, *251*
Two-point position, 241–42
Tying, 26–27

Ulcers, 45, 248
Umbrellas, *198*, 199
"Under" obstacles, *198–99*, 199–200
Under saddle work
   confidence building exercises, 183–84, *183–84*
   considerate riding, 236–246
   Equality, 207
   investigative behavior exercises, 158–161, *162–63*
Unwanted behaviors. *See also* Manners
   overview, 77–79, 89
   assessing, 78–89
   case histories, 22–25
   as communication, 224
   ignoring, 8
   interpretation of, 64–65, 90–98
   rider/handler expectations and, 83–84
   sources of, 18, 46–47, 78, 79–88, 98, 107, 256–58
   things to try, 89
   troubleshooting tips, 225–230, 235

Variety, 117, 185
Veterinarians/veterinary care, 194–95, *194*, 207, 228
Videos, for checking rider position, 246
Vision, in horses, 87, 146–49
Voice, use of, 106, 115, 118, 181
Volunteering of rewarded behavior, 71–72

"Wait a Minute," 210–11, 220
Waldo, Andrea Monsarrat, 234
Walk, 115–16, *115*, 131
Walnes, Kim, 7, 10, 12
Water consumption, 211
Water crossings, 168–69, *169*
Weaning, 40, 45–46
Weaving, 46
Wild horses. *See* Free-roaming horses
Wilsie, Sharon, 63, 110, 126, 215

Xenophon, 10, 116, 128, 238

Young horses, 151, 232. *See also* Foals